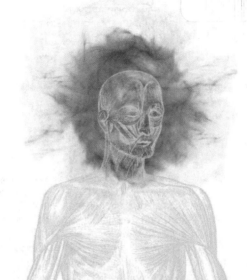

# Migraine Brains *and* Bodies

A comprehensive guide to solving the mystery of your migraines

*Learn* **the truth about common migraine myths**

*Find* **the real causes of individual pain patterns and other symptoms**

*Discover* **effective ways to heal your headaches**

## C.M. SHIFFLETT

Published by Round Earth Publishing, P. O. Box 157, Sewickley, PA 15143

Distributed by North Atlantic Books, P. O. Box 12327, Berkeley, CA 94712

Printed in the United States of America
Cover art by Nium, Inc.
Illustrated by the Author

*Migraine Brains and Bodies: A Comprehensive Guide to Solving the Mystery of Your Migraines* is sponsored by the Society for the Study of Native Arts and Sciences, a nonprofit educational corporation whose goals are to develop an educational and cross-cultural perspective linking various scientific, social, and artistic fields; to nurture a holistic view of arts, sciences, humanities, and healing; and to publish and distribute literature on the relationship of mind, body, and nature. North Atlantic Books' publications are available through most bookstores. For further information, visit our website at www.northatlanticbooks.com or call (800) 733-3000.

MEDICAL DISCLAIMER: The following information is intended for general information purposes only. Individuals should always see their health care provider before administering any suggestions made in this book. Any application of the material set forth in the following pages is at the reader's discretion and is his or her sole responsibility.

Publisher's Cataloging-in-Publication
(Provided by Quality Books, Inc.)

Shifflett, C. M.
    Migraine brains and bodies : a comprehensive guide to
    solving the mystery of your migraines / C.M. Shifflett.
    -- 1st ed.
    p. cm.
    Includes bibliographical references and index.
    ISBN-13: 978-0-9778702-0-2
    ISBN-10: 0-9778702-0-0

    1. Migraine.   I. Title.

RC392.S55 2011         616.8'4912
                   QBI11-600126
1 2 3 4 5 6 7 8 9 Knepper Press 16 15 14 13 12 11

# Contents

---

## Chapter 1    Introduction to Migraine Headaches    **1**

---

## Chapter 2    It's Just Tension!    **33**

## Chapter 6    Triggers and Thresholds  **179**

## Chapter 7    Getting Help  **227**

# Foreword

You may find information here that you have not seen elsewhere, at least not in migraine books intended for the general public.

You should know, therefore, that I am not making this up.

There is a great deal of excellent research on migraine but much of it stays locked in $200 medical textbooks, rarely trickling down to the popular press. You can see it yourself on-line at www.pubmed.com, the medical database maintained by the US National Institutes of Health (NIH). Look for papers by Marcus DA, Bigal ME, Janis JE, Lipton RB, Moskowitz MA, or other researchers mentioned here, or search for any keyword of interest. You will see abstracts stating the high points of the paper. Some include links to full text available on-line.

You don't need a medical degree to read these, although sometimes it may seem so. If you find the text overwhelming, just read the conclusions. Some researchers kindly wrap up these up in beautifully succinct titles.

I've taken these reports and translated them as best I can into everyday English. Some slightly more technical language exists as notes that therapists may find useful. Still, some reviewers have told me that this material is "too technical," while others have warned that "it isn't technical enough."

The first rule of writing is to know your audience.

So who did I write this for, anyway?

Perhaps I wrote it for technical types such as plumbers and electricians, people who work with connections and relationships. I'm certain that anyone who can plumb a house or connect a computer and peripherals can also understand the concept of vascular restrictions and cranial nerves and use that information to get good help.

I wrote it for those of us who have gone through standard medical care and all the standard migraine drugs with little good result, who want to try more, but who are unfamiliar with other options and wary of the pitfalls.

If it helps you, and I sincerely hope it will, then I wrote it for *you*.

# Acknowlegments

Many thanks to Peter Coppola, Emily Dolan-Gordon, Mary Lee Esty, Lawrence Funt, Chuck Gordon, Dale and Franklyn Gorell, Richard Grossinger, Jan Hendryx, Michael Karaffa, Todd Kotyk, Dan O'Block, Emily Perlman, Derek Seimon, Mark Shaw, Devin Starlanyl, Corey Snook, Brian Tuckey, Kim Young, and many many others.

# Migraine Brains *and* Bodies

A comprehensive guide to solving the mystery of your migraines

C.M. SHIFFLETT

# Chapter 1

# Introduction to Migraine Headaches

"I'm very brave generally," [he said] in a low voice:
"only to-day I happen to have a headache."
—Tweedledum, *Through the Looking-Glass* (Lewis Carroll)

There are so many books on migraine that it seems a tad presumptuous to add another to the list. Nevertheless, after many years of advances in migraine research, there still seem to be gaps in the information readily available to the general public.

Migraine tends to be presented as a *neurological disease* but with no explanation of neurology, and as a *vascular disease* with no explanation of what that really means and no way to relate the two. Although muscles are heavily involved in headaches of all kinds, their input is often ignored or flatly denied while many who do acknowledge muscular inputs tend to ignore neurological issues. Despite years of research on the trigemino-vascular system and its critical role in migraine, most migraineurs have never heard it. Most receive little more than a list of forbidden foods and expensive drugs, too often ineffective because they fail to address the root problem.

If your headaches are caused by nerves strained by tight muscles and misaligned bones you must do far more than avoid tyramines. But spinal adjustments will not fix a hole in the heart, and biofeedback is no panacea for bad diet and bad posture. Vasoconstrictive drugs can't help if blood vessels are constricted already and the problem is low oxygen supply to the brain.

I have said little about drugs as they are thoroughly covered elsewhere. Instead, I have tried to emphasize the physiology and body mechanics that trigger the symptoms we call *migraine*.

The first step is understanding what migraine is — and what it is not. To that end, we will explore the anatomy and physiology of migraine. You need not know the names of muscles, bones, or nerves to apply this information. But, understanding something of the relationships will give you the tools you need to understand why you get a migraine one day but not another, why one thing helps but another does not.

Finding your personal set of root causes may involve serious detective work but, in the process, you may heal your pain forever.

# A Beginning of the End of Migraines

While in college, I consulted a campus physician about the flashing lights followed by severe, nauseating headaches lasting for days. I'd had these since childhood, but after marriage and birth control pills they became much worse.

"They are obviously flashbacks from LSD," he said.

"Impossible," I said. "I've never touched the stuff."

"How," he sneered, "do you expect to fool a medical doctor?"

Apparently I had done exactly that.

I knew the light show wasn't from LSD, but all I knew about the odd sparkles and spots was that Bugs Bunny and Daffy Duck sometimes mentioned (or experienced) "spots before the eyes." If only cartoon characters had such symptoms, clearly neither they nor I could be taken seriously. Yet the lights continued, pretty stardust warnings of dark and horrible things to come.

Two years later, I saw an internist. When he found no brain tumor, the headaches that came several times a week were diagnosed as tension. I was offered Valium and a referral for psychological counseling although I didn't feel "tense," loved my job and aside from the migraines, was having the time of my life. When I asked instead to look for root *physical* causes, the doctor threw me out of his office. If I wasn't going to take his advice, he didn't want me as a patient.

Five years after my first try for help, I consulted a crusty Washington osteopath. As I blushed and stammered through my list of symptoms I noticed with alarm that he was becoming increasingly impatient and agitated. But it wasn't with *me*.

"*Scintillating scotomas!*" he roared. "What is *wrong* with these people? Don't they keep up with the literature? Don't they go to conventions?"

He was the beginning of the cure. But it soon became clear that sometimes it isn't so much a matter of keeping up with new information as it is of being aware of the wealth of information that already exists. Migraine and all its symptoms have been in the medical literature for thousands of years.

- The ancient Sumerians wrote of head pain brought by a goddess of wind (and therefore barometric changes).

- The Ebers Papyrus (an ancient Egyptian medical treatise[1]), describes one-sided headaches with vomiting. Not even immortals were exempt: demons once gave the god Horus a headache so severe that he was forced to live in a cave in the dark.

- In 400 BC, Hippocrates, Father of Medicine, wrote about migraine headaches and described aura (visual symptoms), and various triggers. *Migraine* is a version of the original Greek *hemi-krania*, describing the common symptom of "half-headed" pain.

---

1. Dated c. 1,500 BC, but believed to be a compilation of material dating to 3,000 BC.

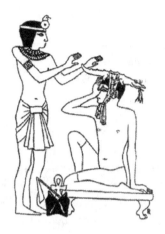 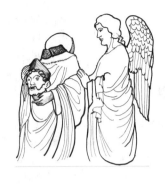 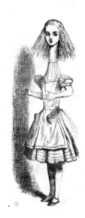

Ancient Egyptians treated migraine with herbs and darkness. A pottery vessel tied to the head and filled with water would have offered evaporative cooling, the only option available in hot and arid Egypt before the mechanical invention of ice.

St. Denis, martyred by having his head chopped off (as portrayed at Notre Dame Cathedral) became the patron saint of headaches.

Distortions in body perception which occur in some migraines are now known as "Alice in Wonderland Syndrome" after the imagery in Lewis Carroll's novels.

**Figure 1.** HEAD PAIN IN HISTORY

- The Western paradigm of the four humours blamed migraines on excess bile. This made sense as victims may vomit and vomiting may end the attack. Attempts were made to speed the process by eliminating the bile via purging and bleeding[1].

- The Eastern paradigm of meridians attributed headaches to the Gallbladder Meridian which correlates well with muscles and connective tissue that the West now associates with head pain.

- In 19th-century Vienna, migraines contributed to Freud's infamous drug addictions.

- In 19th-century England, migraines may have inspired the vanishing Cheshire cat (whose toothy grin remained) and the bizarre changes in body size and shape in Lewis Carrol's *Alice in Wonderland*.

- Throughout the 19th and early 20th centuries, detailed images of auras were published by early neurologists (such as Babinski and Charcot) and by physicians who suffered migraine themselves.

That's the history, but to understand migraine and get to a cure you must also understand what migraine is and what it is not.

---

1. The sometimes fatal consequences of coming down with a migraine are described in Mark Twain's essay, A *Majestic Literary Fossil*, the King James medical manual.

# What Migraine Is Not

Migraine is not imaginary and it is not "just stress." It can be tempting to avoid unpleasantries with claims of headache, but the real thing is rarely "just acting out for Secondary Gain." That's usually just another migraine myth. There are many.

## MYTHS AND MISSES

**EVERYBODY GETS HEADACHES, SO WHAT'S THE BIG DEAL?** Everybody *can* get headaches because every human body has the mechanisms to produce them, but these are not activated in *every body* as often, or with the same degree of severity. They do not produce the same set of consequences. There are great differences between Normals (who never get migraines) and even between migraineurs and other migraineurs.

*Episodic* migraines are defined as occurring on *fewer* than 15 days per month.

*Chronic* migraines are defined as occurring *more* than 15 days per month.

Everyone with migraines does not suffer chronic migraine. Those who do suffer more than pain. Compared to episodic migraineurs, chronic migraineurs are less likely to be employed full time. They have significantly lower incomes, and are more likely to be occupationally disabled (Buse D and others, 2010). They are nearly twice as likely to suffer depression and anxiety, more likely to have depressed immune response and respiratory disorders (asthma, bronchitis, and chronic obstructive pulmonary disease), with higher cardiovascular risk factors including high cholesterol, diabetes, hypertension, and obesity. There is a significantly increased risk of heart attack, stroke, Multiple Sclerosis (MS), and suicide. Any of these can be a very big deal indeed.

**MIGRAINE IS A REALLY BAD HEADACHE.** Migraine is usually thought more severe than "mere" tension headache but there's more to it. Pain that throbs, pounds, and pulses is typical of the dilated blood vessels typical of vascular headaches. To check heart rate a migraineur need do no more than gaze at a clock face and count while the entire vision field pulses. But the *degree* of pain is not necessarily diagnostic. It is possible to have a mild, low-grade migraine and a brutally painful muscle tension headache. Muscles can trigger migraine in many ways, but mention tightness[1] at the back of the neck and a diagnosis of "migraine" may be dropped in favor of "tension headache" and referral for psychiatric counseling. For many, this experience is so emotionally loaded that the preferred term is now "muscle contraction headache."

The best indicator is not the *level* of pain, but *what happens* to the pain. If the pain is pulsing and gets worse with effort (and changes in blood pressure) it is best classed as vascular, as *migraine*. Another symptom of migraine is this: no matter how terrible the pain, the victim avoids crying, because weeping only makes a migraine worse.

---

1. Neck stiffness *during* the migraine is now often mentioned as a side-effect of the migraine ("meningitis-like symptoms"), but it can also be an important initiating factor.

And there's more to it than head pain. Besides extreme sensitivity to light and sound, there may also be frightening visual disturbances, severe nausea, chills, fever, changes in body perception, and / or gastrointestinal (GI) upsets. An arm or leg or entire side of the body may stop working, resulting in staggers, confusion, and slurred speech resembling intoxication or stroke.

**IT'S HORMONES.** Fluctuating hormones make migraine more common in women than men, and especially likely to strike during ovulation and menstruation. Estrogen is huge; men undergoing sex-change with estrogen therapy eventually develop migraines at the same rate as women. Migraines respond to other hormones including thyroid hormone, Vitamin D (actually a hormone), and prostaglandins (which act like hormones). All are important in all humans.

**IT'S A GIRL THING AND IT WILL GO AWAY IF YOU GET PREGNANT.** Migraines improve or vanish in about two-thirds of pregnant migraineurs. In the rest, they get worse, and for some women, migraines appear for the first time during their pregnancies with the additional problem of finding effective treatment that is safe for both mother and child. Some pregnancies may even be migraine-related: estrogen-based oral contraceptives should not be used by women with classic migraine because they increase risk of stroke, a risk that is already elevated in migraine with aura. And when pregnancy is over, the migraines may return to previous levels.

**MEN DON'T GET MIGRAINES.** The strong link between female hormones and migraine has led to the common belief that migraines do not occur in men. Actually they do, but men tend to call them "sinus headaches" and treat them with over-the-counter (OTC) remedies. Men may suffer exactly the same symptoms as female relatives and friends, but hesitate to admit to them or get appropriate medical treatment. Some men see admission of headaches as admission of weakness, and even worse, *female* weakness.

In 1983, I was told by a physician that any man on Workman's Compensation who complained of headaches would automatically be dismissed as *malingering*.

"Men don't get headaches," he said, "or if they do, no *Real Man* would admit it."

In general, men do have fewer headaches than women at a rate of about 1:3. Many men swear that they have never had a headache in their entire life. But many men have. And many a man has blown his head off "while cleaning his guns," often a manly euphemism for suicide when the pain and shame have become too much to bear.

**CHILDREN DON'T GET MIGRAINES.** This long-standing belief has been overwhelmed by modern data on the many children who suffer headaches. In boys and girls, numbers of headaches are the same until adolescence when hormones surge and females come out ahead. But consider the long list of other possible triggers.

Do you know any children with bad posture? Any who must carry heavy backpacks? Who are undergoing dental / orthodontic work?[1] Who have sleep problems? Who are

---

1. See Andrew's story on page 180.

suffering stress or abuse? With asthma, skin, or neurological problems? Asthma and migraine are strongly related and for whatever reason, rates of both are increasing.

What about children with poor diets or food sensitivities? The 1983 Egger study of children with intractable migraines is one of the classics in migraine literature. It was apparently begun with the expectation that it would disprove, once and for all, the notion that migraines were at all related to food. The surprising result of the strict elimination diet was that migraines essentially vanished. So did an amazing range of other symptoms: eczema, seizures, and bed-wetting. There was also an amazingly poor correlation between foods that caused reactions and the standard lists of tyramine-containing foods. The problem wasn't "cheese," it was specifically *cow*'s milk cheese. It wasn't *all* nuts, it was *peanuts*, and it was orange juice and it was wheat.

Older children face other risk factors (Milde-Busch A and others, 2010). High-schoolers with headaches have four outstanding triggers: cocktails and coffee (strongly linked to *migraine*), smoking and inactivity (strongly linked to *tension headache*).

Do children ever sneak booze or cigarettes? Adults may know that caffeine, alcohol and nicotine are migraine triggers. Kids may be unaware of the relationship (or, like some adults, unwilling to admit it) but the resulting headaches are no less real.

**MIGRAINEURS ARE MORE CREATIVE AND INTELLIGENT THAN NORMALS.** This belief seems to have arisen during the Victorian era at a time when migraine was primarily seen as a disease of *men* and attributed to the stress of the business world. It was written about by physicians who suffered migraines themselves. These were intelligent, educated men with the training, opportunity, and income to be creative.

Since then, gender perceptions of migraine have changed radically. And, when Prof. Andrew Levy researched creativity of modern-day migraineurs compared to the general population he found that migraineurs do *not* come out ahead (Levy A, 2009). Many do not make it through the pain. So what of the long lists of celebrities who get migraine? They are reminders that there is life beyond migraine. There may be a hint of the tradition that suffering brings a depth of power and understanding that would otherwise be lacking in the artist and his art, but what creative migraineurs seem to be is *persistent*. They continue to create, not because of the pain, but in spite of it.

A roaring migraine can be so horrific that many first-timers swear they would rather die than endure another. And some really do. Even after adjusting for depression, the suicide rate for persons who suffer chronic migraine with aura (more than seven times per month) is almost double that for persons with other or less frequent headaches[1]. Those who face regular attacks face those same life or death choices on a regular basis.

A bad attack is a life on hold for hours or days or weeks. It *is* a death and a dying. On the other hand, its end offers the opportunity to consider the value of living and what your life will be *for* if you choose to continue on.

---

1. The exception is cluster headache, specifically known as "suicide headache."

**YOU JUST NEED A GOOD PAINKILLER.** Maybe once or twice a month, but more often is a hook into a dangerous drug habit and a vicious cycle of painful rebound headaches, as bad or worse than the original migraine. Worst of all, during the pain of withdrawal, preventive migraine medications do not work. Drugs are enormously useful in their place; they buy us time and space to function. But keep them in their place. Drugging head pain while ignoring the causes is like treating foot pain with painkillers while continuing to wear the shoes that caused the pain in the first place. Finding and eliminating the cause is always better than numbing the symptoms.

**IT CAN'T BE *THAT* BAD!** Oh yes it can. And the suspicions of friends, relatives, and employers just add to the pain. It's hard to convince anyone that migraines are real unless they have experienced something, *anything* like them. Fortunately, simple alternatives for educational purposes are readily available. An ice-cream headache gives a brief glimpse of the pain. A bad hangover from cheap bourbon whiskey or red burgundy at high altitude is another possibility, as is a root canal without anesthesia. This is not exaggeration; the nerves that supply palate and teeth (trigeminals) are the same ones involved in migraine.

We must be thankful on behalf of others who have not experienced and do not know or understand the pain and disability — and we must understand it ourselves.

**YOU JUST NEED TO GET A GRIP.** For chronic migraine sufferers, headaches that last two to four days or even a week or more are not unusual. Their lives are nothing like normal lives. They are more like tales of UFO abductees who go to bed in one state and wake up hours or days later in another, barefoot and disoriented, and having to struggle back home where people demand to know where they have been but don't believe their stories anyway.

Is this stressful? Try it and see. On random days several times a month, have your worst enemy hammer a red-hot railroad spike into your head then dump you halfway across the country. You don't get to plan the trip, you won't be functional while it is happening, and you will be disoriented for a couple days after you get back.

When you do straggle back to Normal Life, you must do what needs to be done *and* all the things that didn't get done while you were away. Meanwhile, you don't know when the next attack will be. When it comes, you don't get to pack beforehand, you don't get to pick the route. You may find that you have no clean clothes, no food, no resources. You may be out of gas and your credit cards won't work because you failed to pay the bills before you were taken. Or maybe there's no money to pay them with because you lost your job and spouse long ago due to "laziness" or "unreliability," or because (thanks to depression and relentless fatigue) you just aren't any fun any more. In such a case it is extremely difficult to "get a grip." Meanwhile, the stress of unmet expectations and demands simply adds more tension and stress.

**IT'S "JUST" STRESS.** Stress is not trivial. It can energize but it can can also kill. Research has repeatedly shown that the worst stress arises from lack of control and predictability. Both are typical of migraine and the social and economic strains of low income or no income which can easily lead to sleepless nights, elevated blood pressure, cholesterol, and obesity linked to migraine and its accompanying diseases.

**THERE'S NO RELATIONSHIP BETWEEN TENSION HEADACHES AND MIGRAINE.** Many believe that tension headaches and migraines are a continuum, but they are still classed as two different conditions. In 1998 researchers discovered a direct anatomical link between a small muscle of the neck (RECTUS CAPITIS POSTERIOR MINOR) and the *dura mater*, tissue that surrounds the spinal cord and brain. When tight, the muscle pulls directly on the pain-sensitive dura, its associated blood vessels, and nerves producing many of the neurological symptoms observed in migraine. Other muscles produce a wide variety of symptoms variously diagnosed as tension headache, sinus pain, bursitis, atypical trigeminal neuralgia, vestibular dysfunction — and migraine.

**THERE'S NO RELATIONSHIP BETWEEN MUSCLES AND MIGRAINE.** The link between muscles, headaches, and many other pains has been thoroughly documented in the medical literature for well over a century. In 1900, Dr. I. Adler wrote a superb article on painful "muscle hardening" and reviewed reports in the German medical literature dating back to the 1840s. 1900 was the same year that Walter Reed confirmed his theory on transmission of yellow fever by mosquitoes, 12 years before the sinking of the Titanic. Both events fired the public imagination. Muscle pain did not, perhaps because, as Adler wryly noted, "No one dies of muscle pain." Many may want to, however.

Adler's "muscle hardenings" are now known as *trigger points*. Nodules, taut bands, and changes in muscle physiology have been documented in thin sections, sonograms, MRI, and EMG[1]. Their reduced blood flow has been tracked with Doppler imaging, deranged electrical signals detected with volt meters. The pain they contribute to many kinds of headaches is now clear, as is relief of symptoms when their input is resolved. Yet muscles and connective tissues are still ignored or denied despite their ability to produce all the neurovascular symptoms typical of migraine.

**IT'S VASCULAR! NO, IT'S NEUROLOGICAL!** Migraines, with their pulsing pain, have long been classed as *vascular* because of the obvious involvement of the vascular system. Today, calling migraine a "neurological disease" seems more acceptable, more respectable. But *vascular* doesn't stop at the head and *neurological* isn't restricted to the brain. Nerves have blood supply, and blood vessels have nerve supply. In the brain, constriction and dilation of blood vessels is controlled by trigeminal nerves. Meanwhile, muscles and connective tissues press, pull, block, and strangle both nerves and blood vessels throughout the body, triggering pain.

Consider *sciatica*, often caused by the piriformis muscle of the hip. The muscle must pass through a narrow bony passage along with nerves and blood vessels that supply genitals and lower limbs. If the muscle shortens and thickens (as it does to turn out feet in ballet) nerves and blood vessels are trapped and compressed; symptoms range

---

1. MRI: Magnetic Resonance Imaging. EMG is Electro-Myo-Graphy, or "electric-muscle-writing," a technique for recording electrical activity produced by muscles.

from hip, leg, and pelvic pain to sexual dysfunction. The problem isn't only vascular or only neurological. It isn't "just" psychological. If your physician precribes muscle relaxants for sciatica, it is because he knows it isn't psychological either.

The odd thing is that pain caused by similar restrictions in the upper body is so often dismissed as psychological simply because it is felt in the *head* rather than in the *leg.*

**MIGRAINE IS A CHEMICAL IMBALANCE IN THE BRAIN.** Very likely, but probably not an imbalance of serotonin re-uptake inhibitors (SSRIs). It can be due to hormones and neurotransmitters but most likely an imbalance of chemicals known as *nutrients,* required for proper brain and body function. Migraine is strongly linked to depression and sleep disturbances. Poor sleep is linked to depression and attributed to an imbalance of *serotonin* required to make *melatonin,* the sleep hormone. But what makes serotonin? B vitamins, magnesium, Vitamin D, and even *light* are all required and all are typically out of balance in migraineurs.

**YOUR ELECTROLYTES ARE WITHIN NORMAL RANGES.** How do you know? If electrolytes were measured using standard blood tests, you don't. Electrolytes in blood are kept within strict limits. The real stores are in bone and tissue; historically, they could only be evaluated accurately via biopsy. Newer tests reveal a clear correlation between disturbed calcium-magnesium ratios in both migraine and tension headaches, but most severe in migraine and menstrual migraine.

Since the early 1980s, migraine rates have risen steadily *in women but not men.* Since the late 1970s, there have been huge changes in food supply, background electrical and light pollution, sleep patterns, stress of the business world,. Another trend since the 1980s is heavy supplementation of calcium urged upon women. Calcium overload is now linked to kidney stones, heart disease, and migraine.

**YOU'RE JUST LAZY.** One unfortunate warning sign of impending migraine is *yawning.* This can be a problem when seen during a staff meeting, especially when the yawner calls in sick the next day. Obviously that person has been staying up late, or is lazy and just sleeping in. Not necessarily, especially if the meeting was held in a stuffy room in a building where energy efficiency is valued over healthy air exchange. Low oxygen can trigger migraines and even seizures.

The traditional canary in the coal mine was there to detect tasteless, odorless, deadly methane gas. Birds have an extremely high oxygen demand. If the bird fell over dead, it was time for the miners to flee to safety. In many modern money mines and cube farms, migraineurs are the canaries, a first alert of Sick Building Syndrome before more subtle signs of fatigue, dizziness, ill health, and increasing absenteeism are recognized in other employees.

**IT'S GENETIC.** There are many possibilities. Familial hemiplegic is a severe version of migraine with aura. Type 1 is caused by a mutation in a gene that handles calcium channels, Types 2 and 3 involves problems with sodium channels.

Celiac disease is a genetic sensitivity to gluten and one of its symptoms is migraines.

Some people have unusually high requirements for individual nutrients. Genetically dark skin greatly increases the need for Vitamin D in northern latitudes while genetically light skin may lead to overuse of sunscreen that blocks all Vitamin D.

What appears to be a genetically reactive nervous system may also be an inherited defect of heart or bone. What about traditional family foods, family patterns of stress and abuse, lifestyles and trades? The soils and water where a family has always lived?

Other genes are believed to cause greater sensitivity to pain and higher reactivity in the system, but it doesn't end there. Drop a brick on a Normal toe and a migraineur toe, and it's possible that the migraineur will fire more nerves, make more stress chemicals, and suffer more severely than the Normal. But the real problem is this: toes don't deal well with bricks. Remove the brick.

The good news is that genes are more likely to create *tendencies* than Sure Things. They are genetic fault lines that can be overcome or worsened by other issues.

**SOON WE'LL FIND THE CURE FOR MIGRAINE HEADACHES.** We will probably never find *The* Cure because migraines are so often *symptoms* that do not arise from *one* thing. Even migraines themselves are not considered to be *one* thing. Migraine with and without aura are very different. There will never be *one* magic bullet because there is no *one* target, no *one* cause that applies to every*one*. We are not all the same. For the individual, a cure may involve serious detective work and many blind alleys. Your best bet? Find the root causes and treat them appropriately.

## DIFFERENTIAL DIAGNOSIS

Headaches are classified as Primary and Secondary, then subdivided by symptoms. Traditionally, migraine, tension, and cluster headaches are seen as *primary*, lone entities unto themselves. *Secondary* headaches are seen as symptoms of underlying pathology such as tumor, aneurysm, hypertension, or other disease. Good differential diagnosis is critical to the process of elimination, to reduce headaches from all the awful things they *could be but are not*, to the things they *are*.

The first step is to see a physician to find and eliminate contributing factors, to ensure that the headaches aren't a symptom of something even more serious. A diagnosis of *migraine* based simply on severe pain or nausea is not enough, especially for head pain of sudden onset. A complete physical and neurological exam should detect:

- *A tumor or cyst.* This is relatively rare, but should be checked.

- *Aneurysm.* With stretching and ballooning of a blood vessel wall, a weak area may burst suddenly (typical of high pressure arteries, resulting in "stroke") or it may leak slowly (typical of low pressure veins). Without contrast, most aneurysms are invisible on CT scans unless very large, calcified, or bleeding.

- *Subdural hematoma.* These form due to broken blood vessels from aneurysm or traumatic head injury. Pooling of blood increases pressure within the confines of the brain, which can result in coma and death. Rate of bleeding determines how fast symptoms appear. A burst arterial aneurysm tends to be quickly fatal, but a slow bleed can kill hours, weeks, or even months later.

- *Carotid artery disease.* Retinal migraine (ophthalmic or ocular migraine) comes with a light show of visual disturbances, often to the point of blindness in one eye. Symptoms are transient and generally considered benign. However, the same symptoms can arise from blocks in the carotid arteries, a serious condition which should be treated.

- *High or Low blood pressure.* Among other ill effects, high blood pressure stresses pain-sensitive blood vessels. Hypertension headache tends to be described as a "hairband" pain, typically worse in the morning. Hypertension can lead to stroke or aneurysm. Low blood pressure with inadequate blood supply to the brain, and to the muscles of neck and head will also cause severe headaches.

- *Infections and disease.* Migraines have been linked to everything from gum disease and impacted teeth to colds, flu, ulcers, and celiac disease. All of these can make you sick and impair muscle metabolism, which in turn can stress nerves and blood vessels.

- *Hypothyroid.* Thyroid has a powerful impact on muscle metabolism. Migraines are a commonly associated with hypothyroid.

If nothing is found, if your headaches are dismissed as "just tension," if you feel there is more going on, don't despair. This is *good* news! Once you have eliminated what the problem *is not*, you can move on to what *it is*. Possibilities include:

- *Cervical Dysfunction.* Misaligned vertebrae strain connective tissue, and / or compress the nerves and blood vessels that travel between them. This can contribute to muscle pain and spasm, but also to high blood pressure and brain slowing. Best checked by osteopath or chiropractor; muscle relaxants alone will not do the job.

- *Nutritional deficiencies.* The biggest possibilities are nutrients contributing to sleep, endocrine, and muscle function. These include Vitamin D, the B vitamin complex, and electrolytes but can also involve overdosing with supplements.

- *Electrolyte imbalances.* Strongly linked to migraine, pre-menstrual syndrome (PMS), and menstrual migraine even when test results are within "normal ranges." Imbalances of calcium and magnesium are especially critical and common.

- *TMJD.* Temporo-Mandibular Joint Dysfunction can cause a host of problems. Jaw joints are stressed by bad bite which directly strains muscles used in chewing. Bite should be checked and corrected by a dentist or orthodontist specifically trained in this area. Bad bite and TMJD can also arise from the muscle strain of poor posture.

- *Sleep apnea.* It can be "obstructive" due to obesity (a major risk factor for migraine) and floppy tissues. It can also be "central" due to brain injury.

- *"Wake" apnea.* Disturbed breathing due to poor posture, restrictive clothing, or stuffy rooms, disrupts oxygen supply to the brain.

- *Head / neck injury, concussion or whiplash.* Pain and dysfunction from unrecognized or untreated injuries can persist for years.

- *Endocrine imbalances.* Common examples involve estrogen from being female, or equal-opportunity endocrine disrupters from food, drugs, and toiletries.

# What Migraine Is

The part can never be well unless the whole is well.

—Plato

Migraine is rarely just one thing, and it isn't limited to the head. It can be a symptom of many conditions and stressors, including poor nutrition, impaired muscle function, infections, autoimmune diseases, sleep disruptions, and more.

*Migraine* headaches are seen as a specific disease. Typically they are painful, one-sided pulsating headaches accompanied by extreme sensitivity to light and sound, often with motor difficulties and vomiting. Many researchers, however, consider the pain of migraine to be a response common to a wide variety of conditions that upset the body's balance, things that the body sees as threats.

## THREATS AND ALARM SYSTEMS

> To be effective, the alarm must detect a predictive signal like smoke. Unfortunately, your alarm doesn't know the difference between the smoke of burnt toast and the smoke of a burning man. Engineers could reduce the likelihood of a false positive (alarming when there is no real fire), but only by increasing the likelihood of a false negative (failing to alarm when there is a real fire).
> —ST Naficy and K Panchanathan, *Buffy the Vampire Dater*

When the fire alarm goes off in an office building, we rarely know the cause. It might be fumes, a grease fire in the kitchen, an electrical fire on the roof. The response is the same: everyone heads for the emergency exits, pours into the stairwells, and exits the building. At least that's the ideal.

If the alarm is perceived as the regularly scheduled fire drill, people can be very casual. Many won't leave until they have saved their work, straightened the desk, and stopped by the restroom. Those with looming deadlines may duck behind a desk in the dark and refuse to leave at all. The stimulus isn't taken seriously, because other things are more important. If, however, there are obvious fumes or smoke, even the most dedicated workers will pour into the stairwells, flooding over the thresholds of the building to the safety of the outlying areas. The alarm bell that triggers this response is the same but the response is more serious.

Body and brain respond in a similar way. Normally we adapt to a constant stream of daily stresses, but if the alarm is big enough and scary enough, the body responds more strongly, bringing more defenses to bear on the problem. Where there have been repeated fires, abuse, or burglars, we are sensitized to ever smaller signals. The merest whiff of smoke, the tiniest flicker of an eyelid, a soft thump at window or door will trigger a serious response.

This reaction resembles that of "defensive" personalities, people notoriously hard to deal with because everything that others say or do is seen as a potential threat. Their responses are meant to be protective, but can go terribly wrong, transforming a simple alert into behavior that family, friends, neighbors, police, and the legal system see as inappropriate overreaction. Similarly, the occasional headache can grow progressively worse. In the brain, increased sensitivity to threats is known as *central sensitization*. Increased sensitivity and defensiveness can transform a simple alert into a full-scale emergency response lasting for hours, days, or weeks at a time. This happens thanks to *facilitation*, any activity which makes things easier to happen again.

Imagine the classic wandering cowpath. Eventually it gets foot traffic and signposts. As population centers develop, the road is straightened, then paved ("set in stone") to speed traffic. Eventually someone notices that it would be more efficient to build a six-lane highway straight from Point A to Point B. Now you can get there faster and avoid any distractions along the way. Your trip has been *facilitated*.

In any condition involving central sensitization (such as fibromyalgia, Irritable Bowel Syndrome, or migraine), *facilitation* is brain plasticity gone wild, the learning ability of the brain hijacked into creating ever more urgent alarms and heightened responses.

## HEADACHES DEFINED

The International Headache Society classifies headaches by characteristics, down to the number of minutes or hours per symptom. See: www.ihs-classification.org/en.

This level of detail is useful for research, but in the opinion of many patients, what a diagnosis of migraine comes down to is this: Headache that is extremely severe (or not) which might be one-sided (or not) with visual disturbances (or not), with nausea and sensitivity to light (or not), or maybe just visual symptoms but no head pain.

In the doctor's office, what it may come down to is: Do you get severe headaches with nausea and sensitivity to light? Did your mother get them too?

If a patient notices that the headache begins with stiffness or pain at the back of the neck and travels upward, the resulting headache may be dismissed as *tension,* the patient referred for psychiatric counseling, or given antidepressants or sedatives.

In my opinion, neither tension headaches nor migraines are necessarily lone entities. Both can be points on a continuum. The beginning of true migraine is the tipping point where muscle problems, food sensitivities or other assaults trigger the trigeminal alarm system which controls the painful expansion of blood vessels in the brain, which in turn produces the sickening pounding of the typical migraine. Other neurological symptoms typical of migraine arise when the vagus nerve is involved. That is:

*Migraine headache is the firing of the trigemino-vascular system, with possible vagus nerve involvement — regardless of initial cause.*

## PAIN AND OTHER SYMPTOMS

Headaches can be of many types and origins (Table 1 ).

*Migraine* headaches (Table 2 ) are seen as very different from other headaches. The division is far less solid than it used to be as researchers have found strong anatomical links between migraines and other head pain. Symptoms can overlap.

**TABLE 1.** HEADACHES, CATEGORIES AND SYMPTOMS

| Diagnosis | Symptoms |
|---|---|
| Anoxia | Related to oxygen / carbon dioxide imbalance, poor breathing, stuffy rooms and Sick Building Syndrome. |
| Barometer | Pain in response to pressure and weather changes. |
| Benign Daily | Daily head pain without tumor or known pathology. |
| Blood Pressure | Headache due to increased arterial pressure. |
| Low blood sugar / hypoglycemia | Pain and weakness due to decreased glucose to fuel the brain. |
| Cluster | Sudden paroxysmal pain typically centered around one eye. Historically more common in men than women at reported ratios ranging from 4:1 to 7:1 but recently on the rise in women who report that it is even worse than labor pains. |
| Effort | Triggered by physical effort; may be related to blood pressure changes, electrolytes and possibly oxygen balance. |
| Hangover | The most familiar example of head pain. Useful for demonstrating migraine to the uninitiated especially if combined with high altitude sickness. |
| Impingement | Can involve everything from muscle and bone compressing nerves and blood vessels, to arteries compressing nerves. |
| Muscle Tension | Deep aching pain which tends to be steady. |
| Orgasm | May be related to blood pressure changes, possibly allergies and oxygen balance. More common in men than women at a rate of 4:1. |
| Rebound | Headaches caused by headache medications. |
| Sinus | Pain in sinus areas. May be undiagnosed migraine, especially in men. Can also be due to referred muscular pain. |
| Trauma | From stretching and tearing of soft tissues (as in whiplash) to subdural hematoma and inflammation. |

**TABLE 2.** MIGRAINE HEADACHES, TYPES, AND SYMPTOMS

| Diagnosis | Symptoms |
|---|---|
| Abdominal | Severe mid-abdominal pain, lasting 1-72 hours associated with nausea and vomiting, but no clear GI pathology or severe headache, but often with a family history of migraine. Most common in children but may also occur in adults. May include prodromes such as flushing, pallor, fatigue and sleepiness. |
| Classic | Pulsing pain preceded by 20-60 minutes of visual symptoms. Pain is typically one-sided with nausea and sensitivity to light, sound, and possibly odors. May continue 1-3 days or longer. |
| Common | Pulsing headache *without* aura, possibly on both sides of head |
| Hemiplegic | Named for the apparent "half-stroke" symptoms of weakness / paralysis appearing on one side of the body. |
| | Includes the usual migraine symptoms of nausea/ vomiting, chills and fever, sensitivity to light and sound, but may go on for days or weeks. There may be meningitis-like symptoms (without infection), confusion, and impaired brain function to the point of loss of consciousness and coma. |
| | Pain tends to begin before the one-sided weakness but may be absent, so attacks resemble stroke even more strongly. |
| Menstrual | Migraine with or without aura during ovulation or menstruation in response to hormone / prostaglandin / electrolyte levels. |
| Ocular | (Opthalmic or retinal migraine). Visual symptoms of migraine but without pain. |

**Migraine Phases**

| | |
|---|---|
| *Prodromes* | Symptoms that "run before" the migraine. May range from high energy, agitation, or euphoria to yawning and fatigue, food cravings or many other symptoms. |
| *Aura* | Diagnostic of "classic migraine" (missing in "common migraine"). Named for visual symptoms, such as *scotoma, flashes of light, areas of darkness, rainbows.* Other symptoms such as tingling, numbness, difficulties with speech and motor skills may also be referred to as "aura." Occurs 20-60 minutes before onset of head pain. |
| *Pain* | Typically a pulsing and pounding sensation that is constant; it does not come and go. Tends to begin in, over, or behind the eyes or in the temple. It may be one-sided, two-sided, or switch sides during an attack or from one attack to the next. May be accompanied by photophobia ("fear of light") or phonophobia ("fear of sound"), possibly with mild to severe nausea. Symptoms can last for hours, days (typically 2-3), or (in status migranosus) for weeks at a time. Vomiting may end the attack. |
| *Postdromes* | Symptoms "running after" the pain has ceased. These may include fatigue, exhaustion, confusion, disorientation. |

### Auras and Visual Patterns

In classifying migraines, a basic division is the presence or absence of *aura*.

*Auras* are effects of light and dark that may precede a headache or simply come and go on their own. They may include shimmering rainbows, rigidly geometric patterns, or glowing lights that appear, then fade away. *Scotoma (*from Gr. *skotos*, darkness) describes the dark or missing areas in the vision field. Auras are not painful. They can be intriguing and entertaining. They can also be terrifying if, besides impairing vision, their onset announces yet another migraine on the way.

In *Alice in Wonderland*, the Cheshire Cat fades away; its grin (and sharp teeth) remain (Figure 2). Author Charles Dobson (Lewis Carroll) is believed to have suffered migraine with aura. Modern migraineurs describe similar real-life experiences. You can see animated examples by artists and filmmakers recreating their experiences at www.YouTube.com. See also www.migraine-aura.org, the website of The Migraine Aura Foundation responsible for the famous Migraine Art project.

### Cold Feet and Hands

The typically cold feet and hands of migraine are considered to be a vascular response to the Autonomic Nervous System (ANS). It can also be a symptom of tight muscles. Muscles in thighs and calves tight enough to block circulation to the feet can actually *cause* a migraine. Restoring circulation can relieve it.

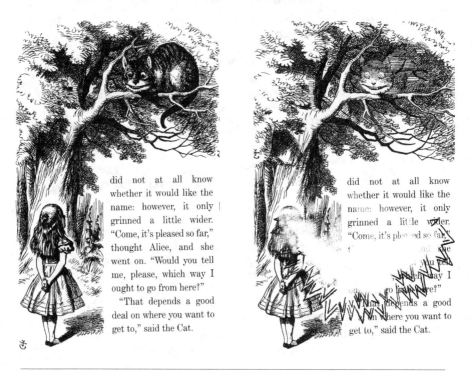

**Figure 2.** Carroll's Cat with Jolly's Scotoma

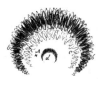

Ruete, 1845

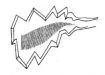

Charcot, 1888

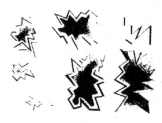

Babinski, 1890

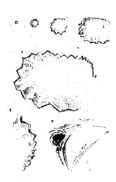

Jolly, 1902

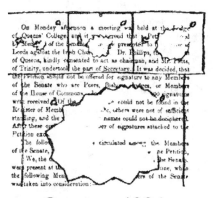

Gowers, 1904

Airy, 1907

**Figure 3.** AURAS AND SCOTOMAS

### Head Pain

You may have noticed that the terrible head pain typical of migraine keeps time with your heartbeat as blood pulses through dilated blood vessels in the brain. Steady, deep, gripping pain is typically of muscular origin. The two can combine. Also vascular constrictions in the lower extremities can cause pulsing pain in the head.

### GI Disturbances and Nausea

We have a brain in the head, but also in the gut and when one is unhappy, the other one is going to hear about it via the vagus nerve behind so many autonomic symptoms. Some of these are protective, but may, from our point of view, go terribly wrong.

When mast cells in the brain are exposed to toxins, they release chemicals that work to flush away the threat via vasodilation. Mast cells in the gut release chemicals that work to flush away toxins via muscle cramps and diarrhea.

### Motor Difficulties

Motor problems may involve everything from a feeling of being weak and clumsy, to confusion and difficulty in forming sounds and words. In basilar migraines, which strongly resemble a stroke, an entire side of the body can be impaired.

### Depression

There is a definite link between migraine and depression. Clinical depression is said to occur in 17 per cent of the general population. Among migraineurs the incidence rises to nearly 50 per cent.

Women with chronic headaches are four times as likely to be depressed as other women. They are also significantly more prone to stomach or back pain, fatigue, and sleep disturbances. Because women tend to suffer depression at rates higher than men, it has long been assumed that the headache and its associated somatic symptoms were due to the depression ("Depression hurts!") but the association remains even after adjusting for depression (Tietjen GE and others, 2007).

All three — migraine, depression and somatic symptoms — can have a common cause.

## MEET YOUR ELEPHANT

> In a knot of eight crossings . . . there are 256 different "over-and-under" arrangements possible. Make only one change in this "over and under" sequence and either an entirely different knot is made or no knot at all may result.
> —Clifford Warren Ashley, *The Ashley Book of Knots*

We tend to think in terms of individual triggers that must be identified and avoided. For many years I used a 10-point scale where 10 was a sure migraine. If hormones were at 6 with a category 5 stormfront, it was no time to add red wine (4) and chocolate (3) to the mix. This system gave some control, or at least, if I had stacked up 23 points of risky conditions, a migraine attack wouldn't be a surprise.

The point system is like a game of blackjack or piling up books. If you can't control the cards you are dealt, or the size or shape of the next book that must go on your stack, all it takes is one more trigger, one more point, to end the game in sudden death.

Despite many possible inputs, migraine headaches are commonly considered to be One Disease. Similarly, a statement by a first-century rabbi ("I and the Father are One") led to many centuries of theological debate on monads, dyads, relative rank, and a great deal of shouting. But join two circles and regardless of which one is higher or lower, greater or smaller, there's that "One" in the middle. Link a third circle and you now have what mathematicians call *Borromean rings*. The Individual rings can bind together into one tightly unified whole, but remove just one ring, change the recipe, and the entire structure (or market) will collapse.

To eliminate migraines, eliminate obvious triggers, but also search for connections and relationships. Change just *one* of the rings, alter just one set of relationships, and everything else may change too. Former triggers may lose their power and one day that elephant may have no place left to stand.

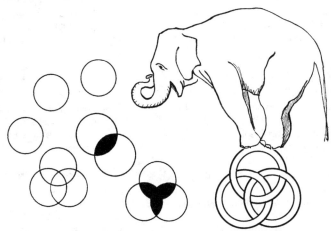

**Figure 4.** RINGS AND SETS

### The Blind Men and the Elephant

—John Godfrey Saxe (1816-1887)

It was six men of Indostan
To learning much inclined,
Who went to see the Elephant
(Though all of them were blind),
That each by observation
Might satisfy his mind.

The First approach'd the Elephant,
And happening to fall
Against his broad and sturdy side,
At once began to bawl:
"God bless me! but the Elephant
Is very like a wall!"

The Second, feeling of the tusk,
Cried, "Ho! what have we here
So very round and smooth and sharp?
To me 'tis mighty clear
This wonder of an Elephant
Is very like a spear!"

The Third approached the animal,
And happening to take
The squirming trunk within his hands,
Thus boldly up and spake:
"I see," quoth he, "the Elephant
Is very like a snake!"

The Fourth reached out his eager hand,
And felt about the knee.
"What most this wondrous beast is like
Is mighty plain," quoth he,
"'Tis clear enough the Elephant
Is very like a tree!"

The Fifth, who chanced to touch the ear,
Said: "E'en the blindest man
Can tell what this resembles most;
Deny the fact who can,
This marvel of an Elephant
Is very like a fan!"

The Sixth no sooner had begun
About the beast to grope,
Then, seizing on the swinging tail
That fell within his scope,
"I see," quoth he, "the Elephant
Is very like a rope!"

And so these men of Indostan
Disputed loud and long,
Each in his own opinion
Exceeding stiff and strong,
Though each was partly in the right,
And all were in the wrong!

Blood vessels are supplied by nerves, nerves have blood supply, and both must pass through bone and connective tissue. Block blood supply and muscles and nerves will scream in pain. Migraine can be *structuro-chemico-musculo-neuro-vascular*. Table 3 lists common migraine triggers and relationships.

| TABLE 3. COMMON TRIGGERS AND RELATIONSHIPS | |
|---|---|
| **Medical** | Infections and disease. |
| | Low stomach acid, impaired nutrient absorption and infections. |
| | Thyroid, autoimmune, gluten sensitivity and celiac disease. |
| **Muscular** | Tightening and swelling with neurovascular impingement on nerves and blood vessels. |
| **Vascular** | Vasodilation and vasoconstriction. |
| | Platelet stickiness and increased clotting. |
| | Decreased blood supply possibly with arterial spasm. |
| | Impaired venous drainage. |
| **Neurological** | Abnormal sensitivity to sensory inputs. |
| | Nerve entrapment / strain by muscles / arteries, edema. |
| | Multiple stimuli (noise, light, odor) overwhelming thresholds. |
| | Brain injury and brain wave abnormalities. |
| | Electromagnetic (EMF) pollution. |
| **Structural** | Poor posture: slumping, Head-Forward, tilted pelvis. |
| | Thoracic Outlet Syndrome (TOS), cervical ribs, extra vertebrae. |
| | Cervical and cranial abnormalities (trauma / birth injuries). |
| | Unequal leg lengths, pelvic bone distortions, foot abnormalities, Patent Foramen Ovale (PFO), Chiari malformations. |
| **Chemical** | Imbalances of nutrients, electrolytes, hormones. |
| | Sensitivity to food, mold, pollen, MSG, aspartame, histamines, nitrates, sulfates, food colorings / flavorings, air / water pollution, toxic personal care products. |
| | Fluctuating blood sugar (skipped meals, sugary foods, diabetes, hypoglycemia), and obesity. |
| | Inflammation / vasodilation (prostaglandins, tyramines. |
| | Impaired breathing and $O_2/CO_2$, acid/base balance. |
| | Stress and strain from overwork, disrupted sleep or digestion. |
| **Environmental** | Damaging work, hobbies, clothing, shoes, furniture. |
| | Barometric changes due to weather or altitude. |
| | Unreliable, unpredictable, abusive home or work environments. |

## TREATMENT CHOICES

In dealing with migraine (or any other disease), you have three basic choices.

**1. DO NOTHING.** A common approach. Reasons for this can range from a belief that it is necessary to resist "weakness" to simple lack of information, perhaps combined with financial issues. At $20-$30 per dose, migraine drugs are *expensive*. If unaffordable, sufferers who lack insurance may assume nothing can be done. Not so!

**2. TREAT THE SYMPTOMS.** Drugs can be the life preserver that keeps your head above water and buys you time to track down the causes. They can save a life, but are a poor way to live a life if there are other options.

**3. FIND, TREAT AND ELIMINATE THE UNDERLYING PROBLEMS.** Do not assume that all headaches are migraines (or sinus infection) and that drugs are the only answer.

Imagine crashing into a tree then trying to fix everything wrong with your vehicle by pouring yet another chemical additive into your gas tank. It may be that fan blades are jammed, the distributor cap cracked, or a spark plug wire was pulled loose in the collision. No drug that treats symptoms only will ever work as well as finding and treating the source of the problem.

After years of mysterious pain, being diagnosed with a Real Disease can be a huge relief. But don't stop there. For many people, migraine meds are just not going to work because *the problem is not just migraine*. Rushing into a diagnosis to medicate it is not the most effective approach.

Drug dependency also risks falling afoul of predatory business models with interlocking products and sales: create a demand, then fill it with a product the victim doesn't really need. At $20-$30 per dose, migraine drugs are extremely *lucrative*.

Currently there is much concern that migraine is "under-diagnosed" and that headache sufferers who should be diagnosed with migraine are too dependent on over-the-counter drugs.

If this is concern for the patient, it is admirable.

If it is merely concern for profits lost to cheaper medications, it is not.

# Personal Evaluations and Testing

Migraine can be a symptom of many things. It is impossible to untangle the many possibilities in a few minutes at the doctor's office. Gather the information that will give you and your doctor the clues you need to end the migraines.

First, how bad, how long, how often are your headaches?

Where are they and how do they progress? How much impact do they have on your life?

## WHAT, WHERE AND WHY?

Migraine symptoms (and their triggers) vary so widely from person to person that "atypical migraine" is amazingly *typical*. So what do *you* mean by "migraine"?

Chances are that your definition won't be exactly the same as anyone else's, yet in online support groups, descriptions of specific location of a headaches is rare. Ask sufferers where it hurts and the standard response is a shocked and somewhat indignant response: "In my *head* of course!"

OK, *where* in your head? There are big differences between headaches in different locations.

Does pain appear:

- In the front, back, temples, and/or top of the head?
- At the front and move back? Or at the back of the head moving forward?
- In your teeth?— which ones? Upper or lower? Front or back?
- With numbness or tingling in legs, arms, or fingers? — which ones? Fronts or backs?
- After a particular type of emotional / physical stress?
- In association with cyclic changes: daily, weekly, monthly, yearly?
- With hunger or after a particular food or drink?
- After a poor night's sleep? With or without leg cramps, numb hands or arms?
- What do you notice first?
- How does it progress, change position, or spread over time?

Observe symptoms carefully over your entire body. Many can be tracked back to root causes and triggers and the areas of brain or body where the symptoms may arise.

## PAIN CHARTS AND DIAGRAMS

Pains caused by disturbance of the second cervical root begin in the suboccipital area, radiating upward toward the [top of the head] and forward behind the [same-side] eye. The patient often feels as if the eyeball is being torn from the socket. The headaches are migraine-like and often associated with nausea, vomiting and blurred vision.

—E Seletz, M. D. (1958)

It is rare for headache patients to actually diagram their pain or for physicians to have them do so. This may be due to the notion that a headache is a headache and whatever it is, it is just *one thing*. That is not the case.

Migraines can progress to full-body pain but they never start that way. Where the pain actually starts and how it progresses is extremely valuable information.

When asked about origins and locations, limiting your answers to "It Hurts Everywhere" isn't useful and at some time it wasn't true. Find the point where your headaches start; put one finger on it if necessary. If it is a vague, hard-to-localize pain deep inside your head, you can still indicate right or left, front or back. Track the pain from *here* to *everywhere that symptoms appear*.

*Everywhere.* Really. If your headache comes with tingly arms and fingers, show where you feel the tingling and in exactly which fingers (fronts or backs). If it hurts right down to your teeth, *which* teeth? If it comes with abdominal cramps and back pain, is it upper, lower, right or left?

Patients often omit critical information for fear of being seen as "crazy." Noticing pain in a shoulder or calf or running down the thumb has nothing to do with "crazy." It just "is" and usually there is a reason for it.

Compare the quote above by a Dr. Seletz in 1958 with the pain diagram in Figure 5. There was a time when pain reported in the neck would eliminate a diagnosis of migraine in favor of "tension headache" and a referral for psychiatric counseling. But nerves in the back of the neck will eventually talk to the trigeminal nerves which are credited with the symptoms of "true" migraine.

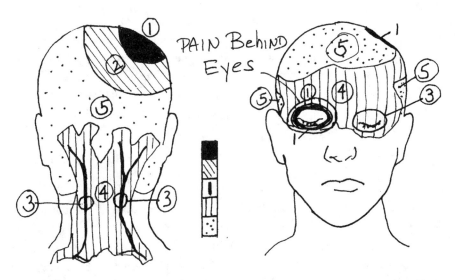

Patient diagram showing beginning and final ("all over") pain — and clues to the source.

**Figure 5.** PROGRESSION OF HEADACHE PAIN

Blocked nerves and blood vessels in neck and shoulder cause the back, arm, hand, and finger pain known as Thoracic Outlet Syndrome. Similar pain is often diagnosed as Carpal Tunnel Syndrome although the carpal tunnel may have nothing to do with it. Arms may "go to sleep" at night (more than you do) but a first sign of outlet problems is often *intractable migraine.* Crampy calves, heel and pelvic pain may also signal reduced blood flow in the lower body. These are important clues. Don't leave them out.

You can also draw the *nature* of the experience. What do you see during an attack? What is the quality of the pain? How does it make you *feel*?

Drawing the migraine was once thought to be an interesting "artsy" thing to do, but it is not a trivial exercise. It is at least an antidote to common migraine images which tend to feature lovely young female models with perfect hair and perfect makeup, delicately touching fingertips to temples.

Images from The Migraine Art Project are not pretty. They are horrifying depictions of pain, frustration, and despair. They have also revealed a wealth of neurological information, and, for both migraineurs and Normals, a window of insight into the migraine brain. See images at: www.migraine-aura.org.

## MUSCLE TESTING

Muscle imbalances are involved in all kinds of headaches. Evaluation can be done manually with Range-of-Motion (ROM) testing. If you must strain to touch your closed jaw to your chest, or if you cannot tilt your head more than a few degrees to the side, you have found an important clue to your headaches. For details see page 69.

A high-tech approach to muscle testing is *electromyography* (EMG). See page 32.

## DIARIES AND LOGS

### PAIN LEVELS

There is no more useful tool for evaluating your migraines than the headache diary, especially if combined with food, medications, weather, and more. Many patients refuse to track their headaches because "Why bother when I get them *all the time?*"

Do you really? Then note when they are worse, when they are milder, when they are pulsing (typical of migraine) or a dull deep ache (typical of muscles), or burning (typical of nerve involvement). Worst case, note when you can sleep, when you need to sleep but can't, what you have eaten, what you have done for the pain, and what does and does not help.

### FOOD INTAKE

Start a food diary at least two weeks before your doctor's appointment. You can do this with pencil and a notebook or far more easily and comprehensively with computerized food trackers. Think of this not as a *diet* (too often an exercise in guilt) but as data.

What have you been eating? What have you *not* been eating? Research has shown repeatedly that the nutritional intake of migraineurs is remarkably poor.

A colleague tells of a woman who consulted him for biofeedback treatment in hopes of relieving her chronic pain. She complained bitterly that none of the many doctors she had seen had helped, nor had the many prescription drugs (which she brought with her in a large shopping bag). When asked what she had been eating it became apparent that her major food source was cinnamon sweet rolls and diet soda.

It is not possible to be healthy or functional on such a diet or to make up deficiencies with supplements. Don't try to fool yourself into thinking it will and don't try to fool your doctor. For details, see "Nutrition Trackers" on page 227.

### TEMPERATURE

Good thyroid function is critical to good health. Low thyroid function is associated with low temperature. Among many other unpleasant symptoms, body temperature that is persistently low by just one degree (and certainly by more), impairs muscle function and poor muscle function is associated with migraine.

Low body temperature is *not* an automatic indication that you need a prescription for thyroid hormone, but it is suspicious and the cause should be examined further. It can result from low-calorie diets, several kinds of anemia, over-use of soy products, endocrine disrupting cosmetics, toiletries, and sedentary life-style. Unfortunately, the side-effect of low temperature is an almost automatic weight gain, commonly dismissed as laziness. Often, a sedentary life-style is automatically assumed no matter how untrue that may be. It is also possible that you do not know how active (or inactive) you really are.

Tracking calorie input and exercise output (with a pedometer) against temperature is a useful test of actual activity. Record your temperature at waking, at bedtime, and before meals. Combine this information with your Food Diary.

## BLOOD PRESSURE

Home blood pressure monitors are easily available and taking your blood pressure at home is far more useful than having it checked occasionally at the doctor's office. Home monitors are not as accurate as professional-quality equipment in the hands of trained medical personnel but you can track trends of high and low pressure and heart rates. All of these can be significant in headache.

## MEDICATIONS

List all medications you are taking including dietary supplements, prescription, over-the-counter (OTC), and herbal preparations, *and their possible side effects*. Notice how often "headache" appears in the list of possible symptoms in products ranging from antidepressants to statins to hair tonics. Be aware of foods, drugs, and cosmetics that impact thyroid. (See "Metabolic Problems" on page 156.) You can get drug information sheets from your pharmacist or from Internet sites such as www.drugwatch.com. Dr. Joe Graedon, a professor of pharmacology, maintains an excellent website at www.peoplespharmacy.com.

## DISABILITY AND IMPACT

The Migraine Disability Assessment (MIDAS) measures and quantifies disability at school / work/ home and social relationships. The Headache Impact Test is a more extensive evaluation. Both are available at www.headachetest.com.

It is useful to re-take the test during the course of treatment to mark progress.

# Medical Evaluation and Testing

## SEEING YOUR DOCTOR

What should you bring to your appointment? The best thing is *information*.

- How do you know you're getting a a headache? What warning signs do you get?
- How many times per (year / month / week / day / hour) do the headaches occur?
- How many minutes or hours do they last?
- Rank pain on a scale of 1-10 (where 0 is nothing and 10 is "Oh God, kill me now!")
- Where do you feel them? Make a drawing of where they hurt and any changes over the course of the attack. Include areas of numbness, tingling, or other symptoms.
- What makes your headaches *worse*? Activity? Lying down? Standing up?
- What makes them *better*? What remedies have you tried (heat, cold, drugs) at what dosages, and how many times? What helps? What doesn't?

This approach helps to *quantify* the problem, that is: How much? How big? How bad? The answers to these questions lead to effective treatment. Saying that you've "tried everything and *nothing* helps!" is never as useful as listing the specific things that you have actually tried and their results. Appointment time is short and precious. Don't waste it. In general, for first appointments:

- *Do* bring your headache diary, pain diagrams, and a one page medical history with dates, surgeries, conditions, diagnoses. This saves the time of trying to reproduce accurate information from memory.
- *Do* bring a list of questions such as medication side-effects and other concerns about treatment. These tend to be forgotten in the stress of an appointment,.
- *Do* get a note signed by your doctor (on the doctor's letterhead or prescription pad) per recommended treatment and dosages should you need to go to the Emergency Room, one of the *worst* possible places for a migraineur. Best case, even if the staff recognizes a severe migraine, you will stay at the end of the line behind the chest pains, asthma attacks, broken bones, and bleeders for hours to come. Migraine is not seen as a life-threatening emergency. Worst case, no matter how bad the pain, the first suspicion will be that you are an addict looking for drugs. A note from your physician shows that you have an actual diagnosis, are under medical care, and will ease the process for every-one involved.
- *Do not* bring books and articles for your doctor to read. Chances are there will be no time to read them and they will not be happy at the prospect of a quiz afterwards.
- *Do not* substitute vague generalities for solid information. When asked how you've been doing with a treatment, "OK I guess" is not useful. What *is* useful is specific information on how symptoms have increased or decreased in number or severity, changed or not changed in duration and intensity. Having this information in a headache diary clarifies the situation for both of you, making it possible to treat intelligently.

# MEDICAL TESTING

When laboratory tests are done, get copies of the reports and get actual numbers rather than statements such as "results are within normal ranges." Different labs use different ranges. Only actual numbers allow an intelligent evaluation of results. Over the years, traditional ranges have changed or been proposed for change, as has happened with thyroid, magnesium, and Vitamin D.

## NUTRITIONAL STATUS

*Migraine can be a symptom of nutritional inadequacies.*

Migraineurs are typically low or out of balance in several critical nutrients. Part of the problem is Fear of Food. Migraineurs are typically given long lists of foods to avoid. Most list foods high in tyramines; some include every food ever known to have caused problems in any patient ever. The message is that if you eat, you will get a migraine and it's your own fault.

But few foods reliably cause migraine in *all* patients. Tyramine-containing foods have long been said to be dangerous but when the tyramine connection was submitted to a double-blind statistical analysis it simply didn't hold up (Jansen SC and others, 2003). Nevertheless, food lists have grown to the point that it may appear that nothing is safe and the problem is worsened through nutritional deficiencies. Tyramine-containing food lists are so very extensive that they are contra-indicated in pregnant migraineurs for exactly that reason.

Several problems commonly lumped as "stress" can be split into several contributing factors. These include sleep and hormone-disrupting schedules such as overtime or split shifts, inadequate outdoor exercise, and fast food diets. When the system rebels, adding antacids to the mix reduces absorption of the nutrients that are available.

Depression is strongly linked with migraine, but over a dozen common nutrients have depression as the first symptom of deficiency. Some directly impact serotonin production and thyroid function.

Vitamin D deficiencies are now so common that testing should be part of every checkup. Electrolytes, specifically calcium and magnesium, are now known to have a powerful effect on migraine even in patients whose blood tests appear to be "within standard ranges." New tests are far more accurate. For details see page 149.

## INFECTIONS

*Migraine can be a symptom of infection.*

The link between migraine and infection is especially strong in migraine *without aura*. Tooth decay is a classic cause of infection that can impact the entire body, to the point of sepsis, cardiomyopathy and heart failure[1]. Tthe trigeminal nerve that triggers migraine-type symptoms is the same nerve that supplies teeth and gums. During dental work, you may notice blips of ache or pain in your head, even after teeth have been numbed by novocaine.

*Helicobacter pylori* is an opportunistic bacterium that and causes ulcers.and thrives with overuse of antacids. And, while migraineurs have long been warned against nicotine due to its impact on vasodilation and constriction, we now know that tobacco in any form is an excellent source of pathogenic soil-borne bacteria.

## ALLERGY

*Migraine can be a symptom of allergies.*

In my experience, migraine is too quickly assumed to be a *primary* condition; the *symptom becomes the diagnosis.* We love to talk about "triggers" but frank *allergies* may not be so quickly investigated before we begin migraine medications. Insurance companies may flatly deny "allergy testing" on the grounds that migraine is unrelated to allergies, insisting that migraine is a *neurological* disease, a neurologist the only appropriate specialist, and migraine drugs the only appropriate treatment.

Your headaches may be migraines but the trigemino-vascular system that makes a true migraine can be triggered by an allergic response. Inflammation and swelling associated with migraine involves the meningeal membranes (surrounding the brain[2]) and mast cells (surrounding the blood vessels in the brain). In response to allergens, stress hormones, and other triggers, mast cells release chemicals (prostaglandins, histamines, and more) that cause vasodilation, inflammation, and greatly increased nerve sensitivity. A first line of defense may be antihistamines and prostaglandin inhibiting NSAIDs (Non-Steroidal Anti-Inflammatories) such as ibuprofen or naproxen. (Not Tylenol; it's not an NSAID.)

If your headaches match the pollen maps, or occur over the same two weeks every May, you have an excellent reason for allergy testing. Avoidance and antihistamines are worth a try before going on to years of costly migraine drugs and their side effects[3].

---

1. Actor Andy Hallet (who played the genial singing demon on the TV show *Angel*) died at age 33, of cardiomyopathy believed to have originated with an infected tooth.
2. These are most familiar in *meningitis,* a deadly inflammation of these membranes. The *dura* is the tough outermost layer.
3. Allergy shots may be worth a trial, but test during the off-season of suspected allergens. Be aware that shots may take *years* to become effective.

## FOOD SENSITIVITIES

*Migraine can be a symptom of sensitivities to food and gluten*

The best way to track food sensitivities is still the food diary. Laboratory tests are notoriously unreliable, with the exception of gluten sensitivity.

Celiac disease is characterized by severe sensitivity to gluten, a protein found in wheat, barley, rye, and other grains. Symptoms include gas, bloating, diarrhea, and *migraines*. Symptoms of gluten sensitivity may be delayed until middle age or later, overlooked because it failed to develop as expected in childhood. This is odd behavior for a condition considered to be genetic, yet celiac disease has increased by a factor of more than 20 since the 1970s (Parker-Pope T, 2011).

Recent studies from the University of Maryland Center for Celiac Research suggests a difference between celiac disease and gluten sensitivity. Both exist on a spectrum of gluten-related disorders, but they not the same. Another issue may be genetically modified (GMO) crops. Travellers from Europe often say that they have gluten problems in the US but not in Europe where GM crops are far less common.

Tests for gluten sensitivity are quick and accurate, but be aware that cutting gluten out of your diet *before* the test will confuse test results.

Meanwhile, read food labels for MSG (and the many names under which it is commonly disguised), aspartame, and other additives. Be aware of the top eight food sensitivities (now required to be stated on packaged food labels): milk, egg, fish, shellfish, tree nuts, wheat, peanuts, and soy.

## HYPOTHYROID

*Migraine can be a symptom of poor thyroid function.*

A healthy, functioning thyroid is critical to general good health. It is part of the feedback loop between the brain and adrenal glands. Their interactions help regulate basic body processes including mood, energy levels, digestion, immune response, sex behaviors, and stress response.

TSH is not "the Gold Standard" of thyroid testing as some claim. It is the tip of the iceberg. Get the full panel, including *free* T3 and T4. Get *figures*, not ranges for "low" or "normal" as these can vary from lab to lab and ranges have been revised several times within the last decade. Too many physicians still base treatment on ranges set when we lived in a very different world. See "Metabolic Problems" on page 156.

## HYPOGLYCEMIA AND DIABETES

*Migraine can be a symptom of fluctuating blood sugar.*

A diet high in sugar and starch (which is broken down to sugar) triggers a rush of *hyperglycemia* ("high blood sugar") which in turn triggers excessive release of insulin which in turn pulls sugar out of the blood. After the initial sugar high, the result is *hypoglycemia* (or "low sugar"). The brain, which runs on sugar begins to starve. Hypoglycemia can cause headache, depression, insomnia, racing heart, panic attacks and more. In diabetics, it is the most common cause of diabetic coma, usually due to faulty insulin management. In Normals, the cause can be as simple as failure to eat regular meals or overdosing on sweets. In general, hypoglyemia is indicated if:

- Blood sugar drop is greater than 100 mg/dl/hr or
- Blood sugar falls below 60 mg/dl at any time during the test.

In diabetes, due to impaired insulin response, blood sugar remains high, either:

- Fasting blood sugar of 126 mg/dl or
- Glucose Tolerance Test of 200 mg/dl 2 hours after the sugar dose.

Home finger-stick blood sugar meters (which sample capillary blood) are useful for tracking blood trends but are unreliable for absolute values. Reliable testing requires venous blood. Hypoglycemia and diabetes are best evaluated by your physician, but keep a log to see how much of your food comes from sugar and refined carbohydrates which contribute greatly to these conditions.

## MRI AND CT SCANS

Imaging can reveal aneurysms, brain bleeds, tumors, cysts, and other problems. These are rare, but of concern if headaches develop or worsen days, weeks, or even months after a traumatic fall or accident. Also of interest are aberrations in the Circle of Willis which can reduce blood flow in the brain or even reverse it. See page 90.

## ELECTROMYOGRAPHY

Electromyography[1] is a means of testing the electrical behavior of muscles.

Needle EMG involves inserting needles into specific muscles. Surface EMG (sEMG) is non-invasive and painless, involving electrodes placed on the surface of the skin.

On a computer screen, EMG reveals muscle imbalances, strengths, weaknesses and improper muscle response. This information guides effective treatment and muscle retraining. See "Biofeedback" on page 258.

---

1. Electro-Myo-Graphy, or "electrical-muscle-writing." For details, see Chapter 8.

---

# Chapter 2

# It's Just Tension!

*Migraine can be a symptom of tight, overstretched, or unbalanced muscles and connective tissue. If you can't touch your chin to your chest without pain or pulling, if one shoulder or hip rides higher than the other, you have a clue to your migraines.*

The one-sided migraine is often attributed to our bilateral symmetry and the paired nerves in the brain. That is, a nerve on *one* side of the brain will produce symptoms on that *one* side of the body. But one-sided pain can also come from one-sided stresses and muscular strains as common and as simple as a heavy purse on one shoulder.

Tension headaches have long been said to be separate from migraine, but this is not necessarily so. In the 1990s the *dural bridge* was found, a direct anatomical link between neck muscles and the pain-sensitive dura surrounding brain and spinal cord. Later, Botox treatments were reported to halt some (if not all) life-long migraines by relieving nerve irritation by muscles in the forehead. Unfortunately, most patients ignore muscular symptoms and most physicians rarely ask about them. If they do, migraineurs tend to respond badly. "Muscle tension headache" may mean "head pain due to tight or dysfunctional muscles." But if muscle relaxants are prescribed but fail to resolve the problem, it has often been a short trip to:

- "You're just stressed," and

- "Have you considered psychiatric counseling?" — too often with the implication that . . .

- The pain is not *real*. YOU are just overly sensitive, acting out, *crazy.*

This approach ignores or trivializes the underlying anatomy and physiology, the pain and the patient. It even trivializes psychotherapy which may offer solutions for contributing issues. Many pains do indeed have psychiatric components, but the psychogenic diagnosis is woefully overdone. Strangely, it is rarely applied to knee pain, toe pain, or shoulder pain, but is used all too often by the practitioner who, when asked for the underlying cause of head pain, cannot bring himself to say "I don't know." And there's a lot to know. More than 20 muscles (primarily of the *neck*) send pain to the *head*, several send pain directly to the *eye*. Several others refer pain to specific *teeth* for reasons that will never be relieved by fillings or repeated root canals.

# Muscles and Trigger Points

Muscles can pull bones out of alignment and compress nerves and blood vessels. This is particularly likely in the neck, head, and upper back, a remarkably complex arrangement of muscle and bone, nerves, and vascular tissue. Many of the structures here are individually known to cause severe pain. In most headaches, regardless of the name given to the symptoms, there is a tremendous amount of *muscular* involvement. Pain from muscles and connective tissue is often dismissed due to unfamiliarity, or to failure to detect taut muscle *in the painful area.* But muscular pain typically appears far from its *source.*

For example, the UPPER TRAPEZIUS muscle of the back produces neck, tooth, jaw, and head pain featuring a fish-hook pattern of pain at side of neck and head, often with nausea, visual, and autonomic symptoms. This pattern is typically diagnosed as *migraine,* especially if one-sided. When the lower part of the same muscle sends pain to the *back* of the neck and head, it is diagnosed as *muscle tension,* shoulder pain as *bursitis,* and jaw pain as TMJD. One muscle, multiple diagnoses. Figure 6 shows pain coming from the TRAPEZIUS muscle. No other pathology (such as a tumor ) is required.

sEMG electrodes at the source (not necessarily where the pain appears) might record something like the pattern shown in Figure 7. UPPER TRAPEZIUS and LOWER TRAPEZIUS are relatively quiet on the left. On the right, they are electrically overactive, under strain,

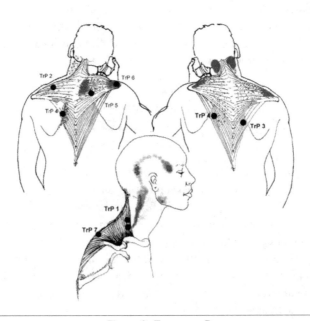

**Figure 6.** TRAPEZIUS PAIN

working much harder than on the left. This patient suffered one-sided headaches on the right side, diagnosed as classic migraine but coming from the right TRAPEZIUS.

Much muscular pain comes from hyper-sensitive spots of shortened muscle fibers. They have been recognized in the world-wide medical literature for centuries, but as a confusion of different names in different languages.

They came to the attention of Dr. Janet Travell in the 1940s in wartime Washington, D.C. While working in cardiology at Georgetown Medical School she saw many men suffering frightening chest pain but found that pressing on nodules and thickenings in chest muscles often sent pain shooting down the arm, reproducing symptoms of angina in men with perfectly healthy hearts.

Around the same time Travell developed a nagging pain in the front of her shoulder. On backing into a coat rack, she discovered that pressure on the muscle at the *back* of the shoulder reproduced the pain in the *front,* then *relieved* it. Intrigued, she planned to write an article for publication, but on reviewing the medical literature, quickly discovered many earlier papers reporting the same phenomenon. Travell dove into intense research in this area, and in doing so, created a whole new field and a standardized terminology. She named these hyper-sensitive nodules "Trigger Points" (TrPs) for their ability to "trigger" pain to other areas, often far from the source.

TrPs represent a local energy crisis in the muscle with abnormally shortened muscle cells and tangles of fascial adhesions. They are like the tangles in a phone cord that is supposed to be 10 feet long but can now stretch only 6 feet (Figure 8). The untangled cells must do all the work that would normally have been done by all the cells working together, thus they are subject to overload and increased strain. And, if the cord or

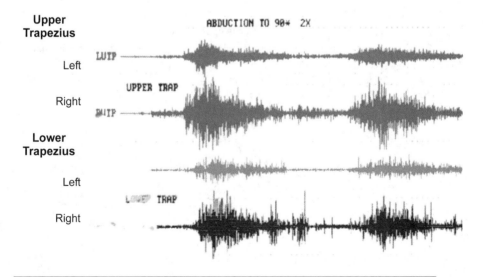

**Figure 7.** SEMG OF A TRAPEZIUS MIGRAINE

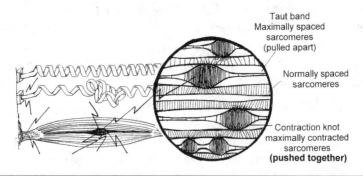

Taut band
Maximally spaced
sarcomeres
(pulled apart)

Normally spaced
sarcomeres

Contraction knot
maximally contracted
sarcomeres
**(pushed together)**

**Figure 8.** TANGLES IN CORDS AND MUSCLES

muscle must stretch a full 10 feet but is too tight to do so, there is the danger that it will rip and tear. To protect itself, a muscle may contract and shorten even *more*.

Shortened fibers block circulation (especially *micro*circulation) and collect waste products. Strain on attachments stimulates reflexes that cause still more tightening to protect the muscle. The result is muscles that are tight and *overshortened* opposing muscles that are *overstretched*. Both can test "weak." With sustained stress, TrPs can provoke inflammation, fibrosis, calcification, severe pain, and even brain injury.

Muscle pain is often considered less *real,* less serious, than that of more obviously life-threatening conditions. But people who have suffered broken bones, kidney stones, *and* myofascial pain can testify that pain of myofascial origin (which includes labor pains and heart attack) can be just as brutal and as "real" as pain from other sources. It can also be just as life threatening. Migraines and other pains of possible muscular origin have led to severe disability, addictions to pain-killing drugs, with all that flows from that, including suicides.

Even TrPs are symptoms. They develop in the course of daily life and work, sports and hobbies, poor food, poor posture, infections, clothing and accessories, musical instruments, colds and drafts.

Combine a Head-Forward posture with a pipe clench-ing jaw and hours of violin played in a cold room and what do you get?

"Elementary!" cries Dr. Watson. "Head pain, back pain, and extreme sensitivity of teeth to heat, cold, and vibration." Avoid "the seven percent solution" of drugs and potions in favor of tracking down the TrPs and clues to their origins.

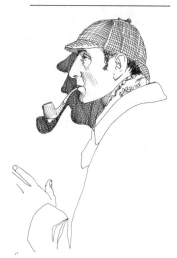

TrPs form at motor end plates (the junction between nerve and muscle) in response to stresses such as:

- Direct trauma, including:
    - Compression, blows, cuts, surgery,
    - Overstraining (heavy weights),
    - Overstretching with protective shortening,
    - Chronic shortening (such as holding a phone between neck and shoulder),

Why does your head ache? It's a mystery!

    - Repetitive motion injuries, and chronic non-motion injuries.

- Suboptimal nutrition, including:
    - Dehydration (too little water, too much caffeine or alcohol).
    - Inadequate/unbalanced nutrition (especially B vitamins, calcium to magnesium. ratios, Vitamin D, and protein), anemia, electrolyte imablanaces.

- Low temperature
    - Local chilling (drafts from air conditioners or wind whipping by a motorcycle helmet).
    - Inactivity, anemia, low thyroid.
    - Metabolic problems (thyroid / adrenal, antibodies, toxins or disease).

- Brain Injury / dysregulation from:
    - Mechanical trauma (including blows, whiplash, birth injury).
    - Emotional trauma.
    - Reduced blood supply or injury/shock to the hypothalamic-pituitary axis.
    - Brainwave slowing.

- Infection, allergy, sleep disorders.

- Low oxygen supply (improper breathing, apnea, circulatory problems, or altitude).

A single TrP is bad enough but more can form by *reference*. When muscles send pain to distant areas TrPs develop in the local muscles which have their own pain patterns. These in turn trigger other muscles and *their* specific pain patterns. All are known as *satellite* TrPs (Figure 9).

For example, TRAPEZIUS refers pain to the temple; the muscle there is TEMPORALIS which sends pain to the upper teeth. TRAPEZIUS also refers pain to the angle of the lower jaw; the muscle there is MASSETER, which refers pain to both upper and lower molar teeth, to the upper jaw, to the ear, and brow where there are more muscles. The domino effect can continue to the point that the sufferer can honestly say "It just hurts *everywhere*!.

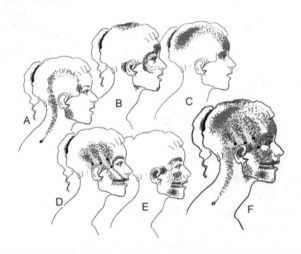

**Figure 9.** SATELLITE TRIGGER POINTS

# The Fascial Connection

> Fascia is the organ of posture. Nobody ever says this; all the talk is about muscles. Yet
> . . . the body is a web of fascia.
>
> —Dr. Ida P. Rolf

How can pain can travel to such distant areas from its point of origin? One reason is fascia, ("FASH-UH") our first nervous system and amazingly strong connective tissue that surrounds and penetrates every structure, every cell of the body.

*Superficial* fascia surrounds the body like a shrink-wrap leotard. *Deep* fascia surrounds and penetrates nerves, blood vessels, bones, and muscles. Fascia in muscles blends to form ligaments and tendons that blend into the *periosteum*, the fascial tissue "around-bone." *Visceral* fascia wraps around individual organs and suspends them in their proper places. In general, fascia stabilizes and supports the body like guy-wires on a radio tower or rigging on a ship. It is the organic equivalent of the steel belting in radial tires, the stabilizing mesh of steel in a reinforced concrete structure.

In the West, this basic body system has been largely ignored for almost 500 years. Early anatomists, such as Vesalius and Leonardo da Vinci, described and illustrated it in great, gory detail. Over the years it vanished from drawings, apparently dismissed as extraneous tissue that had to be stripped away to get to the good stuff, that is, the more interesting individual muscles and organs.

.In the East, fascia appears to be the origin of "meridians." Ancient Chinese medical writers spoke of a "lining" of body and organs called the *Li*. Today *Li* is usually translated as "internal," as a philosophical opposite of "external" in Taoist dualistic thought. But during the Han dynasty (206 BC–220 AD), *Li* indicated very real, specific physical *linings*, apparently what we now call *membranes*.

You will see these membranes on US currency and at the grocery store, separating and bundling individal muscles into groups (Figure 10). You will also find them as sausage casings, the fascial tissue of animal intestines. Pull on a sausage casing or the fascia surrounding a liver, kidney, or other organ, and you will find that it is very tough stuff indeed.

Fascia was the Mylar® of the early 20th and previous centuries, light as tissue paper, able to hold gas, and enormously strong for its weight. Figure 11 shows a bag holding

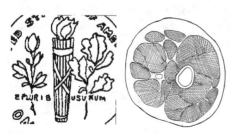

The Roman *fascis* was a bundle of sticks bound together, symbolizing authority and *unity (or at its worst, fascism)*. The Latin phrase *E pluribus unum* means "From many, one."

In the body, fascia binds and supports muscle and bone, joints and organs.

**Figure 10.** FASCIS AND FASCIA

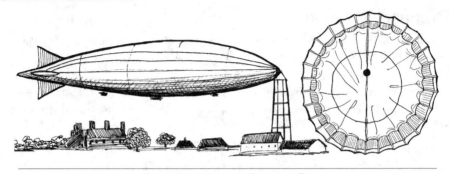

**Figure 11.** INDUSTRIAL-STRENGTH FASCIA

What appears to be a small hole in the bag is actually the opening for a man-sized catwalk.

500,000 cubic feet of gas, one of the many used in a dirigible. The fabric (known as *goldbeater's skin*) was made of fascia stripped from beef intestines[1]. During World War I, in occupied France, sausage-making was forbidden as fascia was critical to the German airships used for observation and precision bombing.

And it wasn't just any fascia, but a specific section of fascia in a specific area of the intestines, all of which were carefully studied and evaluated for permeability and strength. Since then Germany has remained the center of fascial research, now applied to body mechanics, to pain and dysfunction — and to strategies for repairing it.

## PHYSICAL CHARACTERISTICS

Fascia is strong stuff. In the human body, it has an average tensile strength of around 2,000 pounds per square inch (psi), higher in scalp and head. If an evil troll were to tie a ton of concrete to your feet then hang you up by your scalp on a hook on the wall, the amazingly strong fascia of the head would be more than equal to the job, but you would probably have a *terrible* headache afterwards. It might even resemble the severe scalp tenderness reported by many migraineurs after an attack.

Most *nociceptors* ("pain-receptors") are found in fascia and fire the reflex arc of pain and spasm. This is why forcefully stretching muscles shortened with TrPs can make you feel worse: less flexibility and more pain. Fascia "surrounding bone" (*periosteum*) is extremely sensitive to pain. as is the dura (fascia surrounding the brain) as is the *epineurium* (fascia "on" or surrounding and covering the "nerves") as is the *tunica adventitia* (the fascia surrounding blood vessels).

Fascia is also *piezoelectric*. Under pressure or strain, it sends an electrical signal that can run along the entire fascial line sending the pain signal far from its point of origin.

---

1. Natural gut strings for tennis raquets, musical instruments and more, still come from the fascia of beef intestines (not cats).

When a friend struck the top of his head on the corner of a kitchen cabinet it produced a small puncture wound in the scalp. Later there was no particular pain *at the point of impact*, but he suffered several days of blinding pain in his eye, forehead, and at the back of his head. The scalp fascia that he injured is considered to be the connecting tendon of the OCCIPITO-FRONTALIS muscle. (See page 54.)

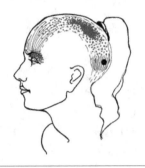

**Figure 12.** MIGRAINE HAIR-ACHE

Pain along this path can explain reports of patients who get relief from migraines *by pulling their hair*. There is no better way to mechanically relax painfully tight fascia of the scalp. But why did it tighten in the first place?

Besides head wounds, another possibility is the "migraine hair-ache" from heavy, tightly pulled pony-tails or corn-rowed hair. Another is dehydration.

Fascia is primarily composed of collagen, a protein. Unlike DNA, the *"double* helix," collagen is a *triple* helix, much of it made up of water. In 1996, German anatomists identified smooth muscle cells (*myofibroblasts*) in fascia. Researchers now believe that these cells enable fascia to contract and relax under the control of the autonomic nervous system, independent of skeletal muscle and conscious control, contracting or lengthening in minutes by regulating water content (Schleip R and others, 2006). This, of course, implies that adequate water is available for "regulation." If not, the inability to re-lengthen contracted tissue may explain some of the pain and dysfunction that comes with dehydration. That is, we dry up and shrivel — and yes, it *hurts*!

Two muscles have unusual densities of fascial myofibroblasts: the TRAPEZIUS muscle of the upper back and the SOLEUS muscle of the calf, both remarkably prone to shortening and stiffening as compared to other skeletal muscles. TRAPEZIUS is the most common site of trigger points in both adults and children (Travell JG and Simons DG, 1992) and it is heavily involved in migraine. SOLEUS sends pain from heel to head, and may also be related to Restless Leg Syndrome (RLS). Restless legs can have many causes ranging from simple muscle strain to electrolyte imbalances and heart disease, but the problem is increasingly linked to simple dehydration.

Tom Myers, a student of Ida Rolf, developed a brilliantly logical fascial support system similar to the rigging on a sailboat (MYERS TW, 2001, 2009). Known as "anatomy trains," 11 basic lines of muscles, bones, and fascial "rigging" working in series or "tracks," explain many odd relationships. For example, Myers' Superficial Back Line (SBL) runs from the bottom of the toes up the back over the top of the head to the eyebrows (Figure 13). It explains why deep massage of the calf can relieve plantar fascitis (inflamed fascia on the bottom of the foot), why massaging muscles at the back of the *neck* improves hamstring flexibility. It also explains why strain at the back of the neck might produce a severe *frontal* headache.

Muscles and fascia unite separate body parts into a marvelously functional whole. They can also lock them into a *dysfunctional* whole, with postural distortions, misalignments, and entrapment syndromes resulting in tissue damage, aches and pains.

Nerves and blood vessels travel along, between, and through myofascial layers. Tight muscles and fascial adhesions can entrap their own nerves and blood supply or that of other more distant structures.

Head pain from connective tissue at the base of the skull is not difficult to imagine. Head pain coming from the lower leg is more of a leap, but it is amazingly common.

SOLEUS is a fascinating example of connection between feet, hips and head. This muscle of the *calf* sends deep aching pain down to the heel, up to the lower back, then to *cheek and jaw*.

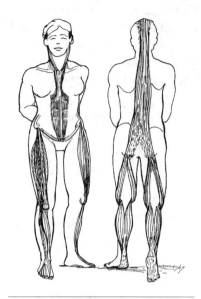

**Figure 13.** FASCIAL LINES

How pain can travel from heels to head.

Simply pointing the toe (shortening the muscle) may be enough to recreate the pain. Hence high-heeled shoes (whether they are called "pumps" or "cowboy boots") can cause head pain, although no *nerve* runs from heel to head. What *does* run from heel to the head? Fascia.

Fascia pulling on the upper jaw changes its shape and therefore tooth alignment. If the responsible TrP in the calf is pressed, patients may suddenly exclaim "My teeth don't fit!" Travell & Simons (1999) reported this as "rare" but in the experience of many bodyworkers, it is no more rare than tight calf muscles in general.

Another point on the lower leg is said to induce labor. Massage therapists are taught to avoid this spot in pregnant women. Controlled studies are inconclusive as to whether it actually induces labor, calling for more studies. On the other hand, if you are female and have all your parts, stimulation of that spot can produce a distinct uterine twinge.

## FASCIA IN BRAIN AND SPINAL CORD

Fascia is continuous with structures of the brain and spinal cord. It stretches up and forward to form the *falx cerebri* (the fascial wall that divides the right and left hemispheres of the brain), and the *tentorium* (a "tent" of fascia that covers the *cerebellum* or "little-brain," dividing it from our big brain).

Brain and spinal cord are surrounded by the meninges[1]. The outermost layer is called the *dura mater*. If you think of the skull as an eggshell, the dura surrounding the brain is much like the tough membrane surrounding the egg inside. Despite its name ("tough mother") the dura is exquisitely sensitive to pain and strain on the dura can start in neck and spine.

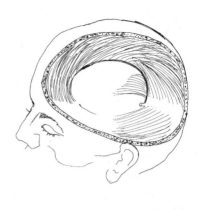

**Figure 14.** FASCIA IN HEAD AND BRAIN

One of the SUBOCCIPITAL muscles at the base of the skull (RECTUS CAPITIS POSTERIOR MINOR) connects directly to the dura via a tough fascial membrane (Hack GD, 1995). This feature, now known as the *dural bridge*, provides a clear link between muscle tension and migraine headaches. That is, *tight neck muscles can yank and pull directly on the lining of the brain and upper spinal cord*. Strain on the meninges may be responsible for many neurological symptoms of migraine including those referred to as "meningitis-like" that occur despite lack of *actual infection* of the meninges.

But the dura doesn't stop there. The brain narrows into *brain stem* then down to the *spinal cord* that travels through the *foramen magnum* ("big hole") at the base of the skull. The dura comes too, enfolding the cord like a glove or a tube. On reaching the spine, the dural tube anchors to the top 3 cervical vertebrae (C1-C2-C3). If these are misaligned, they can pull on the dura, its nerves and blood vessels, stimulating pain receptors (*nociceptors*)[2] and causing severe headaches.

As dura and cord travel down the spine, both structures can (ideally) move freely within the spinal canal for most of the trip. At the end, the dura attaches firmly to the tailbone (*coccyx*). This is *not* a useless appendage, but a critically important attachment for muscles and fascia. Anyone who has damaged the tailbone knows all too well that this seemingly minor injury can be followed by years of pelvic pain and *headaches*. How is this possible?

---

1. (Gr.) *meninx*, membrane. Infection and inflammation of the meninges is "meningitis."
2. In the head, the cell bodies of these pain-sensing neurons report to the trigeminal nerves, those for the rest of the body report to the spinal cord. See Chapter 4.

Because fascia is *piezoelectric*, twisting and pulling muscles and ligaments will send signals from one end of the connection to the other. Because the fascial network runs from head to toe and back again, stress anywhere along the path can show up as pain somewhere else.

I once heard migraines dismissed as "purely psychological" by a lucky fellow who had never had a headache in his entire life. His rationale was this: *brain tissue does not feel pain*. Most brain tissue does not, but much of it does. The dura and tentorium, like other fascial structures, are exquisitely sensitive as are blood vessels that supply every part of the brain. Strain on these structures can cause severe brain aches (Ray BS and Wolff HG, 1940). It matters not whether the strain comes from space-occupying tumors, toxins, inflammation, or the stress of bad shoes, bifocals — or surgery.

Surgery should always be a last resort. Even endoscopic surgeries (done through small incisions) cause internal scarring and disrupt fascial relationships. When individual layers of fascia can no longer slide smoothly past each other, the result can be adhesions and painful restrictions.

Another problem with surgical removal of anything that belongs there is that fascia immediately attempts to fill in the empty space. This is true in procedures ranging from carpal tunnel and thoracic outlet surgeries and appendectomies, to Caesarian sections and more. Problems are often treated with repeated follow-up surgeries, but can be treated or avoided in other ways.

Adhesions are a common cause of post-operative headache following brain surgery. If the bony wall that should separate neck muscles from brain is removed and not replaced (a crani-*ectomy*), fascia begins to fill in. Removing adhesions can relieve the headache but may require repeated surgeries. If the first surgery is done by replacing the bone (a crani-*otomy*) or inserting a plate to *prevent* growth of adhesions, there is a far lower incidence of head pain compared to craniectomy patients overall (Soumekh B and others, 1996; Koperer H and others, 1999).

# Recognizing, Testing, and Treating Myofascial Pain

Muscles are sometimes responsible for severe headaches interpreted as migraines. They can strain the dura and fire the trigemino-vascular alarm system triggering a true migraine attack. Initial pain patterns can help track the resulting headache back to its source.

Pain patterns have been mapped over the years by injecting individual muscles with an irritant such as hypertonic saline solution. Patterns were found to be remarkably consistent. Another consistency is how *rarely* the pain is felt at its point of origin. This is why steroid shots to a sore elbow or knee may be ineffective — over 80 per cent of the time, the pain is from an area *other* than the spot that actually hurts.

Confusingly similar patterns can come from other sources. For example, the gall bladder sends pain to the right shoulder and scapula, abdomen, lower back, and associated muscles. Pain appears in the abdominal and TRAPEZIUS muscles but the pain did not originate there and simply treating these muscles will not fix the problem if the actual origin is a cranky gall bladder or blocked bile duct.

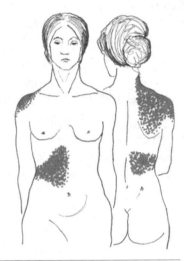

Pain extending from the pelvis down the inner thigh has long been attributed to inflamed ovaries. Many normal organs have been removed but if no pathology is found, the problem has often been assumed to be psychiatric in origin. However, this pain pattern can come *up* to the pelvis from the ADDUCTOR MAGNUS of the thigh

**Figure 15.** GALL BLADDER PAIN

which should be checked *first*, before any surgery. Differential diagnosis is critical.

Pain patterns in the following pages are from Travell & Simons (1992, 1999), Fernandez-de-las-Penas (2010), and other clinicians. Some muscles are easily treated by yourself, or by helpful friends and family[1]. Some are in relatively inaccessible or especially delicate areas and should be treated only by trained professionals.

That said, treating myofascial pain is a six-step process.

1. Identify pain patterns (page 46).
2. Test range of motion (ROM) of possibly involved muscles (page 69).
3. Palpate for taut bands and trigger points (page 79).
4. Break the pain cycle (page 80).
5. Eliminate trigger points (page 82).
6. Stretch (page 84).

---

1. For more detail on self-treatment at home, see *The Trigger Point Therapy Workbook* by Clair and Amber Davies (2006).

## STEP 1: IDENTIFY MUSCLE PAIN PATTERNS

Figure 16 through Figure 37 summarize typical pain patterns from myofascial TrPs. Compare these with your own pain pattern drawings.

- Solid highlighting indicates the most common or most severe areas of pain.

- Less solid, scattered stippling marks the less common or possible "spillover" pain.

- ^^^ indicates areas of goosebumps or other autonomic symptoms.

- ROM refers to Range-of-Motion (muscle-length testing). See Step 2 on page 69.

Too much information? You can ignore the small print. Just look at the pictures and you'll still be ahead of the game.

For *more* detail with superb anatomical illustrations, see *Myofascial Pain and Dysfunction: The Trigger Point Manual*, Volume 1, (Upper Half of Body, 1999, 2nd Ed.) and Volume 2 (Lower Extremeties, 1992) by Travell JG and Simons DG[1]. "Travell and Simons" is the Bible of muscle pain, the source of much of the myofascial information in this book, including specifically numbered TrPs.

Anyone who says they treat trigger points should have a copy of these books, otherwise where did they learn it? These are $100 medical textbooks available through all the usual sources. You can find them in medical libraries or get them through inter-library loan.

---

1. Dr. Travell was professor emeritus of cardiology at Georgetown Medical School in Washington, D.C. Dr. Simons spent years in aerospace medicine followed by rehabilitative medicine for the Veteran's Administration hospitals.

---

**Figure 16.** PAIN PATTERNS: UPPER TRAPEZIUS

---

# Cervicogenic Headache and Migraine

Nerve Supply: Spinal Accessory (CN XI), Vagus (CN X), and Spinal Nerves C2-C4

In both children and adults, the most common muscle with trigger points is Trapezius. Its typically one-sided "fish-hook" headache (often accompanied by dizziness, nausea, visual and neurological disturbances) is commonly diagnosed as "migraine."

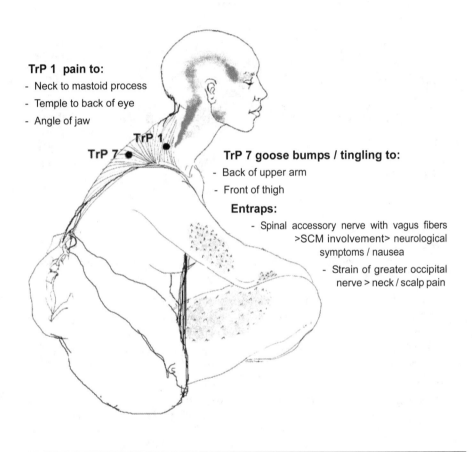

**TrP 1 pain to:**
- Neck to mastoid process
- Temple to back of eye
- Angle of jaw

**TrP 7 goose bumps / tingling to:**
- Back of upper arm
- Front of thigh

**Entraps:**
- Spinal accessory nerve with vagus fibers >SCM involvement> neurological symptoms / nausea
- Strain of greater occipital nerve > neck / scalp pain

---

Both Trapezius and SCM are supplied by the spinal accessory nerve (Cranial Nerve XI) intermingled with fibers of the vagus nerve (Cranial Nerve X) Dysfunction in one muscle can result in pain, weakness with odd neurological and autonomic symptoms, and trigger problems in the other muscle.

Strained by poor posture, stomach sleeping, sustained elevation of arms or shoulders, whiplash, narrow shoulder straps especially with heavy one-sided loads. Cervical joint pain (especially from C4) and gall bladder pain may also radiate to this muscle.

ROM: Cervical Rotation and Cervical Lateral Flexion Tests.

**Figure 17.** PAIN PATTERNS: MIDDLE AND LOWER TRAPEZIUS

# "Tension Headache," "Bursitis," and Chronic Upper Back Pain

Nerve Supply: Spinal Accessory (CN XI), Vagus (CN X), Spinal Nerves C2-C4

Of seven distinct TRAPEZIUS TrPs identified by Travell & Simons (1992), most are in the middle and lower fibers. These points refer pain to back and shoulders. Several TrPs in UPPER TRAPEZIUS may be satellites of TrP3.

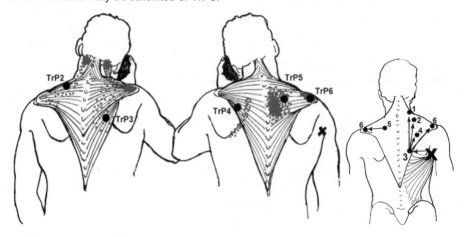

## TrP2

- Pain above shoulder blades, extending up back of neck to occiput

## TrP3

- Pain referred upward to suboccipital area and mastoid process
- Pain from point of shoulder to upper scapula
- Pain between shoulder blades.

## TrP4

- Pain above / between shoulder blades
- Pain to point of shoulder

## TrP5

- Burning pain between shoulder blades

## TrP6

- Aching pain at point of shoulder ("bursitis")

## TrP7

- Goosebumps / tingling to upper arm and front thigh.

## Entrapments:

- Spinal accessory nerve, vagus nerve fibers > neurological symptoms > pain, nausea in both TRAPEZIUS and STERNOCLEIDOMASTOID.

Middle / Lower Trapezius sends pain to upper back and shoulders, up neck to mastoid and occiput, to tip of shoulder and between shoulder blades. It can send satellite TrPs to Upper Trapezius and cause autonomic symptoms including goose bumps on arm and thigh.

Strained by slouching and hunched shoulders. Shortened PECTORALIS muscles should be treated and stretched before treating TRAPEZIUS. TrP3 may develop as a satellite TrP in the referred pain area of Latissimus Dorsi; look for a TrP at X.

ROM: Anterior Cervical Flexion Test (page 71).

**Figure 18.** PAIN PATTERNS: STERNOCLEIDOMASTOID

# Sinus and Migraine Headaches with Neurological Symptoms

Nerve Supply: Spinal Accessory (CN XI), Vagus (CN X), and Spinal Nerves C2-C3

No other muscle displays such a wide range of physical and neurological symptoms including ear, eye, and sinus pain, dizziness, nausea. Sufferers rarely notice problems in this powerful muscle of the *neck;* the pain and dysfunction refer to *head* and gut.

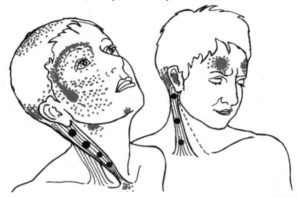

## Sternal Division

### Pain Symptoms

- Eyebrow to lateral cheek
- Top of head
- Occipital ridge behind ear
- Clavicular notch down sternum
- Tip of chin and under jaw
- Back of tongue and throat
- Diffuse pain in jaw joint

### Autonomic Symptoms

- Dry cough, difficulty swallowing
- Sinus congestion
- Tearing, redness, or blurring of eye
- Narrowing of eye (ptosis)

## Clavicular Division

### Pain Symptoms

- In forehead over both eyes
- Deep in ear and behind ear

### Autonomic Symptoms

- Sweating / blanching of forehead
- Distorted weight perception (dysmetria)
- Dizziness, nausea, anorexia
- Distorted proprioceptive/ spatial sense
- Temporary deafness, tinnitus

### Entrapments

- Spinal accessory nerve > perpetuating SCM / Trapezius dysfunction
- Fibers of Nerves: vagus nerve> vertigo, nausea, autonomic and GI upsets

The two divisions have different pain patterns and a wide range of autonomic and neurological symptoms, from nausea and temporary deafness, to sudden sweating of the forehead and emotionless tears. Commonly Injured by whiplash, forced breathing (in asthma or endurance sports), overhead work, gymnastics.

The shared nerve supply between TRAPEZIUS and SCM can produce a feedback loop of pain and dysfunction. SCM can also cause dysfunction of the atlanto-occipital joint at C1 and at the temporal bone (Upledger JE, 1983).

ROM:Cervical Lateral Flexion and Cervical Rotation. Also palpate with pincer palpation.

**Figure 19.** PAIN PATTERNS: MASSETER

# Sinus Pain, TMJ, Tinnitus, and Toothache

Nerve Supply: Trigeminal (CN V)

For its size, the MASSETER is the strongest muscle in the body, the primary muscle that closes the jaw. It works with TEMPORALIS and PTERYGOIDS and is heavily involved in TMJD and sinus pain. MASSETER sends pain to both upper and lower molars causing extreme sensitivity to heat, cold, and vibration.

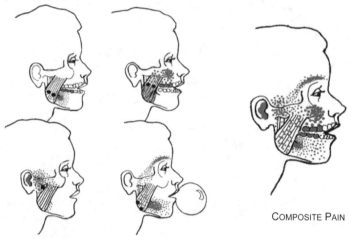

COMPOSITE PAIN

## Symptoms

- TMJ Dysfunction
- Restricted jaw opening ("trismus")
- Pain deep in ear
- Pain in upper or bottom molars
- Extreme sensitivity of teeth

- Tinnitus (without vertigo or deafness)
- Tension headache
- Sinusitis" and maxillary sinus pain
- Baggy eyes

## Entrapments

- Maxillary Vein > Puffy eye on affected side due to blockage of the pterygoid plexus.

Strained by chewing tough foods or clenching teeth (on pipes, cigars, wind instruments), loss of teeth and decreased jawbone thickness, cervical collars or dental work that immobilize the jaw with the muscle in a shortened position. Also strained by tight SCM or UPPER TRAPEZIUS muscles, all strained in whiplash injuries. The anti-depressant Prozac and its relatives such as Paxil, can specifically cause tooth grinding and tension in the masseter muscle, especially when taken at night. With any signs of night-time tooth-grinding, consider taking the medication in the morning rather than before bedtime.

Can refer pain deep inside ear possibly with a dull roaring tinnitus that lacks the vertigo or deafness of true inner ear dysfunction. There may be "sinus" pain over the eyebrow possibly combined with puffy eyes due to blockage of the maxillary vein of the cheek. Gudmundsson G (2010) suggests infantile colic may be a pain syndrome from the masseter, strained by sucking.

ROM: 2-Knuckle and Opening and Closing Tests.

**Figure 20.** PAIN PATTERNS: TEMPORALIS

# Tension, Migraine, and Sinus Headaches, TMJ, and Toothache

### Nerve Supply: Trigeminal (CN V)

Produces severe temporal headache remarkable for "spokes" of pain that radiate from the temple into the teeth. Often tight in association with MASSETER and UPPER TRAPEZIUS, it is heavily involved in TMJD and many unnecessary tooth extractions and root canals.

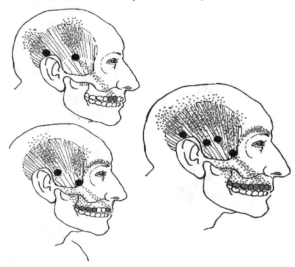

## Symptoms

- Temporomandibular Joint Dysfunction
- Temporal headache
- Slightly restricted jaw opening with lateral deviation

- Pain in cheek, upper jaw, upper teeth,
- Sensitivity of teeth to heat, cold, vibration

## Entrapments

Zygomatico-temporal nerve (branch of trigeminal) > temporal headache

TEMPORALIS lies in the pain referral zone of UPPER TRAPEZIUS and is heavily involved in TMJ syndrome. All but the rear-most fibers refer pain and hypersensitivity to the upper teeth.

Strained by whiplash, blows, tight headbands, chewing tough foods, clenching teeth (on pipes, cigars, or musical instruments), immobilization of the jaw (cervical collars, dental work), and bad bite. Highly sensitive to drafts, B-vitamin deficiency, infections, and low thyroid. Strained by tight TRAPEZIUS and SCM.

TEMPORALIS in turn, strains the weaker hyoids, PTERYGOIDS, and DIGASTRIC muscles. Occasionally fibers of the TEMPORALIS insert into the orbit of the eye producing visual symptoms including eye fatigue, a feeling of pressure in the back of the eye, difficulty focusing, and difficulty seeing at night.

Opening and Closing Test shows lateral deviation of jaw on opening, often due to tightness in the rearmost fibers. Check for TMJ dysfunction and bad bite.

**Figure 21.** PAIN PATTERNS: PTERYGOIDS

# TMJ and Stuffy Ears, with Mouth and Sinus Pain

### Nerve Supply: Trigeminal (CN V)

These relatively weak muscles are intimately involved with jaw and ear and produce a host of symptoms attributed to TMJD: mouth and joint pain with chronically stuffy ears, tinnitus, even peculiar taste sensations. Both PTERYGOIDS entrap nerves. Resulting symptoms may be attributed to sinus or trigeminal neuralgia.

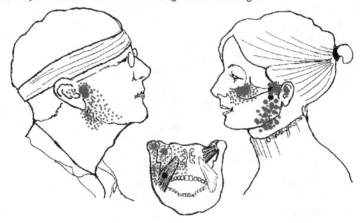

| Medial (Internal) Pterygoid | Lateral (External) Pterygoid |
|---|---|
| - Diffuse pain in mouth to floor of nose, tongue, throat, hard palate | - Pain deep into the TMJ joint |
| - Pain below and behind the TMJ joint | - Pain in / fluid from maxillary sinus |
| - Pain deep inside ear / ear stuffiness | - Tinnitus |
| - Difficulty swallowing | - Clicking in TMJ joint |
| - Lateral deviation of jaw on opening | - Slightly restricted jaw opening |
| - Painfully restricted opening. | - Lateral deviation of jaw on opening |

| Entrapments | Entrapments |
|---|---|
| - Chorda tympani nerve (branch of facial nerve) > bitter, metallic taste on tongue | - Buccal nerve (branch of trigeminal nerve) > numbness /tingling in cheek |
| | - |

*Medial Pterygoid* can be thought of as the Medial (or Internal) MASSETER; the two muscles are fascially continuous, forming a sling to support and close the jaw. This small muscle can send diffuse pain throughout mouth (but not teeth), possibly to base of nose, tongue, hard palate, jaw joint, deep into ear, and possibly to the throat. Can block Eustachian tubes closed, causing chronically stuffy ears.

*Lateral pterygoid* is strained by opening the jaw against the stronger MASSETER and TEMPORALIS muscles and by chewing sticky foods. It causes deep pain and clicking in the jaw. There may be pain / drainage from the maxillary sinus, and sometimes tinnitus.

ROM:Opening and Closing Test. Also test other jaw muscles.

**Figure 22.** PAIN PATTERNS: DIGASTRIC

# Neck, Tooth, and Pseudo-Sternocleidomastoid Pain

Nerve Supply: Trigeminal (CN V, Anterior Section) and Facial (CN VII, Posterior Section)

DIGASTRIC assists LATERAL PTERYGOID in opening the jaw against the counterforce of the powerful MASSETER and TEMPORALIS muscles. Commonly strained in "whiplash" injuries.

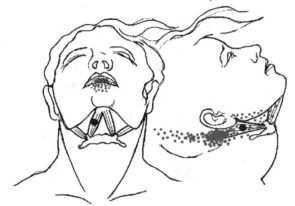

| Anterior Belly | Posterior Belly |
|---|---|
| - Pain to four lower incisor teeth | - Pain to upper STERNOCLEIDOMASTOID muscle |
| - Pain in alveolar ridge | - Pain to throat and possibly to occiput |
| - Pain to throat and to tongue | - Difficulty swallowing |
| - Difficulty swallowing | - Persistent "lump" in throat |
| | - Patient avoids turning head to involved side. |

### Entrapments

- External carotid artery > reduced blood supply to brain > dizziness, depression, headache
- Posterior auricular artery > numbness of scalp behind ear.

Strained by retruded jaw (as in playing reed instruments such as clarinet), chewing with an overbite (especially foods that resist jaw opening, gummy bears versus pudding), coughing, vomiting; by tight MASSETER and TEMPORALIS. DIGASTRIC alone (with *no ossification* of tendon or styloid process) can entrap the external carotid and posterior auricular arteries (Loch and others, 1990). "Lump in throat" and difficulty swallowing occurs with a displaced hyoid bone.

*Anterior Fibers* (below chin): pain to the four lower incisor teeth and ridge; may also refer to throat and tongue and cause problems swallowing.

*Posterior fibers*: Pain to UPPER SCM. Pain at front of the throat and under chin may extend to occiput, ears, floor of mouth.

ROM:Cervical Extension Test with mouth firmly closed. In the Cervical Rotation Test, patients typically avoid turning head to the involved side.

**Figure 23.** PAIN PATTERNS: OCCIPITOFRONTALIS AND CORRUGATOR

# "Migraine Hair Ache"

### Nerve Supply: Facial (CN VII)

Injuries to this two-part muscle or its connecting fascia can cause severe frontal migraine and tension headache possibly with severe eye pain.

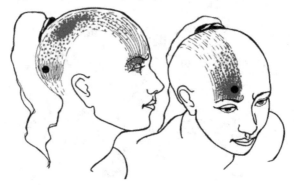

### Occipitalis Pain

- T*hrough* head into eyeball
- In eyelid and behind the eye
- From weight of head on pillow
- From heavy or tightly pulled hair
- Relief by *moist* heat

### Frontalis Pain

- Severe frontal headache
- Migraines relieved by Botox

### Entrapments

- Supraorbital nerve (branch of trigeminal nerve) > frontal / sinus headache

## Corrugator Supercilii

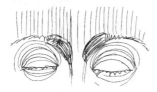

### Entrapments

Supratrochlear nerve (branch of trigeminal nerve) > Migraine headaches

FRONTALIS (at front) raises eyebrows, wrinkles forehead, and assists in opening eyes. Fibers extend to OCCIPITALIS at back of the head. FRONTALIS entraps the supraorbital nerve causing intensely painful frontal headache with neuritic symptoms, commonly diagnosed as migraine.

OCCIPITALIS (at rear) refers diffuse pain across the back of the head and *through* skull causing a deep aching pain behind the eye, into the eyeball and eyelid. There may also be ear ache. Both muscles and connecting fascia are strained by direct trauma, by tightly pulled hair, habitual frowning, squinting, poor eyesight. A wound on top of the head can refer pain in either direction. Strained by tight posterior cervical muscles, POSTERIOR DIGASTRIC, SCM. TrPs and pain in FRONTALIS may be satellites of SCM (clavicular division).

Corrugator strained by habitual frowning that compresses the supratrochlear nerve (a branch of the trigeminal nerve) causing deep aching frontal headaches.

Test for TrPs with flat palpation searching for spot tenderness.

**Figure 24.** PAIN PATTERNS: ZYGOMATICUS & ORBICULARIS OCULI

# Nose, Cheek, and Sinus Pain

Nerve Supply: Facial (CN VII)

ZYGOMATICUS and ORBICULARIS OCULI refer pain to the nose. ZYGOMATICUS produces a hot-spot of forehead pain often mistaken for a sinus condition. Both muscles can be triggered by a blow to the face or strained by facial expressions, ORBICULARIS by chronic squinting or frowning, ZYGOMATICUS by a fixed smile.

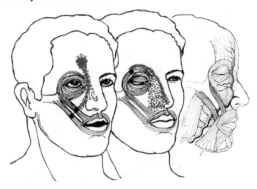

| Zygomaticus | Orbicularis Oculi |
|---|---|
| - Arc of pain alongside nose to mid-forehead | - Pain to eyebrow, nose, and upper lip |
| - Frontal sinus pain | - Visual problems in reading ("jumpy print") |
| | - Droopy eyelid (ptosis) |

### Entrapments

- Facial artery and vein> Pain along path of facial vein and artery > sinus headache.

Zygomaticus draws up the corner of the mouth in smiling, singing, or in playing some wind instruments. Pain follows the track of blocked facial artery and vein, extending from cheek along side of nose to forehead; commonly mistaken for tension headache, sinus pain, or TMJ dysfunction. Test cheek for TrPs with gentle pincer palpation.

ORBICULARIS OCULI surrounds the eye and forms the eyelid; active in blinking and squinting. Strained by blows as in boxing, ill-fitting face masks, habitual squinting.

Pain extends from the lateral side of the eyebrow along side of nose as far as upper lip. Can cause visual disturbances such as "jumpy" print in reading. Orbicularis problems may originate with SCM. The opening between the eyelids may become so narrow and restricted that the sufferer must tilt the head backward to see upward, further straining SCM. This condition resembles Horner's Syndrome but lacks the change in pupil sizes as seen in Horner's.

Test for TrPs by running a fingertip gently across the muscle fibers. TRAPEZIUS/SCM, MASSETER, AND TEMPORALIS all refer pain to this area and should be treated first.

---

**Figure 25.** PAIN PATTERNS: SUBOCCIPITALS

---

# Tension & Chronic Benign Headaches, Occipital Neuralgia

Nerve Supply: C1-C2 (Suboccipital Nerve)

SUBOCCIPITALS are a common source of headache, poorly defined and difficult to localize, but deeply painful, often accompanied by neck stiffness and balance problems.

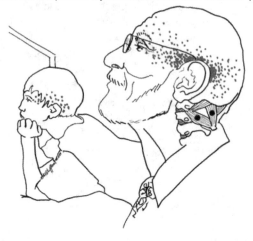

## Symptoms

- Pain on laying back of head on pillow
- Pain on wearing a cervical collar
- Deep aching pain in band from back of head to orbit of eye
- Difficulty rotating head to "blindspot" or rear of car while driving
- Impaired balance and coordination

## Entrapments

- Rarely, greater occipital nerve by inferior oblique > Numbness, tingling and/or burning pain over occipital area to vertex
- RCPm pulls on dura of brain and spinal cord
- Tightness can irritate suboccipital nerve

---

The SUBOCCIPITALS are four pairs of muscles (RECTUS CAPITIS POSTERIOR MAJOR and MINOR, OBLIQUUS CAPITIS SUPERIOR and INFERIOR) that move the head on the cervical spine and are dense with proprioceptors. Tightness or hypertrophy disturbs proprioception > dizziness and balance problems.

Strained by Head-Forward Posture with chin tilted upward.

A vague but deep aching pain extends *through* the head and in a band from back of head to orbit of eye. RCPM attaches directly to the pain-sensitive dura lining brain and spinal cord. Tightness in this muscle can produce odd visual and neurological symptoms to the point of seizures. It can irritate its own nerve supply (the suboccipital nerve) tightening muscles even more in a vicious cycle of dysfunction eventually involving the cranial base, dural tube and upper cervicals (Upledger JE, 1983).

ROM: Cervical Flexion Test. Palpate for tenderness. Persons with shortened suboccipitals tend to carry head tilted and /or rotated to one side.

Local pain in the suboccipital region can also come from SPLENIUS CAPITIS, SEMISPINALIS, and TRAPEZIUS. All refer to the suboccipital area and can produce painful satellite TrPs.

---

**Figure 26.** PAIN PATTERNS: OMOHYOID

# Head, Neck, Shoulder and Arm Pain

Nerve Supply: C1-C3 (Ansa Cervicalis)

This little-known muscle can cause disabling pain after whiplash injury or with vomiting. The pattern of pain is easily confused with that of LEVATOR SCAPULA and SCALENES.

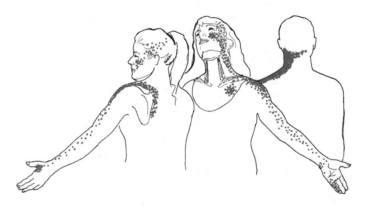

## Symptoms

Pain, sometimes burning:

- Above clavicle (supraclavicular area)

- In inner upper aspect of scapula

- In shoulder / shoulder blade extending to: upper arm, elbow, lateral hand, web between thumb and forefinger

Pain at side of neck, possibly:

- To jaw, possibly into ear,

- To temple producing temporal headache.

- With weakness in arm

## Entrapments

- Upper trunk of brachial plexus> Weakness and/or pain in arm and 4th / 5th fingers

- Jugular vein > reduced venous return from brain.

---

Assists in breathing, swallowing, vomiting, and some actions between clavicle and shoulder blade. Pulls hyoid bone down, necessary for swallowing.

Strained by violent shoulder and neck movements (as in whiplash), sustained contraction, or overstretching. If vomiting is a side-effect of migraine, temporal headache originating from OMOHYOID can appear as continuing migraine or cervicogenic headache.

Pain may extend up neck producing aching pain in jaw and TEMPORALIS pain including toothache. Pain may appear in shoulder blade, especially near attachment at clavicular notch. Impingement on upper branch of brachial plexus can cause pain, weakness, or tingling down arm and hand. Can contribute to an elevated first rib (Thoracic Outlet Syndrome). Intermediate tendon attaches to the fascia of the internal jugular vein; when tight it pulls on and narrows the vessel reducing venous drainage from brain. OMOHYOID pain patterns are commonly mistaken for those of LEVATOR SCAPULA and SCALENES although all may be involved.

ROM:Cervical Rotation Test. Extend neck back and tilt chin up. Rotate head to side *opposite* muscle to be tested. Increase stretch by simultaneously pressing down on scapula.

**Figure 27.** PAIN PATTERNS: LONGUS CAPITIS & LONGUS COLLI

# Eye Pain, Neck Pain, Tension and Cervicogenic Headache

Nerve Supply: Longus Capitis, C1-C4, Longus Colli, C2-C8

These deep anterior vertebral muscles nestle behind the pharynx. Commonly injured in whiplash from rear-end collisions.

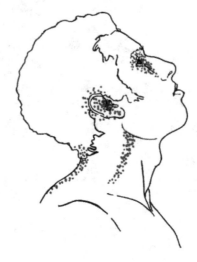

### Symptoms

- Pain on laying back of head on pillow
- Stiff neck (especially on flexion)
- Inability to raise shoulders without pain
- Difficulty lifting head up from supine

- Military neck (reverse cervical curve)
- Difficulty swallowing
- Sore or tickly throat
- Feeling of lump in throat

These two muscles stabilize the neck, preventing it from extending (flopping over backwards) as it would do if the powerful TRAPEZIUS were unopposed.

Strained by poor posture and very commonly in whiplash injuries.

Pain on raising shoulders or difficulty lifting head up from supine position (lying on back). Can reduce normal cervical curve and produce the straight "military neck" or even a reverse curve. Can cause persistent tightness in opposing posterior neck muscles. Swelling and inflammation of LONGUS COLLI can cause severe sore throat and neck pain. Can contribute to T1 dysfunction and Thoracic Outlet Syndrome by helping to raise the first rib.

These muscles lie behind the trachea in the area of the carotid arteries and internal jugular veins. Palpation is not for the untrained.

**Figure 28.** PAIN PATTERNS: SEMISPINALIS CAPITIS & CERVICIS

# Occipital Neuralgia, Tension and Cervicogenic Headaches

Nerve Supply: Semispinalis Capitis, C2 (Greater Occipital Nerve); Semispinalis Cervicis, C1-C8

SEMISPINALIS CAPITIS, commonly injured in vehicular accidents, is a major entrapper of the greater occipital nerve, causing occipital neuralgia and persistent headache.

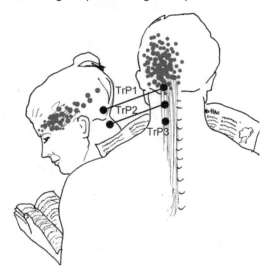

| Symptoms | Entrapments |
|---|---|
| - Pain at back of neck extending to scalp | - Greater occipital nerve > numbness or tingling / burning pain over scalp > occipital neuralgia. |
| - Pain on laying back of head on pillow | |
| - Stiff neck (especially on flexion) | |

Both muscles extend the neck (pull head back) and maintain the natural curve of the neck.

Strained by whiplash regardless of direction of impact, and by a direct blow to the back of the head, as from a fall on ice. Injured daily by furniture lacking lumbar support or armrests, reading materials laid flat on desk requiring neck to support head forward and down. Long flexible "swan" necks are more easily strained than short compact ones. The muscle relaxes when head is erect and balanced on the neck bones, powerfully strained by Head-Forward / round-shouldered postures. These may begin with tight PECTORALIS MAJOR. Similar to SUBOCCIPITALS, pain appears in occipital area of scalp and in a band extending from back of head to the area of the eye.

The greater occipital nerve passes *through* SEMISPINALIS which can entrap its own nerve where it emerges, setting up a painful feedback loop of occipital neuralgia. The nerve also pierces fascia of UPPER TRAPEZIUS which may strain but does not usually compress it.

ROM:Cervical Flexion Test. There may be restriction of several inches and tightness felt extending down the back. Satellite TrPs may arise from the TRAPEZIUS.

**Figure 29.** PAIN PATTERNS: SPLENIUS CAPITIS & CERVICIS

# Computer Neck, Headache, and Eye Pain

Nerve Supply: Splenius Capitis, C3-C4 / Splenius Cervicis, C5-C6

These muscles are consistently injured in auto accidents, often injured in exercise classes, and regularly strained by computer use. A Head-Forward Posture is a constant stress, especially in cyclists when muscles are chilled by wind whipping around a helmet.

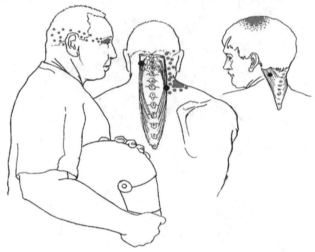

| Splenius Cervicis | Splenius Capitis |
|---|---|
| **TrP 1 (Upper)** | - Pain at top lateral side of head |
| - Pain *through* head to back of eye | |
| - Blurred close vision in same-side eye | |
| **TrP 2 (Lower)** | |
| - Pain at angle of neck, to occiput | |

SPLENIUS CAPITIS is commonly injured in motor vehicle impacts and whiplash regardless of direction of impact. Severely strained by Head-Forward posture especially with head rotated and chin tilted upward; when neck is held flexed in reading/ knitting, by poor-fitting bifocals; chilling or drafts, walking canes or crutches; by tensing the neck while hauling or weight lifting. Often injured by head-rolling exercises.

Pain refers pain to top *side* of head (compare with SCM). ROM:Cervical Flexion Test and Cervical Rotation Test. Restricts less than LEVATOR SCAPULA, but the two combined may leave victim unable to turn the head at all. Evaluate for cervical joint dysfunction, especially C1-C5.

SPLENIUS CERVICIS, TrP1, sends pain through inside of head to back of eye possibly with blurred close vision. TrP 2 causes stiff neck sending pain from base of neck upward in a pattern similar to LEVATOR SCAPULA.

ROM:Cervical Rotation Test. Both SPLENIUS CAPITIS and SPLENIUS CERVICIS cause pain on rotating head to *same* side as the involved muscle and restrict passive rotation *away* from the involved side.

**Figure 30.** PAIN PATTERNS: LEVATOR SCAPULA & ROTATORES

# Stiff Neck and Scapulocostal Syndrome

Nerve Supply: Levator, C3-C4, possibly C5 (dorsal scapular nerve) / Rotatores variable

Levator scapula is the most commonly involved muscle in stiff or "wry" neck. It is the second most common shoulder girdle muscle (after TRAPEZIUS) to have trigger points.

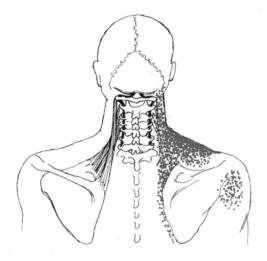

| Symptoms | Entrapments |
|---|---|
| - Pain to angle of neck | - No direct entrapments, but can seriously aggravate cervical radiculopathy via muscle attachments from C1-C4. |
| - Pain to vertebral border of scapula | |
| - Pain to posterior shoulder | |
| - Shortness of breath with involvement of Serratus Anterior | |

Works with TRAPEZIUS to shrug shoulders or support loads on shoulders. Assists in rotating neck to same side. Helps to prevent forward flexion of neck hence strained with other posterior neck muscles in whiplash injuries.

Strained by chronically hunched shoulders (especially if fatigued, cold, or in presence of infections), by swimming when out of condition, by sitting with head turned to one side or by constantly turning head back and forth. Pain appears in angle of the neck and along the vertebral border of the scapula. Pain may also appear in the back of the shoulder.

Cervical Rotation Test is typically painful and limited. In contrast, Cervical Extension is unaffected. There may be a slight tilt to the involved side (a strong tilt is more likely to be due to SCM). Can cause cervical joint dysfunction at the C4-C5 vertebrae.

**Figure 31.** PAIN PATTERNS: SCALENES

# Carpal Tunnel & Thoracic Outlet Syndromes, Swimmer's Palsy

Nerve Supply: Anterior, C5-C6; Medius, C3-C8; Posterior, C6-C8; Minimus, C7.

Scalenes are a leading cause of Carpal Tunnel Syndrome (CTS) and Thoracic Outlet Syndrome (TOS). Intractable migraine can be a first symptom of TOS.

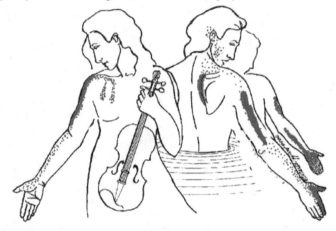

### Scalenus Anterior, Medius & Posterior

- Finger-like pains down into chest
- Pain down front and back of arm
- Pain on thumb side of forearm possibly to thumb and forefinger, arm weakness
- Pain to upper vertebral border of scapula

### Entrapments

- Brachial plexus, subclavian artery and vein > Scalenus Anticus Syndrome, Thoracic Outlet, and Carpal Tunnel Syndromes.

### Scalenus Minimus

- Pain down back of arm
- Pain / edema to back of hand and fingers. Scalenus is highly variable in occurrence and attachment, but when present, it attaches directly to the upper lobe of the lung.

Scalenes attach to the first two ribs. As accessory muscles of respiration they pull the ribs up to make room for expanding lungs. If tight, they may fail to release them for exhalation. They stabilize the neck but can tilt cervical vertebrae forward, causing bulging in the posterior disk. Tightness or adhesions can entrap neurovascular supply to torso and arm.

Symptoms range from slight tingling of thumb and index fingers to hellish pain in chest, shoulder, scapula, and arm. Symptoms may be diagnosed as Carpal Tunnel Syndrome or Thoracic Outlet Syndrome. Radical surgery removes one or two of the three muscles, the first rib and possibly portions of the second rib. (See page 97.)

Strained by turning head forcefully to side while sleeping, swimming, or playing the violin, or by holding a phone between head and shoulder. Injured in whiplash, forced breathing / coughing, and when stabilizing the neck under strain (as in horse-back riding, weight-lifting, and hauling).

ROM:Scalene Cramp or Scalene Relief Tests.

**Figure 32.** PAIN PATTERNS: PECTORALIS MAJOR, MINOR & SUBCLAVIUS

# Chronic Daily Headache, Thoracic Outlet Syndrome, Basilar Migraine

Nerve Supply: Pectoralis Major, C5-T1 / Pectoralis minor, C8-T1 / Subclavius, C5-C6

A wide range of pain and disability, ranging from breast, chest, and arm pain resembling angina pectoris, to shoulder pain resembling bursitis, and carpal tunnel symptoms.

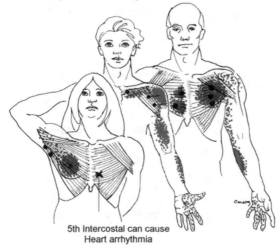

5th Intercostal can cause
Heart arrhythmia

| Pectoralis Major | Subclavius & Pectoralis Minor |
|---|---|
| - Pain in chest, shoulders, arms | - Pain below collarbone, to shoulder |
| - Pain, tingling down underside of arm to 3rd, 4th, 5th fingers. | - Pain down upperside of arm along biceps |
| - Heart arrhythmia (TrP at 5th intercostal) | - Tingling in thumb, index, middle fingers |
| | - Carpal Tunnel / Thoracic Outlet syndromes |

Short pectorals overstretch TRAPEZIUS. Entrapment syndromes range from pain to fainting in Thoracic Outlet Syndrome (TOS) and Military Syncope. Strained by keyboarding (whether piano or computer) and other actions that pull arms together.

*Pectoralis major.* Numbness or pain in chest, shoulders, and arms. Pain down left arm may be mistaken for angina pectoris; in chest, breast cancer. TrP at fifth intercostal can cause heart arrhythmia (Travell & Simons, 1999, p. 822).

SUBCLAVIUS: Compresses subclavian artery / vein. May contribute to aura and basilar migraine, impaired blood supply to or venous drainage from brain.

PECTORALIS MINOR: Compresses axillary artery / vein. Increases entrapment potential of C7-C8 nerve roots that must hook over the first rib; aggravated by tension in biceps brachii and coracobrachialis and weakness (or inhibition) of LOWER TRAPEZIUS muscle. Combined with subclavius, patients may wake at night to find arms still "asleep." Rear auto impacts can produce TOS symptoms via shoulder strap injury to PECTORALIS MINOR. Intractable migraine may appear long before pain recognized as TOS develops in the neck, shoulder, and arm.

ROM:Arm Pullback Test. Wright Maneuver tests for entrapment by PECTORALIS MINOR.

**Figure 33.** PAIN PATTERNS: SOLEUS

# Calf, SI Joint, and Jaw Pain, Jogger's Heel & Plantar Fascitis

Nerve Supply: S1-S2 (Tibial Nerve)

SOLEUS stabilizes knee and ankle and is known as "the second heart" for its role in pumping blood from lower legs. It joins with GASTROCNEMIUS to form the Achilles tendon. SOLEUS refers pain to heel, SI joint, and upward to face and jaw.

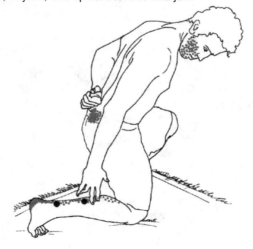

**TrP 1:**
- Pain down the Achilles tendon
- Pain to posterior and plantar aspects of heel, possibly extending to arch of foot

**TrP 2:**
- Calf pain possibly to back of knee

**TrP 3:**
- Pain at Achilles tendon and heel
- Pain at same-side SI joint, referring to same-side face, jaw, and TMJ
- Craniosacral dysfunction
- Malocclusion of teeth (maxilla)

## Entrapments:
-Posterior tibial vein, artery, and nerve

-Popliteal vein and artery (via tendon of plantaris)

Strained by direct trauma, high heels, sitting/sleeping with chronically pointed toes, compression by hard chair edges, long kneeling, stockings or elastic knee braces, shoes with slippery or stiff soles or heels lower than toes, walking up long steep slopes, or trudging through soft sand.

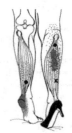

Pain in calf, ankle, heel, possibly down to arch of foot (plantar fascitis) and up to knee; may include foot/ankle edema due to impaired circulation. TrP3 refers aching pain to same-side sacro-iliac (SI) joint. SI pain may then skip to *jaw and cheek*.

Neurovascular entrapments are painful and can be dangerous, leading to Restless Leg Syndrome (RLS) and Deep Vein Thrombosis (DVT).

ROM:Bent-Knee Ankle Dorsiflexion Test.

**Figure 34.** PAIN PATTERNS: ADDUCTOR MAGNUS

# Pelvic, Prostate, Thigh, Groin Pain, Calf Cramps, Cold Feet

Nerve Supply: L2-S1 (Obturator and Sciatic Nerves)

The massive ADDUCTOR MAGNUS muscle refers pain up the leg and into the pelvis and can block circulation to the lower leg.

## Symptoms

- Pain extending down inner thigh
- Pain into pelvis, genitals, GI tract

## Entrapments

- Femoral artery and vein
- Brings thighs together; also serves as a hamstring and can restrict toe-touching more than the hamstrings themselves.

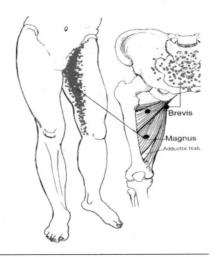

Strained by cross-body motions, climbing stairs, skiing, bicycling, horseback riding, thigh machines, catching falls, walking while taking "giant steps."

Pain refers up the inner thigh and into pelvis. It may be involved in menstrual cramps and vaginal pain in women and the pain of prostatitis without infection in men. In both men and women, it can produce pain and discomfort throughout groin, pelvic floor, perineum and bladder, and a sensation "like a golf-ball" in the rectum (WISE AND ANDERSON, 2008). Satellite TrPs refer pain to the GI tract and genitals.

At the adductor hiatus, ADDUCTOR MAGNUS can block blood supply to lower legs resulting in the calf cramps and cold feet so often observed in migraine. Impingement can be so severe that there may be no pulse at the arteries of foot and ankle (dorsalis pedis and posterior tibial pulses). Test pulses (page 93).

ROM: Adductor Test Position 1.

---

**Figure 35.** PAIN PATTERNS: RECTUS FEMORIS

---

# Thigh and Kneecap Pain, Head-Forward Posture

Nerve Supply: L2-L4 (Femoral Nerve)

The quadriceps muscles stabilize and extend the knee. RECTUS FEMORIS (the only quad to cross the hip joint), can cause anterior pelvic rotation and Head Forward posture.

### Symptoms

- Pain at front of knee-cap.
- Anterior pelvic tilt, kneecap pain, especially while walking *down*stairs/downhill.

### Entrapments

- None known, but TrPs in RECTUS FEMORIS can inhibit the knee-jerk response.

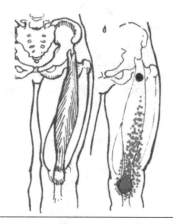

The "four-headed" quadriceps group comprises three vastii muscles (named for their size): VASTUS MEDIALIS, VASTUS LATERALIS, and VASTUS INTERMEDIUS. These attach to the upper thigh bone near the hip joint. The fourth, RECTUS FEMORIS, runs "straight" down the "femur" (thigh bone) from the front of the pelvis to join the other three muscles below the knee. When tight, RECTUS FEMORIS rotates the pelvis forward.

Quads are commonly overloaded by weighted knee extension exercises. Microcirculation is blocked by carrying a child or package on the lap for long periods.Persons who fall asleep in a chair with feet up may be surprised to find on awakening that they can not bend their knees as this position shortens RECTUS FEMORIS completely. Problems may persist for years as this muscle is rarely stretched to its full length which requires *extension* of the hip and flexion of the knee at the same time.

ROM: RECTUS FEMORIS Heel-to-Butt test. Watch for restriction of hip extension by psoas and treat both muscles in association with QUADRATUS LUMBORUM.

**Figure 36.** PAIN PATTERNS: ILIOPSOAS

# Back, Groin, & Thigh pain, Scoliosis & Appendicitis Symptoms

Nerve Supply: L1-L4

### Symptoms

- Pain extending vertically up back (possibly to shoulder blades) and down to SI joint as far as upper buttocks). Psoas minor on right emulates appendicitis.
- Scoliosis from distortion of lumbar vertebrae
- Groin pain possibly extending to scrotum / labia and down front of thigh.

### Entrapments

- Femoral / lateral femoral cutaneous nerves
- Femoral branch of genitofemoral nerve
- Iliohypogastric and ilioinguinal nerves > thigh pain and sexual dysfunction.

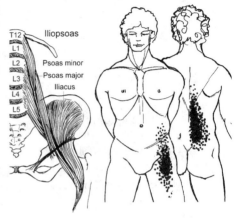

Shortened by long sitting, driving, or sleeping with hips flexed. Strained by tight hamstrings, tight RECTUS FEMORIS, and weak abdominals. PSOAS links the thighs to all lumbar vertebrae and discs of the low back, hence it strains the low back in sit-ups, especially straight-legged situps and especiallywhen PSOAS must substitute for weak abdominals. Oddly vulnerable to developing hematomas in anti-coagulant therapy (blood thinners).

There may be pain and difficulty arising (lengthening psoas) from a deep chair (in which hips are deeply flexed and psoas shortened). Because pain is relieved by flexing the hips, it is easy to fall into a hunched posture with chronic shortening. By necessity, this rounds the upper back producing an automatic Head-Forward posture.

ROM: Psoas tests and Rectus Femoris Heel-to-Butt test. Stretching psoas alone will not suffice. Spinal joint dysfunctions must be corrected first, with treatment of QUADRATUS LUMBORUM, , abdominals, quadriceps, and hamstrings as necessary. In Rectus Femoris Heel-to-Butt ROM test, watch for restriction of hip flexion by PSOAS.

---

**Figure 37.** PAIN PATTERNS: QUADRATUS LUMBORUM

---

# Pain of Lower Back, SI Joint, Hip, Groin, Genitals,Thigh

### Nerve Supply: T12, L1-L4

QUADRATUS LUMBORUM (QL) emulates a short leg by hiking the hip. It can create an apparent short leg which in turn causes postural distortions and strain in muscles of the torso, shoulders, neck, and jaw that can trigger headaches.

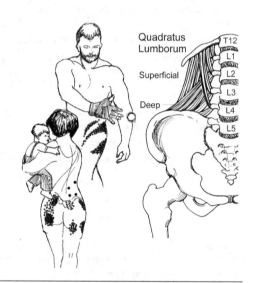

### Symptoms
- Pain to low back, and hip joint
- Pain to groin, scrotum / labia,
- Pain to abdomen, anterior thigh
- Satellite TrPs to gluteal muscles
- Pseudo sciatica.

### Entrapments
- None known.

---

QUADRATUS LUMBORUM hikes the hip and is so critical to walking that if paralyzed, the victim cannot walk even with crutches. It assists in forced exhalation of coughing, sneezing, laughing, and in defecation and lurks behind many failed back surgeries.

Pain referred to lower back (lumbago) is often confused with S1 nerve root pain ("pseudo disc syndrome"). QL is the most common source of low back pain of muscular origin. Fibers are continuous with iliopsoas (Psoas). If shortened by TrPs, the pain from these two muscles can be truly gruesome.

Often strained by simultaneously bending, twisting and lifting, a short leg (a real one, or one created by a walking cast), short hemipelvis, or even short upper arms. Commonly traumatized in motor vehicle accidents, and holding a leaning position over workspaces.

ROM:QL Test.

After identifying pain patterns . . .

## STEP 2: TEST RANGE OF MOTION

The many muscles involved in head pain can be narrowed down via Range-of-Motion (ROM) tests. These are simple tests of muscle length.

Note that it is quite possible to have restricted without obvious pain.

### CERVICAL TESTS

For all cervical tests, anchor arms by sitting on hands or holding onto chair or table. This helps to isolate muscles, to show clearly how far a neck can actually flex down to the shoulder, rather than how well a shoulder can rise to meet the neck.

**To test a partner:**

1. Anchor the arms.
2. Move muscle gently through its range of motion. Stop as soon as restriction is felt.
3. Measure range / degree of inhibition.
4. With any restriction, have patient put one finger where it hurts; mark that point on the Pain Chart.

✓ Indicates PASS.

✗ Indicates FAIL (restricted motion).

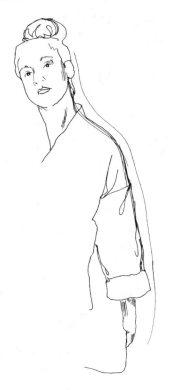

**Figure 38.** ROM TESTING: ANCHOR ARMS

---

**Figure 39.** ROM TESTING: CERVICAL ROTATION

---

Restricting Muscles

**Levator Scapula**
**Splenius Cervicis**
**Splenius Capitis**
Scalenes
Sternocleidomastoid (SCM)
Trapezius

With patient sitting on hands or holding chairseat:

1. Patient rotates head to one side then the other. Do not allow patient to shift shoulders forward, or to tilt head forward or back.
2. Note degree of rotation. Nose should align with point of shoulder (90°).

✓ Head rotates smoothly to align with shoulder.

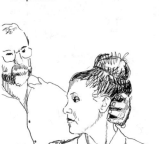

✕ LEVATOR SCAPULA, in combination with TRAPEZIUS, is leading cause of a "stiff" or "crick" neck.

UPPER TRAPEZIUS involvement is most strongly shown by the *Cervical Lateral Flexion* test. TRAPEZIUS also slightly restricts to opposite side, often causing pain at nearly full rotation.

LEVATOR and SPLENIUS CERVICIS restrict on same side.
SCM may restrict last 10° to the opposite side.
SCALENES restrict at end. See *Scalene Cramp* test.

---

**Figure 40.** ROM TESTING: CERVICAL LATERAL FLEXION

---

Restricting Muscles

**Trapezius**
**Scalenes**
Sternocleidomastoid (SCM)

1. Patient attempts to press ear to shoulder. Do not tilt to side or raise shoulder to meet ear.
2. Note distance between earlobe and shoulder.

✓ Ear parallel to shoulder.

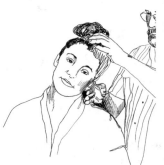

✕ Unable to approach shoulder with ear.

Some people have almost no lateral motion, common, but certainly not "normal." Those who have it are likely to suffer tension or migraine headaches with "fishhook" or other pain patterns typical of the muscles involved.

Upper Trapezius: may limit movement to an angle of 45° or less.

Scalenes: may restrict final 30° of motion. See *Scalene Cramp Test*.

SCM: may restrict about 10° to opposite side.

**Figure 41.** ROM TESTING: ANTERIOR CERVICAL FLEXION

Restricting Muscles

**Suboccipitals**
**Splenius Capitis**
**Splenius Cervicis**
Paraspinals
Semispinalis Capitus
Semispinalis Cervicis
Trapezius
Sternocleidomastoid (SCM)

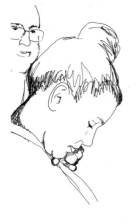

1. Patient clenches jaw and *curls* neck forward touching chin to chest.
2. Observe space between base of chin and chest.
   *Do not* drop open jaw to chest or drop neck straight forward then flex neck.

✓ Chin touches chest.

✕ Cannot reach chest with chin.

Pain from the muscles that restrict this motion may be diagnosed as occipital neuralgia, tension headache, cervicogenic headache, and "chronic intractable benign headache."

These muscles are strained by such everyday actions as watching TV with head propped on elbows and wrists, or by wearing bifocals that require holding the head in a set position to focus.

**Figure 42.** ROM TESTING: CERVICAL EXTENSION

Restricting Muscles

Infrahyoids
Suprahyoids
Digastric

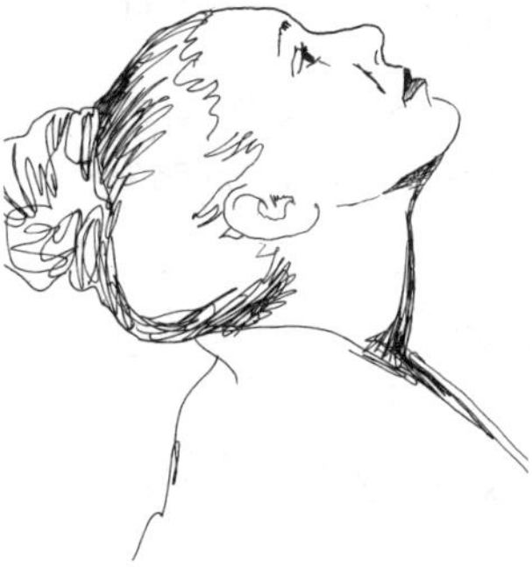

With mouth firmly closed (teeth touching):

1. Patient extends neck to back and looks directly up at the ceiling.
   Caution! Lift chin *up* rather than scrunching *down* to upper back.
2. Observe distance between occiput and back of neck. Ear and eye should be vertically aligned.

✓ Eye vertically aligned with ear, mouth firmly closed and with no neck or head pain.

✕ Unable to extend fully pain-free.

These muscles are commonly injured in whiplash and vehicle accidents. Pain may refer to eye, ear, and neck and cause difficulty opening mouth or swallowing. The feeling of lump in throat is due to shifted hyoid bone.

**Figure 43.** ROM TESTING: SCALENE RELIEF

Restricting Muscles

Scalenes

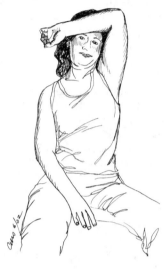

To relieve current scalene pain or to counteract any pain created by the Scalene Cramp Test (below):

1.  Bring forearm up against forehead on symptomatic side.
2.  Rotate shoulder (not just arm!) forward. This movement opens up space for the brachial plexus.

✓ No change.

✕ Decreased scalene pressure on brachial plexus results in decreased pain.

**Figure 44.** ROM TESTING: SCALENE CRAMP

Restricting Muscles

Scalenes

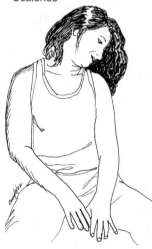

Reproduces suspected scalene pain and /or dysfunction similar to playing the violin and swimming the crawl (and explains why these activities can cause such painful symptoms).

**Do not test** if pain is ongoing or if there is tenderness on the spinous processes of cervical spine. This test can distress a bulging disc or a compromised facet on side being tested. Stop immediately if there is any cervical pain. *Never* test through pain.

Always follow immediately with *Scalene Relief Test*.

1.  Patient turns head to side and pulls chin firmly into clavicle area.
2.  Hold for 60 seconds.

✓ No change.

✕ Pain or tingling in scalene pain reference areas: chest, back, fingers.

---

**Figure 45.** ROM TESTING: OPENING AND CLOSING

---

Restricting Muscles

Masseter
Temporalis
Pterygoids
Digastric (posterior)

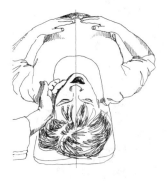

1. Stand behind head as patient slowly opens and closes mouth. Watch for deviation of jaw to side(s). If:
2. Most marked away from affected side as opening reaches full ROM: MEDIAL PTERYGOID. Contralateral deviation: LATERAL PTERYGOID. Zig-zag motion on opening: TEMPORALIS.
3. Listen for popping and clicking. One side or both? Grating sounds require a dental evaluation.
4. Repeat this test supine to eliminate postural muscles.

✓ Jaw opens widely, closes smoothly and evenly, with no sound.

✕ Jaw produces only a narrow opening.

See also the TMJD tests on page 183.

Muscular dysfunction is a far more common cause of TMJD than the joint itself. Muscles move the joint in a balanced, even manner — or not. Surgery is *rarely* the best initial treatment. Better to check muscles and correct dysfunction before damage does occur.

---

**Figure 46.** ROM TESTING: 2-KNUCKLES

---

Restricting Muscles

**Masseter**
Temporalis
Pterygoids

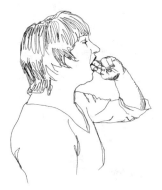

1. Patient inserts 1-2 fingers or knuckles between teeth.
2. Gently adding one finger or knuckle at a time, see how many can fit inside mouth. Do not force.
3. Repeat this test supine to eliminate postural muscles.

✓ Minimum of 2 fingers or knuckles.

✕ Tight MASSETER and TEMPORALIS restrict or deviate jaw opening. See *Opening and Closing* test.

Hypermobility: Suggested by three or more fingers. Referral zones of SCM and TRAPEZIUS perpetuate TrPs in masticatory muscles. See *Cervical Lateral Flexion* and *Cervical Rotation Tests.*

---
**Figure 47.** ROM TESTING: WRIGHT MANEUVER
---

Restricting Muscles

Pectoralis Minor

With patient seated,

1. Check for radial pulse (on thumb-side of wrist). Use your fingers, not thumb.

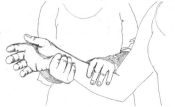

2. Pull shoulder back and raise arm with humerus (upper arm) behind head.

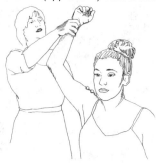

3. Note whether pulse lessens or disappears. In some normal patients, abduction of arm beyond 90° to front of body may cause a false positive. Test *shoulder*, not just arm. Backward movement of the scapula (to which the PECTORALIS MINOR is attached) tightens the muscle over the underlying axillary artery and brachial plexus.

✓ No change in pulse.

✕ Pulse lessens / disappears due to constriction of vascular bundle by pectoralis minor

---
**Figure 48.** ROM TESTING: ARM PULLBACK
---

Restricting Muscles

Biceps
Anterior Deltoid
Pectoralis Major

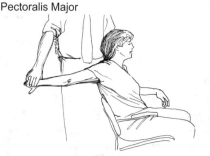

2. Holding shoulders/trunk still, pull arm back aligned with plane of shoulders. Do not rotate trunk. .

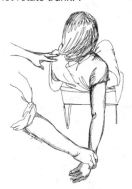

With patient seated, thumb down,

1. Patient raises arm 90° to side.

✓ Arm reaches straight back in a line level with opposite shoulder.

✕ Arm does not reach straight back.

## LOWER BODY TESTS

Lower body muscles (and their trigger points) can contribute to pain in the head and elsewhere because the vascular system does not stop at the neck.

---

**Figure 49.** ROM TESTING: ADDUCTOR TESTS

---

Restricting Muscles

Adductor Longus
Adductor Magnus
Pectineus
Vastus Medialis

Restricting Muscles

Adductor Longus
Adductor Magnus
Gracilis
Pectineus
Vastus Medialis

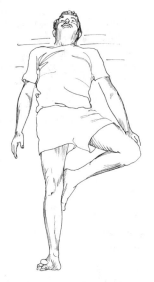

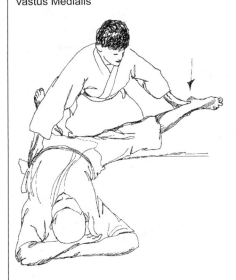

Position 1

This position removes gracilis (the only adductor that crosses the knee joint).

1. Place heel of test leg on table next to knee of other leg.
2. Lower knee to table. Note how close to table it comes. (Sliding heel to crotch can be blocked by vastus medialis, one of the quadriceps muscles.)

✓ Knee drops to table.

✕ Knee fixed above table.

Position 2

This test position includes gracilis.

1. Stabilize hip bone opposite the test leg to keep patient's body from rolling.
2. Raise test leg to 90° (a "hamstring test") then lower at 90° out to side.

✓ 90° angle from body.

✕ Less than 90° from body.

---

**Figure 50.** ROM TESTING: STRAIGHT-KNEE ANKLE DORSIFLEXION

---

Restricting Muscles

**Gastrocnemius**
**Soleus**
Flexor Hallucis Longus
Flexor Digitorum Longus

1. With feet extended over table, and knees fully extended, dorsiflex ankle by pressing on balls of feet.

✓ Ankle dorsiflexes to approximately 20°.

✗ Unable to fully extend knees. Unable to flex ankle beyond approximately 20° and toes curl under.

Flexion of the big toe indicates shortness of flexor hallucis longus. Flexion of the four lesser toes indicates shortness of flexor digitorum longus.

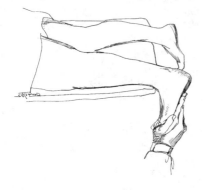

---

**Figure 51.** ROM TESTING: BENT KNEE ANKLE FLEXION

---

Restricting Muscles

**Soleus**
Flexor Hallucis Longus
Flexor Digitorum Longus

This position removes GASTROCNEMIUS to test SOLEUS separately.

1. Bend knee to 90°,

2. Flex ankle by pushing on balls of foot.

✓ Ankle flexes to 20°, toes are relaxed.

✗ Ankle flexes less than 20° and toes curl under. Flexion of the big toe indicates shortness of the flexor hallucis longus; flexion of the four lesser toes indicates shortness of flexor digitorum longus.

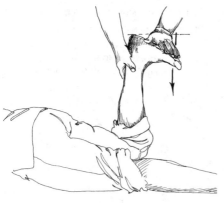

---

**Figure 52.** ROM TESTING: RECTUS HEEL-TO-BUTTOCK

Restricting Muscles

Rectus Femoris

1. Flex one knee to protect back. Drop test leg over edge of table.

2. Place one hand on knee or thigh, one at ankle. Bring heel to buttock with foot neutral (not pointed).
3. Stop when restriction is felt or knee begins to rise.
4. Measure separation between heel and buttock.

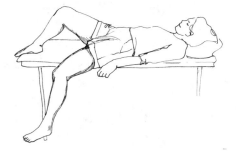

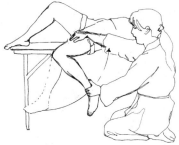

✓ Lower leg hangs straight *down*. Heel can reach buttock.

✕ Lower leg hangs *forward*; heel will not reach buttock. Hip extension may be blocked by a tight psoas.

---

**Figure 53.** ROM TESTING: QUADRATUS LUMBORUM

---

Restricting Muscles

**Quadratus Lumborum**
Abdominal Obliques
Serratus Anterior
Pectoralis Major
Pectoralis Minor

1. On side with upper leg, hips, shoulder and back aligned, lower knee bent.

2. Place one hand on hip to keep patient from rolling.
3. Press shoulder down to table slowly and gently. Note distance from table.
   Substitution: Sliding lower shoulder.

✓ Upper shoulder can touch table.

✕ Upper shoulder cannot touch table.

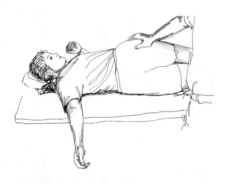

---

**Figure 54.** ROM TESTING: PSOAS

---

Restricting Muscles

Psoas
Tensor Fascia Lata

1. Patient lies on left side, pillow between knees to protect lower back.
2. Stabilize hip with left hand; support right knee and leg with right hand.

3. Gently pull right thigh back until resistance is felt.
   Substitution: Rotating pelvis forward.

✓ Thigh extends 45° at hip.

✕ Extension less than 45°. See also Heel-to-Buttock Rectus Test.

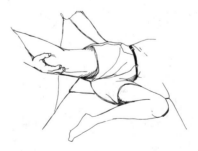

After identifying pain patterns and restricted range of motion, look for the causes . . .

## STEP 3: PALPATE FOR TAUT BANDS AND TRIGGER POINTS

The precise locations of even "classic" trigger points will vary from person to person, hence the need for palpation to actually find the trigger point and recreate the pattern.

*Palpation* is simply "feeling." When a restriction has been identified, palpate across the muscle feeling for taut bands and nodules. You can practice this with pencils and peas (then materials of increasingly smaller diameter) under a bath towel.

*Flat palpation* is done by drawing a finger or fingers at right angles across a muscle. In healthy muscle, it feels like running a finger across piano strings; you can feel the spaces between the strings. Shortened muscle feels like a mass of badly cooked spaghetti all mooshed together. Follow taut bands to find the associated TrPs. These will feel like thickenings or nodules ranging from the size of a pea or a marble or larger. In our example, it is like following the length of the pencil to find the lump of eraser on the end. Taut bands hurt too, but a taut band is not a trigger point!

*Pincer palpation* (Figure 55) is done by squeezing the muscle between thumb and forefinger. This is used with muscles such as the SCM and the upper edge of the TRAPEZIUS at the shoulder. With gloved fingers it is used to check MASSETER and ZYGOMATICUS.

Palpation may reveal a trigger point that needs to be treated, or a taut band that needs relief. But this can't be done most effectively while the muscle is in pain.

What to do? First, stop the pain.

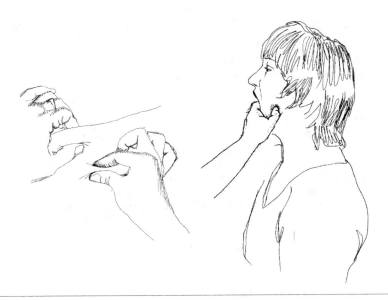

**Figure 55.** PINCER PALPATION

After identifying pain patterns, testing ROM, and palpating for trigger points. . .

## STEP 4: BREAK THE PAIN CYCLE

Tight muscles must be relaxed before healing and active stretching can begin. Detailed treatment techniques are beyond the scope of this manual, but basic tools in the home toolbox are: alternating heat / cold and pressure.

*Cold* shrinks blood vessels, reducing circulation and inflammation; it also blocks pain impulses from muscles. Our bodies consider cold signals more alarming than pain. A cold signal (via fast myelinated nerve fibers) will beat a signal of muscle pain (via slow non-myelinated fibers) to the "gate." Creams that feel cold or hot on the skin work on the same principle; *sensation* follows the same neural pathway as cold. No ice at hand? Use a toothpick, the tip of a chopstick or a retracted ball-point pen, even a feather. Combining cold with tactile sensation (as with the edge of a cold bolt, Figure 57) over-loads sensors even more effectively.

*Heat* expands blood vessels, improving blood flow and removal of toxins and dead cells. It also relaxes muscles before or after treatment. A wonderfully effective hot pack can be made with a sock, dry rice, and a microwave. The rice pack is cheap, flexible, smells wonderful, and it provides moist heat without the drips and tickles of wet towels.

1. Pour 2 cups of dry rice (or more as desired) into a cotton tube sock.
2. Microwave for 3 minutes + 1 minute intervals as needed.
3. Apply as desired.
   With repeated microwaving, the moisture naturally contained in the rice will be lost. The rice will dry out turning all brown and toasty. Replace as necessary.

Cold used to aid stretching is variously known as Stretch-and-Spray (from use with vapocoolant) or Intermittent Cold With Stretching. It is amazingly powerful, and was Dr. Travell's treatment of choice. It may not be as long-lasting as hands-on techniques (it's a tool) but it shows that you can stretch away muscular pain.

With patient seated or lying down and end of limb or muscle anchored:

1. Have patient *inhale* deeply.
2. As patient *exhales,* ice the entire muscle and its pain reference area in sweeping *parallel* lines at a rate of about 4 inches (10 cm) per second.
   *Do not cross the lines.* Don't add frostbite to a migraine. The target is *skin and its sensors*; chilling the underlying muscles causes them to tighten still more, producing still more pain.
3. As patient *exhales*, apply *gentle* passive stretch to increase the range of motion.
4. Apply moist heat to re-warm the skin; re-apply cold only after skin has re-warmed.
5. Repeat cold and stretch followed by moist heat, and passive stretch to proper ROM. Never stretch to full *available* ROM.
6. Have patient move through full range of motion on his/her own.

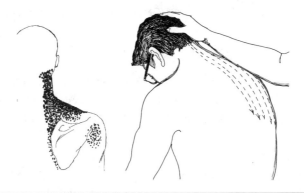

**Figure 56.** INTERMITTENT COLD AND HEAT TECHNIQUE

For cold, you can use the edge of an ice cube held in a cloth, paper cups filled with water and frozen, or stove bolts stored in the freezer until needed (Figure 57). Cold applied via the metal edges is effective, infinitely recycleable, and hypo-allergenic.

An additional technique is known as Strain-Counterstrain. It consists of:

- Gentle ROM stretch, which makes TrPs more obvious. On locating TrP,

- Shorten the muscle (the reverse of the ROM stretch) to find its "position of ease," the position where it does *not* hurt. Treating TrPs in this position avoids resets the alarmed stretch receptors and allows the muscle to relax more easily and completely.

Many aches and pains, particularly acute ones, respond well to this treatment. Chronic problems may be another matter. The muscle may fail to lengthen because it cannot; it is bound up in scar tissue, shortened fascial wrappers, or adhesions. The TrP and fascia must be treated directly.

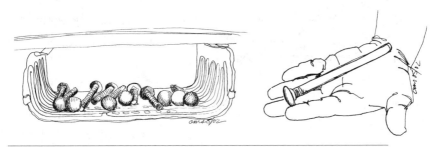

**Figure 57.** STOVE BOLTS AS PAIN RELIEF TOOL

After identifying pain patterns, testing ROM, palpating for TrPs, and blocking pain . . .

## STEP 5: ELIMINATE TRIGGER POINTS

Mental stress and tension can lay down TrPs, but they cannot be released by mindset, meditation, or biofeedback. They don't even go away under deep anaesthesia[1]. Relief of this very real and very physical condition requires real physical attention to the TrPs themselves.

TrPs can be relaxed with needling and hands-on treatment. Legally, needling is limited to medical personnel . Hands-on techniques can be done by anyone, are available from many therapists or your own fingers, knuckles, and elbows. Simple household items such as balls or canes can also be used.

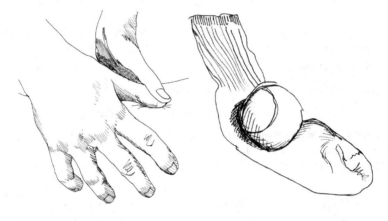

**Figure 58.** TRIGGER POINT TOOLS

- *Tennis Ball.* Lay on the ball or put it in a tube sock or panty hose, hang over shoulder and lean against the wall to reach spots on your own back or neck.

- *Knobble.* Palm-sized wooden tools with projecting "knuckle."

- *Acumasseur.* Like a plastic nutcracker with two golf-balls at the arch. Ideal for round areas such as posterior neck, UPPER TRAPEZIUS, thighs, and legs.

- *Sticks.* These can be leaned into or levered into various positions.

- *Backnobber.* An S-shaped curve that allows you to apply pressure to any point.

- *Theracane.* Extensions along the body provide local pressure or serve as a support in applying pressure to another point.

---

1. First reported by H. Schade in 1919 and verified by M. Lange in 1931.

Pressure techniques were originally thought to work by temporarily reducing blood and oxygen supply to the muscle; without oxygen, a healthy muscle cannot stay contracted. Pressure release allows blood and oxygen to flood back into the muscle.

Another possibility is local lengthening of shortened muscle fibers, rather like untangling and separating individual strands of spaghetti by pressing them gently apart. *Heavy* pressure (with counterproductive pain and bruising) is *not* better than *gentle* pressure. If the patient is holding breath or defensively tightening the muscles you are trying to relax, there's too much pressure. Instead:

1. Find the point where *mild* discomfort begins to be felt.
2. Hold point for 10-15 seconds as necessary until pain drops to mere pressure.
3. Repeat, going in a little deeper to take the point back up to mild discomfort.
4. Hold until sensation drops again to pressure, then move on.

For example, treating the SCM muscle (Figure 59c) ombines direct pressure (at the bump of the mastoid, A) with pincer palpation (of the muscle belly, B), and flat palpation and pressure at the clavicles (the collarbones at base of neck, C). Note that tingling and SCM pain patterns may temporarily reappear.

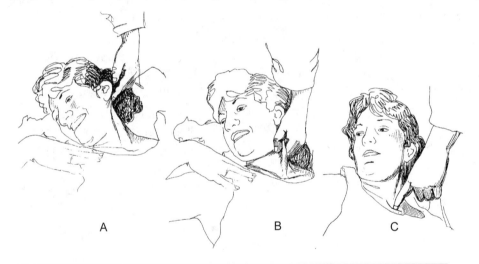

A     B     C

**Figure 59.** TREATING THE STERNOCLEIDOMASTOID (SCM) MUSCLE

After treating,

1. Repeat the ROM test to check for improved (or not) range of motion.
2. With any restricted ROM, ask patient to *point* to any pain or sticking point.
3. Work that point and repeat test.
   After the trigger point has relaxed, do not keep re-treating the same spot. Doing so can irritate the muscle making the problem worse rather than better.
4. Have patient drink plenty of water to help flush metabolic wastes from body.

After treatment, stretching is key to recovery . . .

## STEP 6: STRETCH

*Passive stretching* is done by the therapist after treatment of individual muscles. Chronically shortened muscles can revert to their "normally shortened" state within about 15-20 minutes. To avoid this, muscles are stretched throughout the session.

*Active stretching,* done by the patient alone, follows several rounds of passive stretch. This is continued at home, perhaps in a warm shower or tub with Epsom salts. It should be done about every 15-30 minutes after treatment with gradually decreasing frequency. Do not stretch through pain or exceed normal ROM.

With TrPs, *post-isometric* stretch (stretching against resistance) is most effective. Look again at the over-shortened fibers (nodules) and over-lengthened fibers (taut bands) in Figure 8. Standard stretches can leave shortened areas unaffected while further separating overstretched sarcomeres. This is another reason why stretching as "warmup" can *decrease* flexibility. It is also why "strengthening" exercises can leave muscles weaker. Stretching under load restores both abnormal fibers, pulling overstretched sarcomeres back *together* while pulling shortened ones *apart*.

Stretching is part of whole body health *including brain function*. Stretch receptors are part of our body-brain communication system. They talk to the brain and the brain talks to that area, or at least knows that it's still there. If you don't stretch, you don't fire those receptors. The brain needs to know you're still out there. Keep it posted.

In general, stretch by repeating the ROM tests. Stretching pectoral muscles is more complex, requiring three separate positions to fully stretch all the muscle sections. Place hands as shown and lean through a doorway, or into a corner of room or shower.

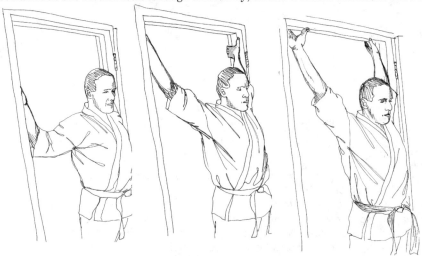

**Figure 60.** DOORWAY STRETCH FOR PECTORAL MUSCLES

# Specific Muscular Issues

## VERTIGO AND VAGUS

We tend to blame dizziness and balance problems on the inner ear , but vertigo (the sense that the room is spinning), can arise from an unhappy vagus nerve. Vagus fibers are commonly entrapped by TRAPEZIUS and STERNOCLEIDOMASTOID. These muscles can produce all the neurological symptoms of migraine: dizziness and nausea, chills. The vagus nerve talks to the hypothalamus. The hypothalamus talks back.

Suboccipital muscles are rich with sensors that monitor the relationship between head and spine. (This is so critical to balance that if these muscles are anaesthetized in monkeys, they fall right over.) The smallest, RECTUS CAPITIS POSTERIOR MINOR, is the most important in tilting the skull backwards. It also forms the dural bridge (page 43) and if strained, pulls on brain and spinal cord with painful results.

Some therapists have begun injecting SUBOCCIPITALS with Botox in hopes of relieving migraine symptoms. Patients report pain relief, but may find that they can't raise their heads without help from a hand. Injecting Suboccipitals with Botox takes them offline, just as forehead muscles are out of action for months when Botox is injected for an "instant facelift." When you need to tilt your head, adjacent muscles will attempt to fill in, but with less mechanical advantage they are subject to strain and can trigger their own pain patterns. Procaine rather than Botox can provide a quick test for pain relief, but the muscle is best treated with hands-on manual methods.

## MUSCLE RELAXANTS

Muscle relaxants work best on healthy muscles. Muscles with trigger points (TrPs) are not healthy.

Although these drugs are commonly prescribed, many doctors and patients will say their biggest benefit appears to be that when *all* muscles are made non-functional, patients can't run around when they should be resting in bed. Another downside is that when muscle relaxants don't work for a problem seen as muscle tension, the problem may be seen as emotional, or *psychiatric*. Poor nutrition is not improved by muscle relaxants, nor are the causes of genuine stress.

Muscle relaxants do not relieve TrPs, but neither does deep anaesthesia or even coma. Muscle relaxants do have one advantage: because they relax all healthy muscles but not TrPs, they can serve as contrast medium, like barium in an X-ray. When normal muscle tone collapses and becomes flaccid, TrPs remain and are even easier to find. They also offer relief when TrPs are combined with fibromyalgia pain. For relief of *local* muscle problems, alternating local heat and cold with TrP release and gentle massage is almost always more effective.

# Chapter 3

# "It's Vascular!"

*Migraine can be a symptom of impaired circulation and high or low blood pressure. Why cold feet and crampy calves are possible causes, rather than mere symptoms.*

Arteries and veins are the plumbing of the body, delivering nutrients and removing waste materials from every cell of the body.

For many years, migraine has been understood in terms of painful expansion of blood vessels (vaso*dilation*) possibly triggered by initial vaso*constriction.* Treatment for migraine has long focused on ways to avoid radical swings between constriction and dilation and means of squeezing swollen blood vessels back down to normal size.

With recent brain research, this model has fallen out of favor[1] but basic physiologic issues still apply. In the brain, there are no valves as there are in legs and arms. Vessels shrink and swell in response to heat and cold, signals from the autonomic nervous system, hormones, oxygen (or lack of it) and balance between $O_2$-$CO_2$ and other chemicals (including sugar, caffeine, nicotine, nitric oxide, and toxins from infection).

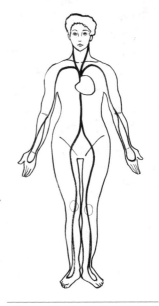

**Figure 61.** MAJOR VESSELS

Blood vessels can be lumped into two large groups: "Up" (to arms and head) and "Down" (to trunk and legs). That's too broad for practical use, so just as segments of continuous highways are named for local towns and highway commissioners, blood vessels are named for local landmarks. For example, as the the aorta from the heart passes "under the clavicle/collarbone" it becomes the *subclavian* artery, the *axillary artery* as it passes through the armpit (*axilla*) then the *brachial artery* (of the "arm"), and finally the *radial artery* at the radial bone of the forearm.

---

1. See "Cortical Spreading Depression" on page 130.

# Circulation

Blood pumped from the heart travels through the body and returns via the veins all within about 20 seconds.

Arteries are the supply system. From heart and lungs, they distribute blood, carrying oxygen and other nutrients to body and brain. The main supply line, direct from the heart, is the *aorta*. This branches and narrows into individual arteries which branch and narrow into *arterioles* ("little arteries") which branch and narrow further still into *capillaries* ("hair"-sized blood vessels, just one blood cell wide).

Veins are *drains*. Or should be.

Major veins travel with major arteries and can be blocked by the same structures.

Veins are not designed to handle high-pressure fluids. Their walls are thinner, stretchier, and floppier than those of the more robust arteries. Unlike arteries, veins collapse when empty or under reduced pressure. The difference between the two is very roughly the difference between an airless bicycle tire (which keeps its shape) and an airless latex balloon (which does not).

Like arteries, veins can stretch and expand to accommodate elevated pressures when necessary, but overstretching can thin the walls so that waste products, toxins, and fluids leak through, accumulate, and cannot be removed efficiently. Resulting edema and swelling exposes pain-sensitive tissues to pressure and pain[1].

Normally, arterioles blend into *venules* ("little veins") which blend into larger veins which eventually dump into the *vena cava* (the big cavernous vein that goes straight to the heart.

---

1. One toxin is blood, perhaps surprising, but as analogy, think of your brain as the driver of your Earth vehicle. Things are fine if everything stays in its place, but if hoses break, spraying the driver with anti-freeze and gasoline, things are not fine. One problem is that when blood leaks or pools, blood cells break down freeing iron from the hemoglobin molecule that should contain and control it. The free iron breaks down blood vessels still more.

## ARTERIES OF THE UPPER BODY

Aorta > (Brachiocephalic) > Subclavian > Carotid > Vertebral > Basilar Arteries

### AORTA AND UP

The *ascending aorta* is the main "up artery" that comes directly from the heart. On your right side[1] a branch forms the *brachiocephalic artery* ("arms and head").The first branch forms the *subclavian artery* (that goes "under the clavicle"). On your left side, the subclavian artery comes directly off the aorta.

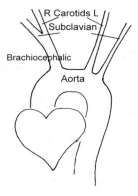

The subclavians branch to form the vertebral arteries and the carotid arteries which supply blood to the brain. The SUBCLAVIUS muscle can compress the subclavian artery, reducing blood flow to all of these.

**Figure 62.** "UP" ARTERIES

### CAROTID ARTERIES AND CEREBRAL ARTERIES

The *carotid* arteries are the main blood supply to neck, head, and brain. The common carotid splits into two branches. The *external* branch supplies structures *outside* the brain, including muscles of the face, mouth, throat, tongue, ear, scalp, glands (including thyroid) and the dura mater of the meninges. The deeper branches (*internal* carotids) supply structures *inside* the brain, eventually becoming the cerebral arteries. Their various branchings supply most of the brain.

### VERTEBRAL ARTERIES > BASILAR ARTERY

Branching from the subclavian arteries, the vertebral arteries tunnel up through the edges of the cervical vertebrae. At the *atlas* (the first cervical vertebra or C1) they join to form the basilar artery which supplies the brain stem (breathing and the most basic life support), the cerebellum (balance and coordination), and the occipital lobe (the visual cortex) of the brain. Blood supply can be reduced by spasm or blockage in the basilar artery or its suppliers. These areas are responsible for many symptoms of migraine including aura.

The DIGASTRIC and Stylohyoid muscles of the neck can compress the external carotids[2]. The SUBOCCIPITALS at the base of the skull can compress the vertebral arteries, or yank on the dura and its associated blood vesels in the brain. Any of these can cause symptoms that linger after whiplash accidents.

---

1. In anatomy, "right" and "left" are from the point of view of the person.
2. They can also compress the posterior auricular artery, a branch of the external carotid that supplies the flap of the ear and the scalp behind it, causing aching pain in these areas.

## CIRCLE OF WILLIS

The Circle of Willis connects the arteries from the carotids to the basilar and vertebral arteries. This provides redundancy of the brain's blood supply. In theory, if one artery is narrowed or blocked, blood travels via alternate vessels. Unfortunately, the textbook circle and redundancies are often missing. Dr. Willis (who also named the cranial nerves) identified this structure in the 1600s, and most anatomy texts have shown it as a circle ever since. But not even Dr. Willis' original illustration showed a circle, and it turns out that the perfect circle is relatively rare, found in only about 40 per cent of humans. Figure 63 shows the classic textbook form with variations, each appearing in about 10 per cent of the population[1] (Clemente CD, 2011).

Why do we care? Because Options A-D with their narrowed connections, could cause problems. These may be perfectly adequate configurations under normal conditions. They might also make a person more susceptible to side effects when something does go wrong.

Anything that decreases circulation in the brain is a potential problem. When circulation to and from the brain decreases, individual modules of your on-line computer will slow and begin to drop off-line. Eventually, tissues will begin to signal their pain. If blood slows long enough, clots may form.

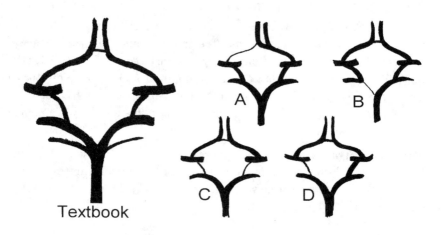

Textbook

**Figure 63.** CIRCLE OF WILLIS VARIATIONS

1. For details, see plates 582 of Clemente CD.

## BRAINS AND PAINS

Problems arise with:

- Inadequate blood flow to muscles and brain or

- Slowed return of blood *from* muscles and organs to heart and lungs.

When we think of blockages, we think of atherosclerosis, blood clots, and stroke. But as we have seen, it is also possible to block or reduce blood flow by compression[1]. Tight muscles and trigger points will do the job (Sikdar S and others, 2009)[2]. Muscles of calf and thigh (especially SOLEUS and ADDUCTOR MAGNUS) can block blood to and from the legs, SUBCLAVIUS below the collarbone can block blood flow to and from the brain, and OMO-HYOID (a muscle of neck and shoulder) can reduce blood flow through the jugular vein. When blood stays and pools, several things happen.

- Blood is not returned to the lungs for a fresh supply of oxygen.

- "Old" blood, depleted of oxygen and nutrients, cannot be replaced by fresh blood.

- Swelling, edema, and increased pressure inside vessels or pressing on the vessels, can impede circulation even more.

When muscles and brains are deprived of adequate oxygen and nutrients they hurt. Think of the pain of walking on a foot that has "fallen asleep." Now think of that pain in your head.

Functionality may also be reduced. If blood supply in the cerebral arteries is reduced, starving the neurons of the brain, the problem may be vascular in origin, but it has now become neurological. Arteries pulsing on nerves may also trigger a response.

If a migraine involving these areas strikes while you are in your car, you may be pulled over because you were driving erratically. You may be unable to walk the white line thanks to balance problems arising from a blood-starved cerebellum or legs that just won't work.

Strangely enough, migraines can also come from the *lower* body.

---

1. So will a variety of clothing and accessories. (See "The Fashion Migraine" on page 216).
2. The carotids derive their name from (Gr.) *karotides,* related to *karos,* deep sleep, reflecting the ancient realization that pressing on these arteries could render a person unconscious. Judo players do this regularly, matter-of-factly choking each other out as part of their art. Do not try this at home.

## ARTERIES OF THE LOWER BODY

Descending Aorta > Iliac > Femoral > Popliteal > Tibial Arteries

### HIP AND THIGH

The *descending aorta* is the major artery travelling "down" from the heart to the abdomen. There it splits, creating a branch for each leg. While in the pelvis, these are known as *iliac* ("hip") arteries. When the same vessels reach the *femurs* ("thighs"), they become the *femoral* arteries.

On nearing the knee, femoral artery and vein pass through the *adductor hiatus*, a gap in the massive ADDUCTOR MAGNUS muscle of the inner thigh. In some people, this gap is a potential trouble spot, small enough to block blood supply to the lower legs. It can become smaller still if the muscle is tight and shortened.

### KNEE AND LEG

On leaving the hiatus, the femoral artery becomes the *popliteal artery*, named for its position in the "back of the knee." Traditionally, bodyworkers are solemnly warned *never* to work in the popliteal space for fear of compressing the artery, but knee-high stockings, elastic knee braces and vollyball pads, driving for hours, or sitting in an office with knees draped over the hard edge of a chair are more realistic and daily opportunities to block circulation to the lower leg.

The attachment of the GASTROCNEMIUS can also entrap the popliteal artery (and venous return) behind the knee. Locking the knees combined with a shoulders-back posture can impair circulation enough to reduce blood supply to the brain. In the armed services this is known as Military Syncope. In civilians, as "fainting."

As the popliteal artery descends below the knee to the area of the tibia (shin bone) it splits into what are locally known as the *tibial arteries*. These supply SOLEUS and GASTROCNEMIUS, muscles of the calf which merge to form the Achilles tendon[1]. SOLEUS is known as "the second heart" for its action in helping to pump blood back to the heart. It cannot do its job if tight and inflexible from high heels or cold and stiff from upstream blockage. When blood supply drops, calf muscles cramp and can tighten around their own blood vessels and nerves, including the posterior tibial vein, artery, and nerve[2] (Travell & Simons 1992, p. 448).

Restless Leg Syndrome with night-time calf cramps, is known to raise blood pressure. This makes its own contribution to headache but the most obvious result may be icy cold feet so often seen in migraine. Muscles can compress circulation so severely that

---

1. If overstressed, the tendon can become painful or even rip loose from the heel (especially if weakened by cortisone shots, given in an attempt to ease the heel pain referred by these muscles). A torn Achilles tendon is usually the last gasp of chronically tight calf muscles.
2. And possibly around the popliteal vein as well via the plantaris muscle, a slip of the SOLEUS.

the arterial pulses in foot and ankle may vanish, but can be restored by working the ADDUCTOR MAGNUS and calf muscles[1].

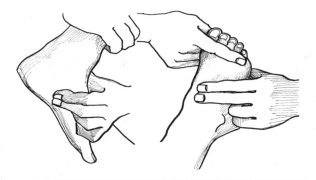

**Figure 64.** CHECKING PULSES IN FOOT AND ANKLE.

Warming the extremeties via biofeedback training is considered a first step in learning to control migraines. The intent is to learn to *restore* circulation by relaxing muscles that block circulation. Learning this skill can produce a remarkable decrease in the frequency of migraines. Students usually start with hand-warming, then move on to warming feet. Changes in temperature can be remarkable, but few migraineurs (especially beginners) can abort a full-blown migraine with this technique alone. Body workers, however, can do the same thing *mechanically*, and stop a migraine in minutes *if* these lower-body muscles are involved.

If feet are cold, find the lowest *warm* spot (where circulation is unimpaired, possibly in the groin) and work down from there. The apparent cause doesn't seem to matter; reported triggers have ranged from income taxes to noise, to peanut butter to perfume. How can this possibly work?

The relationship between blocked circulation in the *legs* and what happens in the *head* is supported by *pneumatic anti-shock trousers*. These are essentially blood pressure cuffs that fit over legs and abdomen, modeled after flight suits designed for jet fighter pilots. The original intent was to prevent the pilot from blacking out when subjected to powerful G-forces; compressing the legs forced blood to remain in the abdominal area and head rather than pooling in the legs, but pilots who crashed wearing this gear had higher survival rates than pilots who crashed without it.

---

1. Pulses at foot and ankle are checked with patient lying on back and having been at rest for at least 5 minutes. Studies have shown that the dorsalis pedis and the posterior tibial pulses cannot be palpated *at all* in some 8% and 3% (respectively), of healthy individuals (McGee SR and others, 1998). Absence of *both* pulses correlates all too well with peripheral arterial disease, of which cold feet and migraine may be just one related symptom.

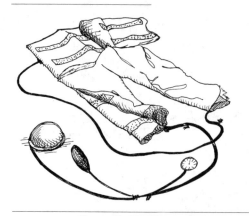

**Figure 65.** MAST TROUSERS

This observation led to their use in emergency medicine where they are now known as Medical Anti-Shock Trousers (MAST) and used to block or reverse symptoms of shock. Because MAST increase blood flow to the brain and other vital organs, they are not used if there is serious trauma to chest or *head*. Patients sent to the ER in MAST must be decompressed slowly; rapid decompression is equivalent to losing a liter or two of blood.

As with too-rapid decompression of MAST, treating the lower body of a migraine patient with cold feet due to muscle contraction can abort a headache but leave the patient dazed and disoriented. Give the patient support when leaving the table and appropriate time to recover. Do not allow the patient to slide off the table unassisted, or stagger out to the car and into traffic.

Over the years (dating back to when men weren't even supposed to get headaches), I met several men who swore they had never had a headache in their entire lives — until they caught shrapnel in the calf or ripped an Achilles tendon playing ball. These men suffered persistent migraines following their *lower leg* injuries.

Both MAST and myofascial constrictions have the potential to block blood from lower extremeties and keep it in the brain. Sometimes this is helpful and life-saving. Sometimes it is not. It is *not* helpful when normal drainage from the brain is blocked.

## VEINS OF THE UPPER BODY

### FACE AND HEAD

Many headaches are assumed to be sinus infections, but *true* sinus infections (with foul greenish discharge swarming with pus and bacteria) are relatively rare. Sinus pain usually originates with something other than infection, very often blood vessels blocked by tissue swollen from allergies or TrPs and muscle problems. When blockage, inflammation, or TrPs fire off pain-sensing nerve endings, the resulting sinus pain (sensed and propagated by the trigeminal nerves) can be every bit as "neurological" in origin as a migraine.

For its size and weight, MASSETER (Figure 19) is the strongest muscle in the body, with pain power to match. When tight it can entrap the maxillary vein which drains fluid and waste from head and face. The resulting swelling and edema contribute to many headaches, including pain in the maxillary sinuses of the cheek. It can also cause tooth and ear pain (that may include a roaring tinnitus) and baggy eyes.

STERNOCLEIDOMASTOID (Figure 18) can cause severe pain in frontal sinuses. ZYGOMATICUS (Figure 24) can produce more frontal sinus pain by blocking the facial artery and vein.

During a migraine, do you prefer to lie down or sit up? Your preference may offer another clue.

Normally jugular veins drain into the subclavian veins and back to the heart. Any blockage along this route can cause back pressure and pain. Researchers demonstrated this by manually pressing on the jugular veins of 25 patients in the throes of a migraine attack. Pain increased in 68 per cent of the patients who were lying on their backs. Only 24 per cent reported more pain when this was done while they were sitting up (Doepp F and others, 2003).

Besides changes in body position, jugular flow can be reduced and back-pressures increased by:

- *Jamming of skull bones.* If temporal and occipital bones are jammed together (as can happen in birth and traumatic head injury), the vein may be squeezed at the jugular foramen where it exits the skull.

- *OMOHYOID tightness.* OMOHYOID attaches directly to the fascia of the jugular vein. A pull on the jugular can narrow the vessel greatly slowing and impeding drainage (Rajalakshmi R and others, 2008).

- *Constriction by SUBCLAVIUS.* Blood gets through the jugular, but slows on its way through the subclavian vein due to compression by the subclavius muscle.

# Specific Vascular Issues

In conditions which alter the normal blood flow to the brain, headaches may be the first sign of problems, appearing long before other more classical symptoms.

Hypertension, Thoracic Outlet Syndrome (TOS), Patent Foramen Ovale (PFO, a hole between the chambers of the heart), Subclavian Steal Syndrome (SSS), all may result in intractable migraines or even seizures due to reduced oxygen supply to the brain.

*If your migraines originate with conditions of reduced blood flow, they can't possibly respond well to vasoconstrictive migraine drugs which reduce blood flow and oxygen supply even further.*

## BLOOD PRESSURE, HIGH AND LOW

*Hypertension* is defined as blood pressure of 140/90 or above[1]. It is traditionally thought of as a disease of older adults and now suspect in much cognitive decline traditionally attributed to aging. It is now seen in children and teens, especially the overweight ones.

Hypertension does its damage by weakening blood vessels to the point of rupture causing stroke, aneurysm, heart attack, disability or death. Very high blood pressure may cause headaches and nosebleeds, but more subtle symptoms such as shortness of breath and cognitive decline are commonly overlooked or attributed to other factors.

It can reduce attention, learning, memory and decision-making skills through constant stress on the brain including small strokes. Brain changes appear on MRIs as lesions in the white matter (the nerve fibers that link neurons together) in the brain. Damage to these communicating structures impacts all brain function and the ability to function well in life. Meanwhile, brain tissue may not feel pain, but the dura and blood vessels do.

*Hypotension*, usually defined as below 100/40, starves the brain of needed nutrients.

---

1. The first number is the *systolic* pressure (Gr.*systellein*, to contract) a measure of the force of blood pushing against artery walls when the walls of the heart squeeze together. The second number, *diastolic* pressure, is the pressure during relaxation of the heart when the walls of the chambers move apart (Gr. *dia*) and fill with blood.

# THORACIC OUTLET SYNDROME

> Literature review and commentary makes it clear that surgeons are frustrated because only about half of operative interventions for TOS are successful. Some are dramatically successful and some are disastrously unsuccessful. There is little agreement as to how one can reliably predict the postoperative outcome. Apparently a piece of the puzzle is missing.
>
> —Travell & Simons (1993)

The *thoracic outlet* is the opening between neck muscles and the rib cage, in the area of the collarbones. It's a hallway, a tunnel, for passage of major blood vessels and nerves. Neurological symptoms are attributed to inadequate space in this area, but having passed through the outlet, nerves and blood vessels must still navigate under the SUBCLAVIAN muscle and PECTORALIS MINOR muscles, make their way through the armpit, and down the arm and elbow to the hand.

Early TOS symptoms include hand weakness and numbness and tingling in the palm side of the fourth and fifth fingers, and inner forearm. (Symptoms in thumb and first two fingers are usually attributed to Carpal Tunnel Syndrome via compression of the median nerve at the wrist, but can come from the neck, chest, or elbow). *The first symptom of TOS may be intractable migraines.*

A hand-held Doppler unit (for checking vascular function) can detect problems in seconds. The simplest home method is hand temperature. Migraineurs frequently suffer cold hands, usually attributed to dysfunction of the Autonomic Nervous System (ANS), but if one hand is warm and the other hand is cold, something else is involved. This is especially likely if you get headaches on the same side as the cold hand, if you play violin, tennis, or swim the crawl or suddenly developed problems at age 40. Entrapment at the outlet decreases blood supply. Block blood flow to the arm and you will get arm pain. Block it to the brain and you will get head pain.

The first suspicion in TOS is often an extra cervical rib, but these do not suddenly develop in adults. More likely candidates include shoulder injury from falls, overuse, or poor posture resulting in inflamed narrowed spaces, myofascial strain and imbalances. Involved structures include:

- SCALENES. These muscles connect neck vertebrae to the first and second ribs pulling the ribs upward on inhalation to make room for expanding lungs.

- *Misaligned cervical vertebrae.* Vertebrae can be pulled out of alignment by SCALENES, LEVATOR SCAPULA, and LONGISSIMUS CAPITIS and other muscles, compressing discs and nerve roots.

- *SUBCLAVIUS / PECTORALIS MINOR.* When these shorten and bulge (typical of a round-shouldered posture), they can compress blood and nerve supply to arm and fingers.

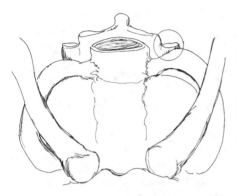

A raised left first rib in a patient with left-sided symptoms. (It appears on the right in the picture, but this is the patient's *left* side.)

Compared to the rib on the patient's right (symptom free) side, the left rib is higher, narrowing space available for blood vessels and nerves to pass through.
(After CT scan in Lindgren KA and others (1995).

**Figure 66.** HIGH FIRST RIB IN THORACIC OUTLET SYNDROME

First treatment should be myofascial therapy or appropriate physical therapy applied to these structures. Where this has failed (perhaps due to traditional "strengthening" exercises) the next step is often surgical removal of one or two scalene muscles with the first rib and possibly part of the second). In a report dealing specifically with TOS and migraine, NH Raskin and others (1985) reported a successful series of TOS surgeries. Of 30 patients, 26 reported headaches long before (or in place of) the classic TOS symptoms of neck and shoulder pain. Only 11 developed neck and shoulder pain in addition to the headaches. In 21 patients, headache was one-sided migraine; it was continuous and unrelenting in 14 patients. Some had been given standard vasoconstrictor migraine medications which gave no relief. *Migraines due to low blood supply won't be helped by drugs that reduced blood supply even more.*

After surgical removal of entrapping scalenes and first rib, 11 previously disabled patients returned to work; 13 were completely headache free, while 11 others reported benefit from the same medications that had failed to help before the surgery. Surgeries for cases reported here were successful. Still, there are other options. The missing piece involves the interplay between muscles and movement, correcting impaired relationships rather than cutting them out. Less invasive options can address the root problem: *constricted scalenes and a first rib stuck in the raised position, narrowing the space available for nerves and blood vessels.*

In healthy breathing, it is normal for SCALENES to pull up the first rib, narrowing the outlet, but allowing room for lungs to expand. Problems arise when muscles remain too short, thick, or tight to allow a raised rib to drop down again. This happens in chest breathing (see page 169) as do shifts in the thoracic outlet "frequently seen in young women" (Lindgren KA and others, 1995).

Figure 66 shows a non-surgical maneuver that treats tight SCALENES and an elevated first rib. There are several versions of this, but all require a therapist who knows how to palpate a first rib, who has the time to allow muscle to relax, and who has the training and skills to release shortened fascia.

*Manual Release of First Rib*

L=Left / R=Right

**Therapist will:**

1. Support patient's head with L arm.
2. With R thumb, push TRAPEZIUS posteriorly to palpate head of first rib.
3. With L hand, gently bend patient's neck to L side until slack in neck is taken up and head of first rib begins to rise against R thumb.
4. With R thumb, press down gently against first rib to stretch scalenes. As therapist eases patient's head to L side,

**Patient will:**

5. Press against resistance supplied by therapist's L hand (using only about 25% of strength to resist).
6. Breathe *in*, looking *up* and R.
7. Relax by breathing *out* while looking *down* and L.

**Therapist will:**

8. Gently rotate head and neck into the positions that challenge each of the three main scalene muscles while maintaining pressure on first rib. This locates specific areas and directions of shortened fibers.
9. Take up slack by gently stretching to the new "length barrier" of the involved muscles.
10. Repeat 3-5 times as necessary.

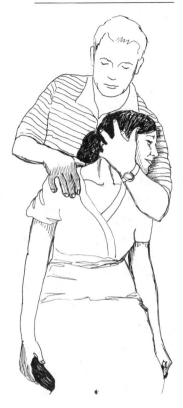

**Figure 67.** MANUAL RELEASE OF SCALENES AND FIRST RIB

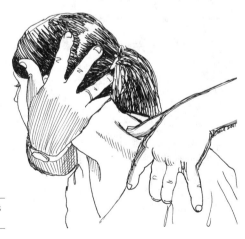

**Figure 68.** MANUAL RELEASE OF SCALENES AND FIRST RIB (DETAIL)

## WASH-BASIN STROKE

Vascular accidents or reduced blood flow can occur when the neck is sharply *extended* (the head tilted toward the back), strongly rotated, or the two motions combined.

Vertebral arteries travel through the tips (processes) of cervical vertebrae, making a 90-degree turn when they reach the upper surface of the atlas. Tilting the head back (extension) can compress the arteries between the skull and upper surface of the atlas vertebra. Blood flow may drop by as much as 30 per cent. Neck rotation adds to the strain as the artery must stretch, possibly decreasing blood flow still more. Fixing the head in extension ( in front-row seats or extreme Head-Forward posture), or rotation (as in stomach sleeping) can decrease blood flow for hours.

When flexibility of these vessels is lost with age or adhesions, risk of rupture increases. "Washbasin stroke" can occur when the neck is sharply extended over the edge of a sink at beauty parlors, especially in persons over 50. In high risk groups, simultaneously extending and rotating head and neck can be risky even in such seemingly innocent maneuvers as head rolls in exercise class, sleeping on the stomach with the head rotated strongly to one side, or even backing a car while looking over the shoulder with chin tipped up. Ordinarily the arteries stretch very well. The temporary decrease of blood flow on one side is handled by the Circle of Willis — in theory. But in some people, theory does not match anatomy.

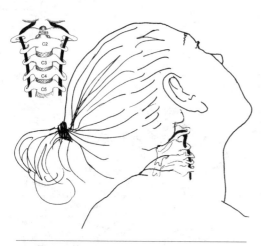

**Figure 69.** VERTEBRAL ARTERY COMPRESSION

What actually happens is uncertain. A recent review evaluated 20 studies reporting blood flow in vertebral and basilar arteries with cervical spine rotation (Mitchell J, 2007). Methods between the different studies were found to be so non-standard that *no* overall correlations were found between rotation, blood flow, and vetebrobasilar ischemia (VBI) that leads to stroke. Results ranged from significantly reduced blood flow (with or *without* VBI) to no detectable changes at all. One reason may be variations in plumbing, the different versions of the Circle of Willis (see Figure 63 on page 90), perhaps another genetic pattern in migraine.

# EXTREME SLEEPING

Posture is important even in sleeping.

When physicians examine the carotids they are careful to compress just *one* at a time.

Judo players are careful to compress *both* with the specific intent of decreasing blood flow to the brain causing unconsciousness[1].

Sleepers may inadvertently do this and more, especially if sleeping on the stomach or draping the neck over a hard pillow.

Stomach sleeping requires turning the head strongly to the side in order to breathe. In some people, this can reduce blood flow through the vertebral artery on one side.

Tilting the head back, as when propped up on a pillow, can compress the vertebrals between skull atlas.

Add some pressure on the carotids from firm pillows or pre-existing tightness in some muscles (such as OMOHYOID, DIGASTRIC, and SUBLAVIUS) and blood flow to the brain can be reduced for hours at a time.

Keeping the head directly affects muscles that produce migraine symptoms, shortening them on one side, overstretching them on the other. Any or all of these can produce severe headache.

If you regularly wake up in the morning with headache, take a long hard look at your sleeping arrangements and positions.

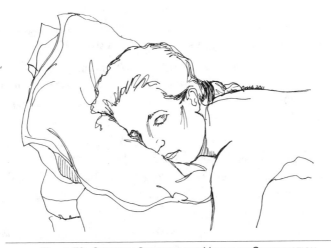

**Figure 70.** STOMACH SLEEPING AND VASCULAR CONSTRICTION

1. Pressure required is a mere 300 mm of mercury (about 6 pounds per square inch) (Koiwai EK, 2002).

## SUBCLAVIAN STEAL SYNDROME

In Subclavian Steal Syndrome (SSS) blood flow can actually *reverse*.

Normally, blood flows from the subclavian artery to the branchings which form the carotids and the vertebral artery to supply the front and back of the brain.

The direct low resistance path along the subclavian artery to arms can become a high resistance path (with reduced blood flow) if the artery narrows (as in atherosclerosis) or is squeezed (by the SUBCLAVIUS muscle or rib dysfunction).

When this happens, thanks to the Circle of Willis in the brain, the path of least resistance around the blockage becomes the vertebral arteries and internal carotids.

Blood travels up one of the other blood vessels to the brain (the other vertebral or the carotids), reaches the basilar artery or goes around the Circle, and descends via the same-side vertebral artery back down to the subclavian artery, but on the other side of the blockage to deliver blood to the shoulder and arm.

It is a beautiful example of redundancy and back-up design and can be life-saving in a stroke. In daily life (or a game of tennis) flow from brain to arm is considered a *steal* because blood intended for the brain ends up in the arm instead. Symptoms include:

- Headaches, dizziness, and vertigo.
- Faintness or fainting due to reduced blood supply to brain and/or brain stem,
- Blood pressure and temperature differences between right and left arms.

The left subclavian artery is more likely to be clogged by plaque than the right one, producing steal syndrome 3 times more often on the left than the right. But it's still rare and not diagnosed unless there are neurological signs and symptoms of low blood supply to the brain brought on by using the arm on the blocked side.

In one large study, (Fields WS and Lemak NA, 1972) found that 17 per cent of 6,534 patients (1,110 patients) had evidence of clogged (by greater than 30 percent) or blocked arteries. Of these, only 168 patients showed actual symptoms of subclavian steal syndrome.

Another study (Berguer R and others, 1980) found that only about half of patients with significant subclavian blockage actually showed reversal of blood flow in the same-side vertebral artery. In another variation reported by Bergman RA and others (1995), both anterior cerebral arteries are supplied by a single internal carotid artery. If that is blocked, you're in trouble.

Rare, but it happens. Problems can be diagnosed via Doppler and CT angiography.

# Headaches from the Heart—Patent Foramen Ovale

Physicians have long seen a disturbing link between migraine and stroke. Not only is the rate of stroke higher in migraineurs, but so is the occurrence of "paradoxical stroke," that is, stroke which occurs outside of all the usual known risk factors in young and seemingly healthy persons.

A small congenital heart defect has been found to play a surprisingly big role in stroke *and* migraine. About half of stroke survivors who have a history of migraine also have a *Patent Foramen Ovale,* or PFO, an "open oval hole" in the heart. The migraine-PFO connection was first reported in 1999 by neurologist Roman Sztajzel in a patient who had suffered two strokes of *cryptogenic* or "unknown origin"; that is, with no sign of the usual precipitating factors. She did, however, have a PFO. After the hole was surgically closed, the patient reported a surprising side-effect; her migraines vanished (Sztajzel R and others, 2002).

Before a baby is born, its oxygen comes from the mother through the umbilical cord. Blood bypasses the lungs via the "oval hole" in the wall dividing the two upper chambers of the heart (the *atria*). At birth, the bypass is no longer needed and the hole should close. When the newborn child begins to breathe air directly through the lung:

- The right chamber of the heart has low oxygen blood returning from veins.
- The left chamber of the heart has oxygen-rich blood from the lungs.
- The two are not intended to mix.

A condition similar to PFO is *Atrial Septal Defect* (ASD) in which the "wall" (*septum*) between two upper chambers (*atria*) fails to develop properly. The difference between the two is that ASD is a continuing problem. A PFO can act like a valve; sometimes blocked with adhesions or a clot, sometimes open.

In both PFO and ASD, blood can travel (or "shunt") between the two chambers of the heart. Right-to-left shunts are the most dangerouse. Increased pressure in the chest

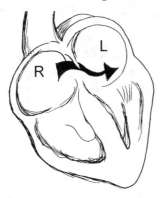

**Figure 71.** Blood Flow in Normal and FPO Hearts

/ pulmonary artery and vessels (a cough, a sneeze, or strenuous exercise) can force the valve open. Low-oxygen blood that should go to the lungs is misdirected to the brain or other body parts causing a host of symptoms. Problems arise when:

- Blood passing through the tunnel of the PFO slows and clots. When a clot pops loose, it enters the arteries that supply the brain, risking a stroke.

- Gas bubbles pass through the tunnel and enter arteries to the brain as "paradoxical embolisms," in turn causing "paradoxical" or "cryptogenic stroke," that is, stroke of unknown origin that occurs despite lack of normal precipitating factors.

- Blood chemicals that should be filtered out by lungs end up as toxins in the brain.

Persons with PFO may have symptoms *sometimes*, but not *always*, maybe just when combined with enough stress, strain, or fatigue to earn reputation for "convenient" migraines and laziness. But research on PFO explains:

- Extreme sensitivity to low-oxygen environments and resolution by oxygen therapy.

- Extreme sensitivity to food / allergen triggers.

- Tendency of migraines to run in families.

- High prevalence of migraine with aura among stroke patients, especially in men.

- Extreme sensitivity to pressure changes.

- Autonomic symptoms related to the hypothalamus which lacks a blood-brain barrier.

When migraines run in families, what is inherited may be more than a sensitivity; it may be a septal defect that causes sensitivity (Wilmshurst PT, 2004). A study of 20 patients with large PFOs or ASDs included 71 relatives including 4 families with 3 generations, 14 families with 2 generations, and a pair of siblings.

PFO was clearly linked to the family tendency to migraine. For patients who had migraine with aura and an atrial shunt, 15 of 21 (a whopping 71 per cent) of their first degree relatives with significant right-to-left shunts also had migraine with aura. In those lacking a significant shunt, only 3 of 14 (21 per cent) had migraine with aura.

PFO incidence is also high in divers who suffer unusually high rates of decompression sickness ("the bends") compared to other divers. Sudden changes from high pressure to low pressure (as when ascending too quickly from deep water to the surface), allow gases such as nitrogen to bubble out of the blood, just as carbon dioxide bubbles out of soda when the can is opened and pressure drops. These gases should go to the lungs for removal, but with PFO they can be shunted directly to the brain (Holmes DR and others, 2004; Wilmshurst PT, 2000).

The connection between PFO or ADS and decompression sickness is considered so solid that it is no longer rare for surgeons to treat professional divers by closing the holes in their hearts. Again, these patients reported an immediate decrease in headaches and migraine; not the presenting condition for which they were being treated.

Migraine sufferers typically have a higher-than-normal risk of stroke. Studies of stroke survivors suggest that half those with migraines have PFOs. And the rate of PFO is unusually high in migraineurs as a group.

In a 2006 review of stroke patients, 140 migraine patients were compared with 330 stroke patients (130 "young" and 200 "elderly"). The odds of finding PFO in migraine patients with aura was roughly *twice* that of patients without aura, and even higher in young "cryptogenic" stroke patients (Carod-Artal FJ and others, 2006).

PFO is diagnosed via contrast electrocardiography, echocardiograms, or Doppler sonography. Multiple studies show that closing a PFO either eliminates migraines or reduces their incidence. Best results are seen in migraineurs with aura, the group most likely to have a PFO and least likely to have responded favorably to migraine drugs. Most studies showed that PFO surgery *completely relieved* migraines with aura in about half the subjects. In general, an additional third noticed *substantial* improvement. But the picture is not altogether positive.

When a heart defect is found, most surgeons limit repairs to patients who already have a history of serious cardiovascular problems (such as stroke) in addition to severely disabling headaches. Others are advised to wait until more data is available. Compared to the risks of cardiovascular disease and open-heart surgery (or early retirement from one's diving career), migraine is considered relatively trivial.

On the other hand, surgical techniques have been simplified to the point that the hole is closed by threading a catheter through a vein in the groin, with local rather than general anaesthesia and on an outpatient basis.

Sounds great! But before you demand this procedure remember that "simple surgery" usually means "simple for the *surgeon*" — not for the patient. In some cases, closure via the "simple" trans-catheter approach has made the frequency and severity of migraines worse for months afterwards. Side effects included aura and severe and unrelenting migraines, or *status migrainosus*[1].

Symptoms were relieved by adding a stronger anti-coagulant to the follow-up treatment which had originally involved only aspirin (a mild anti-coagulant). Wilmshurst PT and others (2005) suggest that platelet stickiness may play a role in migraine, possibly related to serotonin[2]. Whatever the cause, this paper suggests that there's something different about the "safer" trans-catheter surgery. You might want to watch and wait for further improvements.

---

1. Latin for "the migraine never stops." Many migraineurs get to this state all by themselves. They need not go through the pain, expense, and risk of surgery to achieve it.
2. Serotonin is related to depression and migraine but platelet clumping is also related to iron and magnesium, known factors in migraine.

## DEEP VEIN AND AIRLINE THROMBOSIS

"Airline Thrombosis"is a new name for an old affliction, in the medical literature since first systematic assault of civilians by the aircraft industry: the Nazi Blitzkrieg against England in WWII. After the bombs and returning safely home, many civilians, (usually middle-aged or older) died from pulmonary embolism (Simpson K, 1940). Whether in the airplane or below it, long stressful periods of sitting can cause blood to pool in the legs, the perfect environment to form a clot (a *thrombus*). With renewed activity, the clot can break loose to travel (as an *embolism*) through the bloodstream to lungs, brain, or heart causing death hours or days later.

Problems arise with anything that blocks circulation. The classic example is the pregnant woman sleeping on her back with a 7 pound baby and 2 pound womb pressing on the inferior vena cava; she wakes up with leg clots. Alcohol, heroin, barbiturates, or other painkillers, can also cause death by blood clot in persons who pass out with legs crossed. "It's the semi-comatose insensitivity to pain, plus inability to wake up, that leaves legs crossed so long that blood flow slows. Clots form and drunken reveler dies," says forensic pathologist Wendy Gunther, who has seen this on her slab.

Air travel gets all the press, but desk work is far more likely to kill you (Beasley R and other, 2005). Hours at a computer terminal can do the trick, even in conscious workers

## IS THERE A BLOOD TEST FOR MIGRAINE?

Many migraineurs have low levels of *free* magnesium in combination with relatively high levels of calcium. This will not appear in a standard blood test however. See the Exatest on page 153.

Calcitonin Gene-Related Peptide (CGRP) is a potent vasodilator. It helps transmit pain signals and increase nerve sensitivity. During migraine attacks, high levels of CGRP have been found in blood leaving the brain via the jugular vein. Injecting it back into the now headache-free migraineur reproduces the migraine.

Factor V Leiden is a genetic blood-clotting disorder in which blood clots form all too easily in veins. It is extremely rare in Asians, most common in Northern Europeans or their descendents. It is present in about 5 percent of Caucasians in North America but it shows in up to 30 percent of patients with Deep Vein Thrombosis (DVT) or pulmonary embolism. Women with the disorder have a greatly increased risk of clotting and preeclampsia during pregnancy (and while on estrogen-containing birth control pills or hormone replacement).

Relationship to migraine is controversial, high in some populations, insignificant in others. However, because of the strong correlation between migraine and stroke due to blood clots, you might consider testing if you are of Northern European heritage (especially Scandinavian).

# Chapter 4

# It's Neurological!

*Migraine can be a symptom of nerve overstimulation or compression. If you've ever hit your funny bone, suffered sciatica or an ice-cream headache and can imagine that pain in your head, you have a clue to your migraines.*

Nerves are the electrical wiring of the body and brain. Even nerves have nerves in the fascial covering "on the nerves" (the *epineurium*).

Nerves may be traumatized by everything from simple impingement (squashing) to chemical toxins, to heat and cold. A familiar example of referred neurological head pain is the ice cream headache ("brain freeze") that develops within seconds of eating icy cold foods. It comes from nerves in palate and throat, but typically appear at the temples and back of the head[1].

Because ice-cream headaches can be triggered on demand, they can be used to give physicians, family members, and other civilians a close-up personal experience of migraine and cluster headaches. A researcher found that applying crushed ice to *one* side of the palate produced one-sided pain at the side of the head and around the eye. Icing the midline produced the same pain on *both* sides of the head. (Hulihan M, 1997).

Many apparent *sinus* headaches are actually *migraine*. This is especially true in men for whom "sinus" is a more acceptable diagnosis than the seemingly more feminine diagnosis of "migraine." Because the same nerves involved in migraine supply sinus tissue, a "sinus" headache can be be every bit as "neurological" as migraine headache.

Understanding the nerves behind the pain helps in understanding why neurological stress can end in tension and sinus and migraine headache, why these are related, and how to prevent them.

But first, a look at the brain.

---

1. Strangely, persons subject to migraine do not tend to be as subject to ice-cream headaches. Even stranger, some claim that purposely triggering an ice-cream headache can abort a migraine, like a reset button. Doesn't work for me, but might be worth a try.

# Brain Organization and Function

The brain is divided into two hemispheres with different functions and even different personalities. They talk via the *corpus callosum* ("beautiful body"), a wide, flat bundle of white matter. Unless the corpus callosum has been surgically cut (as done in some cases of intractable seizures) there is no such thing as a purely left-brained or right-brained person although there are patterns and tendencies.

The left hemisphere is cheerful and optimistic, responsible for social approach behaviors. It can talk and manipulate words and grammar (speech areas are usually on the left). It is commonly credited with math and logic, but its skills are *linear* math and logic. That is, it can add and subtract, reason from point A to point B, and measure space and time with great precision but it can't do calculus or play basketball. It is extremely literal, controls the Go Button and can cheerfully rationalize and justify its behavior, no matter how absurd. It is the Extroverted/ Sensing/ Thinking/ Judgmental (ESTJ) aspect of the Meyers-Briggs Personality Indicator.

| Left hand and body | Right hand and body |
|---|---|
| Approach behaviors, cheer | Avoidance behaviors, depression |
| Words, writing | Foreign languages |
| Confabulation | Rhyming |
| Sequential math (arithmetic) | Tone and rhythm |
| Splitting and linear thought | Unconscious emotion |
| Conscious emotion | Body language |
| | Insight and holistic thought |
| | Facial expression / recognition |

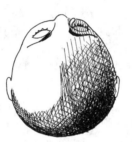

The right hemisphere is more holistic, that is, it connects *all* the dots. It is cautious and hesitant, responsible for social avoidance behaviors. It controls the *Pause* and the *No* Button. It communicates with images and movement, recognizes faces and places, and interprets the facial expressions, emotions, and body language in others, while keeping the left brain emotionally and procedurally on target. Verbal skills may be limited to what we experience in dreams, but it can learn foreign languages which, in adults, require awareness of tone, accent, rhythm; these may remain after a left-sided stroke that would silence a person with just one language.

The right hemisphere is as mathematical and logical as the left, but its skills are the spatial skills of calculus, estimating, geometry, and leaps of insight. It is "the zone" in sports, the bringer of dreams in sleep. It tends to assume and plan for the worst, to the point of being depressed and fearful Unbalanced by the Left Brain, it can slip into paranoia and nightmares. It is the Introverted/ Intuitive/ Feeling / and Perceiving (INFP) aspect of the Myers-Briggs Personality Indicator.

Over this general map are installed individual areas of specialization[1].

# FUNCTIONAL AREAS

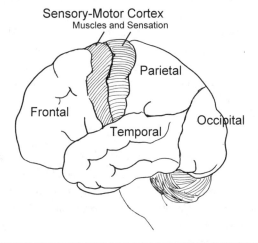

**Figure 72.** FUNCTIONAL AREAS OF THE BRAIN

### FRONTAL / PREFRONTAL LOBES

The most "human" part of the brain, the frontal lobes control impulses, emotions, and judgement. They also serve as the managers of movement, planning the movements carried out by the motor strip. The left frontal lobe handles "executive" function: organizing, ordering, and sequencing.

### SENSORY MOTOR STRIP

The sensory motor strip crosses the brain from ear to ear. Problems with motor function (from ability to speak coherently to handwriting and bowel function, with sensory disruptions and bizarre alterations in sense of touch) can come from this area.

### TEMPORAL LOBES

These lobes, on the temples (sides of the head), are home to the auditory cortex and important in forming long-term memories including verbal memory. They contain the hippocampus critical to transferring information from short to long term memory.

Damage on the left impairs language comprehension; words just don't make sense. The person may have a hair-trigger temper falling into a rage for the smallest (or even no) provocation. Damage on the right may impair recognition of tones and musical notes but remove inhibition of talking.

---

1. This pattern is true for about 90% of humans but may be reversed in about 10%. Second languages, learned via tone and intonation, are handled by the opposite hemisphere. Multi-lingual persons who suffer left-hemisphere stroke may lose their first language while healing, but retain languages learned in adulthood.

## PARIETAL LOBE

The parietal lobe handles position in space and integrates other information. Lewis Carrol is believed to have suffered migraines in large part because of the bizarre imagery in his books. Today the neurological condition known as "Alice in Wonderland Syndrome" includes perceived changes in body size, shrinking, growing, or the impression that one's feet are miles away. Damage to the parietal lobes can result in difficulty naming objects, reading, writing, doing math, problems with spatial relationships (from drawing to telling left from right) and eye-hand coordination.

## OCCIPITAL LOBE

The occipital lobe contains the visual cortex. Your eyes may be in the front of the head, but the connections are here. The occipital lobe doesn't just handle the physical vision; it is also responsible for dreams and hallucinations. Slow waves spreading from this area are believed to be associated with the aura typical of classic migraine. See "Cortical Spreading Depression" on page 130. Figure 72 shows the general wiring diagram and source of various symptoms.

If blood supply is reduced affecting the motor cortex, you will have problems with muscle movements. If the left hemisphere at Broca's area, there will be problems finding words. Slowing in the occipital lobes will cause aura and vision problems.

# DEEP BRAIN STRUCTURES

The following structures produce specific symptoms during migraine attacks.

## HYPOTHALAMUS

The 1997 movie *Men in Black* featured a tiny alien prince enthroned within the control module of his human transport vehicle. He was a brilliant parody of the diencephalon and hypothalamus of the brain. In real humans, the hypothalamus sits at the center of the brain, controlling :

- Autonomic nervous system (nausea, vomiting, constipation/diarrhea, flushing/pallor, sweating / chills / fever / changes in heart rate,
- Sleep-wake cycles and the circadian clock,
- Osmoregulation: the balance of water and mineral salts in the blood,
- Hunger and lack of appetite,
- Hormone balance (thyroid, sex hormones, kidney function),
- Sensory triggers, both visual and olfactory.

When these responses (or deranged versions of them) show up before or during migraine, the hypothalamus is thought to be involved.

To do its job, the hypothalamus must constantly monitor the blood for sugar, hormones, electrolytes, and other blood chemicals. By necessity, parts of the hypothalamus have *no blood-brain barrier between the hypothalamus, the blood, and anything that is in the blood.* As a result, the hypthalamus is painfully aware of allergens, toxins, and the molecules of emotion such as stress and fear, sending and receiving information via the vagus nerve. It is also aware of light, which it uses to trigger processes associated with being awake, such as rise in temperature and hormones like cortisol. All of these can combine to send the hypothalamus into a tizzy. But is the problem with the hypothalamus? Or with the chaos of conflicting messages, warning lights, biological sirens, and red alerts, that it must try (and fail) to manage?

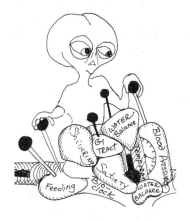

**Figure 73.** A MASTER CONTROLLER

One odd symptom of migraine is altered patterns of urination which in turn may be due to attempts by the hypothalamus and pitutitary to deal with dehydration.

CEREBELLUM

Behind the big brain is the *cerebellum*[1] or "little brain" or , responsible for smoothly coordinated physical movement. If it goes off-line, movements become clumsy and uncoordinated. This can happen when blood supply to cerebellum and brain stem is interrupted or decreased as happens in basilar migraine. The problem isn't just on one side of the head, it's on one side of the body. A left arm can't dial the phone, a left leg collapses.

Basilar migraine is one of the most frightening versions of migraine. Not only does it resemble a stroke, but can set the stage for a real one. A more immediate result may be stumbling and staggering that has landed hapless migraineurs in the drunk tank. With luck, they may land in the ER being evaluated for stroke, which may be better than being evaluated for migraines which are taken far less seriously.

Vasoconstrictive drugs can't be used in basilar migraine. When blood flow to brain stem and cerebellum is reduced, constricting those vessels still more is a bad idea.

---

1. In *Men in Black*, the back of the Prince's chair is a parody of the cerebellum.

# Nerves Involved in Migraine

Nerves are divided into two types: cranial nerves and spinal nerves. Cranial nerves emerge from within the cranium (skull). Spinal nerves come from the spinal cord.

Cranial nerves are like the connections that come directly off the computer box (the "brain" of your system) and provide instructions to "peripheral" equipment such as video cameras and public address systems. Imagine a dozen plugs on the box.

Spinal nerves can be thought of as the connections further down, perhaps coming from a USB port on the peripheral or via a USB hub.

Nerves can be painful on their own, or send confused signals to muscles. Muscles can then tighten, entrapping their own nerve supplies or hapless bystander nerves that were just passing through minding their own business. Nerves can even be irritated by the pulsing of neighboring arteries that have sagged or been pushed together by swelling and inflammation. Similarly, if overstimulated, a nerve may scream at other "customers" along its route just as pounding on wire with a hammer can produce static further down the line.

## CRANIAL NERVES

There are 12 cranial nerves in all. Numbers 5, 7, 10 and 11 are heavily involved in migraine. These are also known as CN V (trigeminal), CN VII (facial), CN X (vagus), and CN XI (spinal accessory nerve).

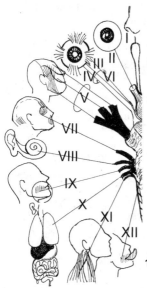

1. **CN I - Olfactory:** smell
2. **CN II - Optic:** vision
3. CN III - Oculomotor: eye motion
4. CN IV - Trochlear: eye motion
5. **CN V - Trigeminal:** head and jaw muscles, teeth and all muscles involved in chewing.
6. CN VI - Abducens: eye motion
7. **CN VII - Facial:** facial muscles, taste, salivary glands.
8. CN VIII - Vestibulocochlear: ear (hearing) and balance
9. CN IX - Glossopharyngeal: muscles of throat, tongue,
10. **CN X - Vagus:** autonomic nervous system, organs, throat muscles, "ear cough" reponse.
11. **CN XI - Spinal Accessory:** Sternocleidomastoid and Trapezius and muscles
12. CN XII - Hypoglossal: muscles of the tongue.

**Figure 74.** CRANIAL NERVES AND CONNECTIONS

## CN I: OLFACTORY NERVE

The *olfactory* nerve (from L. *olfacere*, to smell) can trigger migraines as a response to perfumes and other odors. There has been little research on this input but it is an extremely common trigger especially via synthetic fragrances.

## CN II: OPTIC NERVE

The optic nerve (from Gr. *optikos*, pertaining to vision) is extremely important in migraineurs who can be extremely sensitive to light (*photophobia*). You can often recognize migraineurs (or head injury patients) on the street simply by their very large and very dark sunglasses. Light travels along the optic nerve to the hypothalamus affecting wake sleep cycles.

## CN III: OCULOMOTOR NERVE

The oculomotor nerve is named for its function of "moving the eye," which is done by CN III, CN IV, and CN VI. Straining the muscles supplied by these nerves can cause eye pain and headaches, but problems will probably not be caught on an a standard eye exam. If you can trigger a headache just by looking to one side, let your doctor know.

## CN IV: TROCHLEAR NERVE

The trochlear nerve (from L. *trochlea*, a set of pulleys), is one of several cranial nerves responsible for eye movement. It supplies the superior oblique muscle of the eye. In some people, straining this muscle can trigger a migraine. Problems will not show up in an eye exam unless the examiner watches carefully for jumpy eye movements.

## CN V: TRIGEMINAL NERVE

The trigeminal nerve is the major nerve involved in migraine. The trigeminal is named for its three-way split ("three-twins" into upper, middle, and lower branches: opthalmic, maxillary, and mandibular (or V1/V2/V3). These are mostly sensory, but the lowest portion has motor nerves to control the muscles of the lower jaw (mandible).

CN V controls vasodilation, vasoconstriction, vessel permeability. It is the nerve that controls all the things that make migraine a "vascular" headache. It also supplies tissues of the face, jaw, and teeth, the sutures between the individual bones and joints of the skull, and is a major part of the Reticular Activating System (RAS) that triggers the alarm when something goes wrong with any of these. The combined effects and responses are referred to as the trigemino-vascular system, that is, control of the brain's *vascular* system by the trigeminal *nerve*.

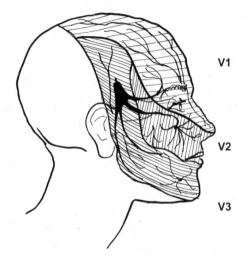

**Opthalmic (V1)**: eyes, nose, sinuses, scalp, forehead, and *meninges*.

**Maxillary (V2)**: lower eyelid, cheeks, nostrils and membranes of the nose, the upper lip, upper teeth and gums, roof of mouth, sinuses, and *meninges* including the pain-sensitive dura mater.

**Mandibular (V3)**: lower lip, lower teeth / gums, tongue, chin and jaw (except angle of jaw).
Motor branches go to to muscles used in chewing: DIGASTRIC (front section), MASSETER, PTERYGOIDS, TEMPORALIS, and to the mylohyoid which forms the floor of the mouth.

**Figure 75.** TRIGEMINAL NERVE

Why forehead, eye, nose, teeth, sinuses, jaw, scalp, brain and ice cream all hurt.

The trigeminal nerve talks to teeth, gums, tongue, and the muscles for chewing. It also supplies forehead, scalp, the sinuses, and the blood vessels and membranes (meninges) that wrap around the brain. Ordinarily this system provides wonderful abilities, from sensing the soft touch of a hand on a cheek to chewing the food that fuels the body. But if something goes wrong, these nerves sound the alarm with stunningly painful consequences.

The auriculo-temporal ("ear-temple") nerve is a branch of the trigeminal. Janis JE and others (2010) found a major trigger in this nerve and the superficial temporal artery. Normally these two structures run together in the soft tissue of the temple, forward of the ear[1]. But when the two entwine together (found in over 30 per cent of samples) the pulsing of the artery can trigger the nerve.

Teeth are a common trigger. It may seem odd that teeth are so sensitive, but they need to be. For example, it is difficult to chew a delicate food such as lettuce with dentures; the wearer can only locate the lettuce with the tongue because the false teeth offer no sensory input. (On the other hand, full plate dentures that cover the roof of the mouth, protect against ice cream headache.)

---

1. These may be compressed by eyeglass frames. See page 220.

The ice-cream headache is thought to come from cooling and vaso*constriction* followed by rewarming and painful rebound vaso*dilation*. But that's vascular, right? Again, it is *trigemino-vascular*, control of the brain's vascular system by trigeminal nerves.

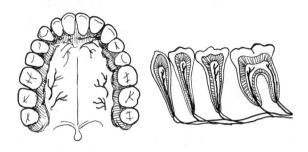

**Figure 76.** NERVE PAIN FROM JAW AND TEETH

The three branches of trigeminal nerves join at the trigeminal ganglion.

Doing bad things to one branch and expecting no consequences is like doing bad things to one brother of triplets and expecting that the other two won't hear about it. They surely will, and they may even talk to the neighbors about it because the trigeminals are close friends with the occipital nerves (down at the corner of C2-C3) who supply the back of neck and head. Strain the neck, and the trigeminals will hear about it as will their buddies the facial nerves.

Terminal fibers of trigeminal nerves near blood vessels (and cells on the trigeminal ganglion) release peptides responsible for inflammation and pain. These include Substance P (the "Pain" peptide) and Calcitonin Gene-Related Peptide (CGRP). Both can dilate blood vessels then transmit the resulting pain. Substance P shows up in migraine (and fibromyalgia and other painful conditions). Neurons that respond to Substance P produce sensations of burning pain.[1]

---

1. Pain exactly like biting into a hot pepper. Capsaicin, the active ingredient in hot peppers and arthritis creams containing hot pepper oil, causes a flood of SP to be released. This is painful at first, but the end result is to deplete supplies of SP between neurons. When it's just not there to be released, the pain threshold rises.

Triptans interrupt this process at various levels but to avoid pain from this source, avoid triggering the mechanisms that control it. Tight FRONTALIS and CORRUGATOR SUPERCILI muscles entrap branches of the trigeminal nerves that were just passing through. This can also be done with tight headwear, cold muscles (you might want to rethink winter surfing), and frowning.

When warned not to frown, many people protest that they frown because they hurt, but frowning may be the actual trigger. In biofeedback,

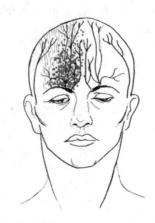

**Figure 77.** TRIGEMINAL FRONTAL HEADACHE

a basic starting point is learning to relax the frontal area to reduce mechanical strain. This affects more than the front. Electrodes placed on the forehead can pick up local electrical impulses of muscle activity and impulses running along the fascia from the back of the head and neck.

Botox makes it impossible to frown by paralyzing the CORRUGATOR muscles. They have also been cut out with mixed, often with striking initial relief followed by gradual return of the pain. This may be due to regrowth of fascia and scar tissue filling in the empty space as happens in any surgery. Or, it may be because these muscles were indeed triggers, but a bigger one lies elsewhere. Surgery should never be considered until a trial of Botox has provided extended relief. Perhaps best to relax your face, dress warmly, wear hats and helmets that fit properly — and smile.

## CN VI: ABDUCENS NERVE

The abducens nerve supplies a muscle on the side of the eye that *abducts* the eyeball (moving it outward). See CN III.

## CN VII: FACIAL NERVE

The facial nerve (CN VII) controls muscles of facial expression. This includes the rear portion of DIGASTRIC, not usually considered a muscle of expression, but it helps to open the jaw in shocked surprise or to put in food. The facial nerve also supplies the salivary glands and the sense of taste to the front of the tongue.

These muscles don't usually produce symptoms interpreted as migraine, at least at first. Pain is more likely to be attributed to sinus or TMJ dysfunction. Two exceptions are OCCIPITOFRONTALIS and CORRUGATOR SUPERCILLII, which can trigger migraines by entrapping branches of the trigeminal nerves. This happens with habitual frowning or exposure to cold that tightens these frontal muscles. Fibers of the facial nerve also blend and link to the trigeminal alarm system[1].

## CN VIII: VESTIBULOCOCHLEAR NERVE

The vestibulocochlear nerve (once known as the auditory nerve) sends information on sound (from the cochlea) and balance information (from the vestibule of the inner ear) to the brain. Note that while any dizziness problems tend to be attributed to inner ear (and possibly issues with this nerve), the suboccipital muscles can be heavily involved.

## CN IX: GLOSSOPHARYNGEAL NERVE

The glossopharyngeal nerve is the nerve of "tongue and pharynx," responsible for the tongue and swallowing actions in the throat. This nerve exits the skull through the jugular foramen in company with CN X (vagus) and CN XI (spinal accessory nerve). Problems with all three can suggest a problem at the foramen.

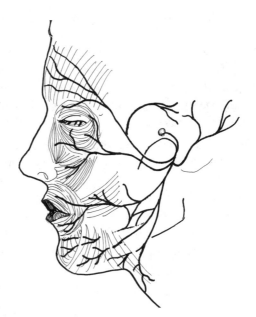

Digastric

Buccinator

Platysma

Occipitofrontalis

Corrugator Supercilii

Zygomaticus

Orbicularis Oculi

**Figure 78.** FACIAL NERVE

---

1. Fibers of the chorda tympani nerve (a branch of the facial nerve) blend with the lingual nerve (a branch of the trigeminal nerve). Both of these are strained by TMJD.

## CN X: VAGUS NERVE

The *vagus* nerve is named for its "wandering" path through the body, from its beginnings in the brain stem, through the dura, to the intestines. In the course of its travels it supplies parasympathetic fibers to *all* the organs (except adrenals) hence its old name: the *pneumogastric* ("lungs 'n stomach") nerve.

---

**TABLE 4.** VAGUS NERVE AND SYMPATHETIC / PARASYMPATHETIC EFFECTS

| Parasympathetic | Organs | Sympathetic |
|---|---|---|
| Constricts pupils | **Eye** | Dilates pupils |
| Stimulates salivation | **Salivary Glands** | Inhibits salivation (dry mouth) |
| Slows heartbeat | **Heart** | Speeds heartbeat |
| Constricts bronchi | **Lungs** | Dilates bronchi |
| Stimulates peristalsis | **GI Tract** | Inhibits peristalsis |
| Releases bile | **Liver** | Glycogen > glucose / Adrenaline and noradrenaline |
| Contracts bladder | **Bladder** | Inihibits bladder contraction |

---

Vagus is the messenger of the hypothalamus, and essentially the parasympathetic nervous system. It is behind the cold sweat and pounding heart, the queasy stomach and GI tract that works or doesn't, nausea, and vomiting. Vagus also talks to tissues of mouth and throat. Under stress your mouth may be dry and vocal cords freeze to the point that you can't even swallow[1]. A branch of the vagus innervates the ear canal causing some people to cough or gag when it is doused with cold water or tickled with a Q-tip (a response known as the "ear-cough").

The vagus nerve leaves the brain and passes through the skull via the jugular foramen in close company with the spinal accessory and glossopharyngeal nerves, and of course, the jugular vein. Fibers of the vagus intermingle so thoroughly with those of the spinal accessory nerve that it is almost impossible to separate them in dissection. This is why some anatomists consider the two nerves (X and XI) to be *one* nerve: the *vago-accessory nerve*. It is also why SCM and TRAPEZIUS can produce such a range of bizarre neurological symptoms: both muscles receive fibers from both these nerves.

---

1. Vagus also supplies the palatoglossus muscle which raises the back of the tongue to help start a swallow (or *not*, if vagus is unhappy). Anatomists are still arguing over which nerve supplies that muscle. Some swear it's the spinal accessory nerve, which suggests that many of us are wired differently.

The jugular foramen is just a wide spot in the road, an opening in the suture between occipital and temporal bones. The vagus, spinal accessory, and glossopharyngeal nerves must all squeeze through this small hole.

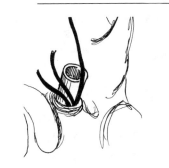

Symptoms relating to all three nerves suggest a problem of bone, blood, and nerves at the the foramen, . A blow to the back of the head can slam the occiput into the temporals, narrowing the space, compressing nerves, impeding drainage, and mimicking symptoms usually attributed to infections and tumors.

**Figure 79.** JUGULAR FORAMEN:

Jugular Foramen Syndrome (Vernet's) includes:

- Hoarseness, difficulty swallowing, and loss of gag reflex.
- Drooping of the soft palate and deviation of the uvula towards the *normal* side.
- Numbness at back of tongue.
- Dry mouth (decreased saliva production).
- Weakness or spasm of STERNOCLEIDOMASTOID and TRAPEZIUS muscles.

## CN XI: SPINAL ACCESSORY NERVE

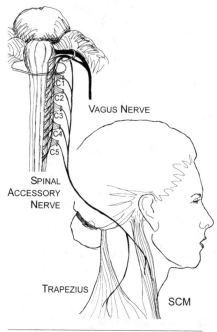

**Figure 80.** SPINAL ACCESSORY NERVE

The spinal accessory nerve supplies TRAPEZIUS and STERNOCLEIDOMASTOID (SCM) muscles, both heavily implicated in tension, sinus, and migraine headaches. It is one of several reasons why neck and posture are so heavily involved in *all* kinds of headaches and their autonomic symptoms. (Another is because the dura attaches to C1-C2-C3.)

This is the oddball of nerves, more *spinal* than *cranial*. Rather than starting inside the skull, 5 out of 6 of its roots erupt from between the vertebrae of the neck. It travels from neck to brain through the "big hole" (*foramen magnum*) at the base of the skull.

*Inside* the skull, it joins an actual cranial nerve root, blending with fibers of the vagus nerve (CN X). (Remember that the vagus talks to the stomach and gut.)

The entire assembly then travels back *out* of the skull through the jugular foramen in company with the jugular vein, and the vagus and glossopharyngeal nerves.

The link between cranial nerve fibers and spinal nerve fibers provides an enormous amount of information for balance and posture which are heavily controlled by SCM and TRAPEZIUS. But if anything goes wrong between these two powerful and opposing muscles, problems in one can trigger problems in the other. Tension, tightness, and injury to either muscle can produce severe headaches with nausea, vertigo, goose bumps, and other distressing autonomic symptoms. (See a long list of these in the SCM pain diagram, Figure 18 on page 49.)

## CN XII: HYPOGLOSSAL NERVE

The hypoglossal nerve supplies all the muscles of the tongue (except palatoglossus). This is the nerve the doctor is testing if you are asked to press your tongue against either cheek or stick it straight out. If there's a problem, the tongue will press weakly, or drift towards the affected side.

## SPINAL NERVES

Spinal nerves extend from the spinal cord through openings between *cervical, thoracic, lumbar, and sacral* vertebrae ( bones of neck, trunk, lumbar region (lower back), and the sacrum of the pelvis. They are named for their neighboring vertebrae. Spinal nerve C1 emerges from under the first cervical vertebra (the atlas); C2 from under the second, and C3 from under the third.

Many headaches and neurological problems are *cervicogenic,* "coming from the neck,"especially the upper three vertebrae. All of these nerves may be compressed ("pinched" or even *strangled*) by misaligned vertebrae and or tight muscles.

### C1

C1 (at the first vertebra, or atlas) gives rise to the suboccipital nerve which supplies the SUBOCCIPITAL muscles (Figure 81) One of these muscles in particular (RECTUS CAPITIS POSTERIOR MINOR) can entrap its own nerve supply, producing visual and neurological symptoms ranging from vertigo to seizures thanks to its direct attachment to the pain-sensitive dura that lines brain and spinal cord.

Irritation of its nerve can tighten RECTUS even more producing a vicious cycle of pain and dysfunction. This typically produces a vague but deep aching pain that extends *through* the head and in a band from back of head to orbit of eye. This pattern may blur into that coming from SEMISPINALIS and SPLENIUS CERVICIS.

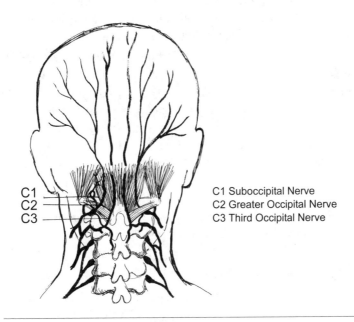

C1 Suboccipital Nerve
C2 Greater Occipital Nerve
C3 Third Occipital Nerve

**Figure 81.** SUBOCCIPITAL NERVE

## C2

A branch of the second spinal nerve (C2) forms the greater occipital nerve. It arises from between the first and second cervical vertebrae, along with its smaller brother, the lesser occipital nerve. It travels along the INFERIOR OBLIQUE (one of the SUBOCCIPITAL muscles) passing *through* SEMISPINALIS CAPITIS (which it supplies) and *through* the fascia of TRAPEZIUS, traveling up the neck to innervate the scalp from the back to the top of the head. Scratch the back of your head and it's the greater occipital nerve that sends those pleasurable impulses to your brain.

If this nerve is unhappy, the impulses can be extremely *un*pleasant. It is the source of much "suboccipital neuralgia," ("nerve pain at the back of the head.") It may be interpreted as "migraine" pain on its own, or it may fire off the trigemino-vascular system triggering a true migraine. As the suboccipital nerve passes through SEMISPINALIS (often tightened by a Head Forward Posture) the muscle will bite the nerve that feeds it, entrapping its own nerve supply. It can be compressed by vertebrae and other muscles, including TRAPEZIUS, straining the nerve where it passes through the fascia.

How often might this be a problem? One study of 20 cadavers without *known* headache problems, found that the nerve penetrated TRAPEZIUS in fewer than half, but penetrated SEMISPINALIS in 90 per cent of bodies. Rarely (8 per cent), it also penetrated the INFERIOR OBLIQUE of the SUBOCCIPITALS. *Almost as rarely, it curved around* SEMISPINALIS piercing only fascia near the attachment, an arrangement shown in standard anatomy texts (such as Netter), but found to be unusual in the subject group. On observing "possible compression" in 11 cases (28 per cent) with no reported history of headache, the authors concluded that nerve compression may be of minor importance since it seemed to exist in the absence of headache (Bovim G and others, 1991). However, this idea does not seem to have been tested against cases with *known* history of headache.

Surgical release of the greater occipital nerve has been shown to reduce or eliminate chronic migraine in *some* (but not all) patients. In studying 50 heads, Janis JE and others (2010) found that the greater occipital nerve and artery crossed each other 54 per cent of the time. The relationship varied from a single crossing to a twining. In either case, pulsing of the artery could irritate the nerve and provide a possible explanation (and a possible genetic pattern) for migraines triggered in the occipital region.

## C3-C5

The primary muscle of breathing is the *diaphragm*. It is primarily supplied by the phrenic nerve (from C4, with contributions from adjacent nerves at C3 and C5).

If you have sleep apnea, you may not know it. But if you do know that you suffer headaches and fatigue and never seem to get enough sleep, it's always worthwhile to check.

The condition is named for abnormal breathing during sleep. Pauses between breaths (known as *apneas*, or periods of "no-breathing") may last for 10 seconds to several minutes, occurring up to 30+ times per hour. Or, breathing may be regular but so slow and shallow that it qualifies as *hypopnea* ("under-breathing"). The person is breathing regularly, but getting inadequate oxygen which starves the brain. Sleep apnea is strongly linked to headaches and linked so strongly to heart problems that multiple studies have found some form of apnea to be common in heart failure patients.

Sleep apnea is tested with an overnight sleep study (a *polysomnogram*). Clinicians look for 5 or more episodes of either apnea or hypopnea, neurological arousal, 3 per cent or greater drop in blood oxygen, or a combination of both arousal and low oxygen.

What is meant by *neurological arousal*? Essentially it means that your brain realizes it is suffocating and struggles awake — out of the deep slow brainwaves (delta or theta) to brainwaves that are faster by 3 Hz or more (rising to theta or alpha) — to deal with the situation. The constant arousal blocks deep restorative sleep, contributing to hyptertension and daytime fatigue.

There are two types of sleep apnea: *Obstructive Sleep Apnea* (OSA) and *Central Sleep Apnea* (CSA). The two can occur together (as "complex" or "mixed" sleep apnea). The obstructive form, with its snoring, choking, and sputtering, gets most of the press. It is caused by physical blockage to the airway, by overweight or floppy tissues, by simple congestion, or even by TrPs in the respiratory muscles.

Central sleep apnea is rarely mentioned, but is even more insidious. It isn't a matter of obstruction or blockage; the sleeper simply seems to "forget" to breathe. The problem is often associated with brain injury, but disturbed breathing may be another reason to check for nerve impingement in the cervical vertebrae.

What happens if the nerve that stimulates breathing is compressed? There is tantalizing evidence of what happens if it is *stimulated*. In a preliminary study involving 13 heart failure patients with central sleep apnea, stimulating the phrenic nerve decreased apnea symptoms by 91 per cent and increased oxygen uptake by 55 per cent (Ponikowski P, 2010).

## C3-T2 AND SHOULDER, ARM, AND FINGER PAIN

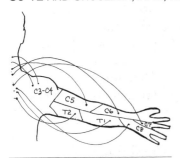

**Figure 82.** NERVES TO ARM

When making a pain chart for *headaches* you may wonder why you should bother to map pain in *arms*.

It is because nerve supply for arms also comes from the neck, thus pain in arms or fingers can reveal problems at individual vertebrae. This is why neck problems are a far more common cause of Carpal Tunnel Syndrome than the often innocent carpal tunnel. Normally there's plenty of room there.

While symptoms can arise from tightness and inflammation in the forearm muscles, they can also come from the neck providing a clue to the cervical dysfunction and tissue strain lurking behind many headaches.

# The Electric Brain

*Migraine can be a symptom of abnormal electrical activity in the brain. If you are foggy even on headache-free days, have trouble organizing, can't sleep even when desperately fatigued, or have a history of falls, auto accidents, or high fever, you may have found a clue to your migraines.*

The brain runs everything, with the tools and resources it is given. Sometimes it runs things well, sometimes not so well. And sometimes it all goes to pieces.

Like other computers, the brain gives off tiny electrical signals. When recorded on EEG[1], the raw signal can be separated into waves of different frequencies: *beta* (fastest) to *alpha*, *theta*, and *delta* (slowest). In general:

- Faster waves should be stronger at front and left.

- Slower waves should be stronger at right and back.


What happens if these relationships change? If slow waves are strongest at left and front, the result can be fogginess, fatigue, impulsiveness, and depression.

If fast waves are strongest at right and back, the result is anxiety and racing thoughts, possibly with paranoia, sleep disruptions, nightmares and night terrors.

A "backwards brain" (slow waves dominating at front and left, fast ones dominant at back and right) will be depressed *and* anxious, desperately fatigued and yet strangely unable to sleep.

Brainwave *slowing* is typical of head injury. But so is brainwave *speeding*. Both can be the result of trauma that creates an imbalance in functionality. Healthy frequency and power depend on healthy blood and nutrient supply with intact interconnecting pathways. Faster waves may be concentrated outside of the injured area simply because that is where nutrient supply and network connections are unimpaired. Whatever the cause, the discrepancy can impact sleep, mood and other functions. Sleep problems are considered to be a sign of depression which they may be, but the answer isn't always anti-depressants, especially in a Backwards Brain. Speeding up the slow left brain may be great for depression. But drugs are not hemispherically specific. When an already faster right speeds up too, you may be scraping the patient off the ceiling. Anti-anxiety meds and sedatives to counteract the anti-depressants make it easy to get caught in a see-saw of depression, anxiety, and associated side effects.

Inattentive ADD and associated learning disabilities are also associated with brainwave slowing and often occur after a head injury. It isn't that slow waves are bad, it is that brainwaves must also be *flexible* rather than stuck at one speed.

---

1. Electro-Encephalo-Gram, that is, an "Electrical-Head-Recording."

## BRAINWAVES AND FUNCTION

Flexibility in daily life functioning, the ability to shift at will between tasks, is a characteristic of a healthy brain. For example , a healthy brain can shift focus from a learning task to an interesting conversation and back again, or from a relaxed meditative state then back to writing a report. A brain that can't do this has a problem.

With high frequency and power in the left hemisphere you may have a wonderfully energetic person who is an excellent organizer and speaker. But turn the dial up to 11 or damage the moderating right hemisphere and these good qualities may segue into a personality that can't hear NO and has no awareness of consequences. You may see a once-respected athlete now unable to understand that assaulting female fans is unacceptable behavior, or a cheerful psychopath who is maxed out on his credit cards.

Strong low frequency waves in left frontal regions may be associated with fogginess, anxiety, and inability to organize. Hoarding may appear after traumatic brain injury, stroke, and some degenerative brain diseases. In one study of 87 patients, only 13 developed hoarding behaviors, but *all* 13 had damage to the pre-frontal area responsible for executive decision making and impulse control (Brown WA, 2007).

## ON BRAIN INJURY

It is difficult to overstate the degree of ignorance about brain injury. Our concepts are based more on cartoons, The Three Stooges, and the performance art known as Professional Wrestling than on Reality. The sad result is that brain injury is often missed or misunderstood by the victim, family members, employers, and even medical professionals who may all assume that you really ought to be better by now.

It is certainly misunderstood in Hollywood. Characters are constantly knocked unconscious yet never suffer ill effects. In *The Wedding Planner,* the hyper-organized Jennifer Lopez is "saved" from a runaway dumpster by a young doctor who knocks her to the ground, smashing the back of her head into the pavement. She awakens in his hospital where he announces that X-rays and MRI "are

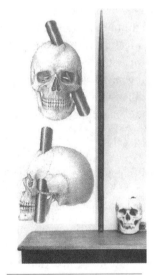

**Figure 83.** PHINEAS GAGE

clear" and therefore she "does not have a concussion" (despite remaining unconscious throughout all these tests). In the Real World, she would almost certainly find that she could no longer organize, read or sleep well, nor continue work as a planner. She would find that she had indeed suffered a brain injury.

In the Real World, we do not smash our laptops together on football fields or hurl them through windshields or walls then be surprised that they don't work well afterwards.

We are strangely able to believe that doing the same thing to a massively powerful computer — with the consistency of custard pie, its parts joined by billions of spider-web connections — should have no consequences. The corollary to this is the equally absurd medical belief that if the victim of a head injury did not lose consciousness, then no real harm was done. Not so. Loss of consciousness suggests shock or injury to the brain *stem* which controls consciousness. One can suffer severe brain damage but remain fully conscious; this does not mean there is no damage elsewhere. Vivid proof of this lies in the tale of the unfortunate Phineas Gage.

In 1848, Gage, a highly regarded young man working as a foreman on railroad construction, was tamping blasting powder. The powder sparked, blowing the 14-pound tamping rod under his left cheekbone and launching it through his brain and out the top of his head to land some 30 yards away. Eyewitness accounts differ on whether Gage lost consciousness at all. Some claimed he never did; others thought he might have been unconscious (or merely dazed) for a few minutes. But all agreed that he was conscious and sitting up in the wagon when taken to a nearby hotel to await a doctor. Gage had suffered severe injury to the left temporal and frontal areas. He lived for another 12 years but with radical changes in behavior, personality, and complete loss of social skills. He died, friendless and alone, of a massive seizure in 1860.

Less dramatic injuries can ruin lives, from birth, falls and sports injuries, to vehicular trauma including thrill rides and roller coasters. Damage may also occur through infection, fever, stroke, or environmental toxins. Even hypertension can reduce learning, memory and decision-making ability through constant stress on the brain including small strokes. MRI reveals lesions in the brain's white matter (the spider web of nerve fibers that link neurons). Damage to these communicating structures impacts all brain function and ability to function well in life — conscious or not.

In daily life, brainwaves slow in response to neuronal damage from decreased blood and nutrient supply. This can arise from low blood sugar ( poor diet and missed meals) to sleep apnea or deranged breathing during waking hours. It can occur with mechanical blockage of blood supply to the brain, whether through myofascial compression, or by plaque and arterial narrowing (with results known as *vascular dementia)*.

Many resulting symptoms are attributed to age but many are due to having reached an age at which injuries and insults have had time and opportunity to develop through behavior that we would (I hope) deny to our own children. Perhaps an age old enough to drink and drive, to live on junk food and antacids, to spend hours on the computer, slouch all we want and never have to eat vegetables.

| TABLE 5. QUICK TEST FOR BRAIN DYSFUNCTION | | | |
|---|---|---|---|
| **Symptoms** | **Scale (1-10)** | **Sudden Onset** | **Seen in Parents** |
| **Sensory and Emotional Issues** | | | |
| Extreme sensitivity to lights or sound | | | |
| Loss or change in sense of smell | | | |
| Problems focusing / converging eyes | | | |
| Problems with sense of touch | | | |
| Sudden, unexplained changes in mood | | | |
| Loss of sense of humor | | | |
| Loss of former interests / recreations | | | |
| Impulsivity | | | |
| **Memory and Focus** | | | |
| "Fogginess" and confusion; lack of clarity | | | |
| Forgetting what you are doing | | | |
| Difficulty concentrating and focusing | | | |
| Difficulty learning new things | | | |
| Difficulty learning from experience | | | |
| Difficulty reading or comprehending text | | | |
| Problems following conversations | | | |
| Not understanding what was said or asked | | | |
| Problems with sequencing and prioritizing | | | |
| Procrastination / lack of initiative | | | |
| Not finishing projects | | | |
| Disorganization (room, office, paperwork) | | | |
| Getting lost in daydreams | | | |
| Problems with speech or finding words | | | |
| **Pain and Physical Dysfunction** | | | |
| Fatigue during the day | | | |
| Unexplained local pain or weakness | | | |
| All-over body pain; fibromyalgia symptoms | | | |
| Nausea, dizziness, car-sickness | | | |
| Insomnia or disturbed night-time sleep | | | |
| Headaches | | | |

## THE BRAIN AND SLEEP

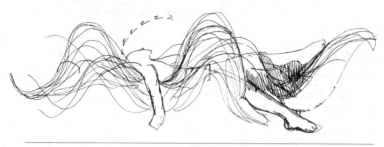

**Figure 84.** SLEEPING IN DELTA

There's far more to sleep than simply passing out[1]. The process of falling asleep involves slow waves, generated by the brain stem, moving from the back of the brain to the front. When all goes as it should, the the result is sweet restorative sleep. When it does not or can not, you will not sleep well, wake well, or work well.

Disturbed sleep is a well-known trigger for migraine. It may come from family demands, erratic work schedules, physical conditions such as apnea, disturbed cortisol cycle, stress hormones, or even a bed partner who snores.

It can also be a symptom of the migraine life-style. That is, if treatment strategy includes caffeine-containing drugs or sleeping off the migraine whenever it occurs, it may be difficult or impossible to sleep again at a regular hour. Schedules and body rhythms may be disrupted for days to come.

Unfortunately, lack of sleep, especially REM sleep, greatly increase nerve sensitivity[2]. For example, rats deprived of REM sleep for three consecutive nights showed changes in proteins that suppress and trigger pain by changing the sensitivity of the trigeminal nerves so heavily involved in migraine (Durham PL and others, 2010).

Sleep disruptions are extremely common after brain injury If, for whatever reason, a brain is running fast frequencies at right and back, sleep simply does not come. It is common to see brain-injured people who cannot sleep despite heavy dosing with pills and "night-time cold medicines." I've seen clients who were drinking a fifth of whiskey a night in a desperate bid for a few hours of unconsciousness. "Iron Mike" Webster, damaged by years of football injuries, also resorted to shocking himself unconscious with a Taser gun. Singer Michael Jackson, unable to sleep, resorted to having himself injected with coma-inducing drugs which eventually killed him.

---

1. See Chapter 5 for hormonal and nutritional inputs.
2. REM, the deepest and most restorative stage of sleep, is named for its characteristic Rapid Eye Movements associated with dreaming.

Fast dominant waves at right and back can block all sleep, or keep the brain on the razor's edge between sleep and wakefullness, ready to go on alert at the slightest sound. This is comonly seen in people suffering from the hyper-vigilance of Post-Traumatic Stress Syndrome (PTSD) but is not limited to veterans and victims of assault. Others may train themselves into this state. A father may have had hypervigilance issues left from his Marine Corps days, but more recent and more compelling was his concern for a daughter born with cystic fibrosis. Failure to wake and respond when she was in distress could have meant death for a beloved child.

Waking at 2-3 AM appears to be a normal part of our sleep cycle, a time-out to check for saber tooth tigers or folks who might have wandered into the wrong house when the pubs let out. Now blamed on stress or modern lighting, Robert Louis Stephenson mentioned this in *Travels With a Donkey*, a report of his pre-electric trek through the desolate French Cévennes in 1879. The problem isn't so much awakening as inability to return to sleep.

For good or ill, brains adapt, but sleep loss is a serious stress. It destroys cognitive function, muscle function, and even contribute to obesity, all risk factors for migraine. Nedeltcheva AV and others (2010) researched sleep deprivation and weight loss[1]. Both men and women lost 55 per cent *less* fat and were hungrier when restricted to 5.5 hours of sleep, compared to test periods allowing 8.5 hours of sleep.

During both 2-week periods, participants averaged 6.6 pounds of weight loss, but what was lost was very different. With *adequate* sleep, losses averaged 3.1 pounds of fat and 3.3 pounds of fat-free mass (mostly protein). During *restricted* sleep, fat loss dropped to 1.3 pounds and fat-free losses rose to 5.3 pounds with a near10-point rise in the appetite hormone *ghrelin* — with corresponding hunger and insulin resistance[2].

This may be an evolutionary adaptation to hard times, the hope of surviving a seige of your city or castle, and looming starvation where fat stores and willingness to eat (even putrid animal parts or vending machine food) may be more critical than muscle power. Today's seige mentality can come from long commutes where many workers have a 4 am appointment with traffic on I-95 and a 24/7 society where sleep deprivation is actually considered a point of pride, proof of dedicated professionalism. But sleep deprivation increases ghrelin which triggers hunger for food to support "growth." Unfortunately one of the growth areas is abdominal fat, linked to Metablic Syndrome, heart disease, Type II diabetes, heart attack, and stroke.

---

1. The title of their research paper sums it up nicely: "Insufficient sleep undermines dietary efforts to reduce adiposity." That is: "Mess with sleep, blow your diet."
2. The "Stop!" and "Go!" hormones of appetite. *Leptin* (Gr. "slender") signals you to stop eating; GRELin (GRowth Hormone RELeasing), secreted by stomach and hypothalamus, triggers release of growth hormone and the increased food intake to support that growth.

## CORTICAL SPREADING DEPRESSION

Cortical Spreading Depression (CSD) is an electrical phenomenon involving depolarization of brain cells[1]. It moves like a wave from the rear of the brain (visual cortex) to the front. It is believed to be responsible for the aura of migraine. It also results in breakdown of the blood-brain barrier, leaking plasma proteins resulting in brain edema and possible stroke lesions (Gursoy-Ozdemir, Yasemin and others, 2004). It releases nitric oxide which can trigger migraine pain. Infusing 12 migraineurs (with aura) and 14 controls (Normals) with nitrate produced headache in *all* subjects but pain was worst in the migraineurs. In the Normals, the pain gradually faded away; in migraineurs, it peaked hours afterwards (Christiansen I and others, 1999).

In CSD, slow waves from brain stem and rear brain spread forward. Why this happens is not entirely clear. It may include injury to the hypothalamic-pituitary (HPA) axis through infection, high fever, or traumatic brain injury. It may be due to injury to the occipital lobe itself.

It can certainly involve poor nutrient supply[2] which may involve tight muscles, clogged arteries, or poor posture. A drop in blood sugar alone slows brainwaves and may trigger CSD resulting in migraine or seizures. Fried R (1993) considers these as symptoms of improper breathing and low or unbalanced oxygen supply.

The visual aura grows and spreads as slow waves spread forward over the cortex. But this can produce more than visual symptoms alone. When specifically asked, migraineurs (72 per cent migraine with aura, and 49 percent without aura) reveal many other symptoms including:

- Inability to recognize faces and objects,

- Alterations in color perception,

- Memory problems in general, including inability to remember names of people and things and even how to use everyday tools or objects.

In a 40-year-old woman, Wernicke's aphasia[3] appeared as a migraine prodrome, first mistaken for stroke. MRI showed none of the vascular lesions of stroke, but EEG showed slowing (delta and theta) over Wernicke's area in left rear temporal lobe (Mishra NK and others, 2009). Whatever the cause, CSD is clearly linked with migraine and the aura typical of classical migraine. Correcting this problem may explain the quick response (in *some* patients, if not *all*) to oxygen, better nutrition, sleep, and treatment with neurofeedback, found effective in both migraine and epilepsy.

---

1. *Depolarization* is a drop in voltage across a cell membrane.
2. The most urgent one is oxygen, of which the brain needs a constant supply and lots of it. The three-pound brain uses about a quarter of the body's oxygen supply.
3. Broca's aphasia features extreme difficulty in finding words. Wernicke's is characterized by fluent speech that makes little sense and degenerates into "word salad." There are several video examples of the disorder available on www.Youtube.com.

# Specific Neurological Issues

## ATTENTION DEFICIT DISORDER AND HYPERACTIVITY

Attention Deficit Disorder (ADD) alone and combined with hyperactivity (ADHD) is the most prevalent psychiatric condition diagnosed in children, but also common in migraine and brain injury. Many wonder if it is real.

In children, some diagnoses of ADD and ADHD correspond all to well with elimination of physical education, music, and art in schools. Children are expected to sit quietly in crowded classrooms. Those who wiggle and squirm are drugged into passivity and silence. But other factors are also involved.

ADD is very real and it is not new. It appeared in the medical literature in the 1930s as Minimal Brain Dysfunction (MBD), based on clinical experience of the 1920s based, in turn, on damage from the flu pandemic of 1918. Today, ADD, chronic fatigue, and fibromyalgia are commonly reported following viral infections or high fever. They may also appear after mechanical injury to the head and neck.

A bright but hyperactive 9-year old, with a known head injury, had earned failing marks since first grade in his Catholic school class of 10. There was no recess or gym class and "Calvin" couldn't sit still. His teacher insisted that he be evaluated for ADD/ADHD and drugs. After the required psych exam "They handed me a 6-inch thick stack of scrips," said his mother, "warning that the drugs would stunt his growth and he would need regular liver scans. I went out to the car and cried. Then I tore up the scrips and went looking for other options."

Calvin's father emphasized his sleep problems, certain his son would do better if only he could *sleep*. Dad was right. Mapping showed a probable site of injury and reasons why sleep would be difficult. After two weeks of biofeedback this child was sleeping normally — and bringing home A's[1].

ADD is not merely a disorder of children. Sub-normal levels of dopamine have been documented in adults with ADHD (Volkow N and others, 2007) as has high rates of use of tobacco, alcohol, marijuana, cocaine, "meth" and other drugs compared to Normals. All of these drugs increase dopamine levels in the brain.

Dopamine is involved in movement, attention and focus, but also "reward centers," hence it controls the ability to control behavior, to pay attention, and to feel pleasure. The temptation of dopamine-enhancing drugs is not a mere "high". The temptation — and the reward — is the ability to feel and function like Normals do on autopilot, at least temporarily.

---

1. His teacher seemed indignant that Calvin was not on drugs as she had demanded. "During the Adoration of the Eucharist," went her worst complaint, "he *fidgeted*."

This explains why *stimulant* amphetamines would *calm* ADD/ADHD. If you're out late driving, tired, and far from home, what do you do? Roll down the windows, scream along with the radio, pound on the steering wheel, and bounce in your seat.

Similarly, a child may wiggleand chatter, pull his sister's hair, kick the cat. What he gets with each of these actions is a little spurt of adrenalin, helping to stay awake.

Normalize the brainwaves, normalize the behavior.

# MIGRAINE OR TRIGEMINAL NEURALGIA?

> Whether the pitcher hits the stone or the stone hits the pitcher,
> it's going to be bad for the pitcher.
> —Sancho Panza in *Man of La Mancha*

*Trigeminal neuralgia* (TN) means "nerve pain from the trigeminal." It is one of the most painful afflictions known, characterized by sudden shocks of pain lasting a few seconds to a few minutes. Its old names, *tic doloreux* ("painful twitch") and *neuralgia epileptiforme* ("epileptic nerve pain") described the tendency of victims to wince or jump. But the wince is neither a tic nor a seizure; it is a natural reaction to being hit with the neurological equivalent of a cattle prod to the face. Nevertheless, TN can be treated with anti-seizure drugs such as Tegretol® or a later metabolite, Trileptal® (oxcarbazepine), and Dilantin®.

It is commonly said that TN is similar to, co-exists with, and is mis-diagnosed as, *migraine.* As in migraine, TN pain is usually one-sided and afflicts women nearly twice as often as men. In contrast to migraine, first onset of TN is more frequent in older patients, typically in their 50s or 60s. The rate rises in in people over 70. Attacks may be triggered by sensory stimulation as mundane as eating and chewing, drinking, brushing teeth, combing or washing hair.

It is often said that sufferers endure years of suffering and incorrect treatments before receiving the *correct* diagnosis of trigeminal neuralgia. *Wrong* diagnoses are said to include dental and sinus infections, TMJ, eye disease, inflamed temporal arteries, *migraine,* and *myofascial pain* treated with tooth extractions and root canals, sinus and other surgeries.

The similarities between TN, cluster, and migraine are because all can arise from the trigeminal system. Most TN attacks are now believed to be caused by compression of the trigeminal nerve by a pulsing artery at the point where the nerve root enters the brain stem[1]. A pulse may seem a small thing, but if it hits a nerve over and over . . . over time it can irritate the nerve to the point of hypersensitivity and over-reactions.

As analogy, there is nothing obviously harmful about humming a tune, but if a cubicle mate or spouse hums the same tune over and over . . . you may want to scream, and someday you may do that or worse. It may be seen as an inappropriate over-reaction, but it is an understandable one.

TN has been relieved by microvascular decompression, pioneered by Dr. Peter Janetta of Pittsburgh's Allegheny Hospital. The operation relieves pressure on the nerve root by placing a protective Teflon sheath between nerve and artery. But why the age disparity between TN and migraine? "As we get older," says Janetta, "things sag."

---

1. The perpetrator is usually the superior cerebellar artery.

Whether blood vessels sag into the trigeminal nerve root, or the nerve sags and drapes over the vessel, there will be trigeminal pain.

The difference between the trigeminal pain of TN versus the trigeminal pain of migraine may be the different, more local point of contact. In standard TN, unlike standard migraine, the vascular system is not so ferociously stimulated. The nerve response to compression at the root is very different from how it behaves on receiving multiple messages from the field screaming that the entire precinct is under attack. Perhaps the nerve recognizes this as a local problem. It may register protest at the ongoing abuse, but it does not mobilize the entire trigemino-vascular emergency network (typical of migraine) to flush out system-wide attackers if the problem is only the annoying co-worker from the next cubicle.

Perhaps we call it *migraine* when compression or other trauma occurs far away from the root, out at the terminations. And the fact that TN can be triggered by stimulation of the outlying nerve endings suggests that trauma "out there" adds to the stress at the nerve root.

# Chapter 5

# It's Chemical!

*It isn't just serotonin. There are many chemical imbalances behind headaches, everything from food and water, to sex and stress hormones, fresh air and sunlight. All play a role in headaches.*

Good water, good food, and good sleep are basic requirements for good life and good health. Consider the painfully obvious: If you're living on junk food, high-fat, low-fat or other unbalanced diets, dehydrated and constipated, sleeping poorly, it's no surprise that you might get headaches.

## Chemical Nutrients

Patients with chronic myofascial pain are a select group which . . . has a remarkably high prevalence of vitamin inadequacies and deficiencies. When the patient fails to respond to specific myofascial therapy or obtains only temporary relief, vitamin deficiencies must be ruled out as a major contributing cause and, if present, corrected.
— Travell & Simons (1983), *Myofascial Pain and Dysfunction*

I think so Brain, but if they called them SAD meals, kids wouldn't buy them.
—*Pinky and the Brain*

When I was a kid, the Standard American Diet (SAD) was very different from today. By amazing coincidence, rates of asthma, allergies, and obesity were far lower.

Easter Eggs were hard-boiled *eggs*, and candy, ice-cream and other sweets were *treats*.

The joke about Chinese food (heavy on bean sprouts and vegetables) was that you would be hungry again an hour later. Today it would make a Colonel proud[1].

Coffee was for adults, not children, "because it would stunt our growth." Today I see children ordering caramel machiatto (iced espresso with caramel sauce) at Starbucks.

---

1. You will not find General Tso's Chicken (heavily battered, fried chicken with a sugar sauce) in any classic Chinese cookbook. Now a staple of Chinese restaurants in the US, it first appeared in New York City in the 1970s.

Fish were caught by fishing. Today they are raised in fish farms fed on cheap corn and soy and other materials producing fish with nutritional profiles very different from the original.

Seasonal vegetables were seasonal. It was a huge event when the first asparagus or strawberries appeared in the market. Now these items are available year round from tropical growers.

Milk cows were pastured and every spring the milk tasted of green onions. Today most cows are confined to barns and fed on grain (the high carbohydrate diet is bad for the cow but increases milk production). Protein may come from chicken manure.

When I was in college in strip-mined southeastern Ohio, we were sorry for the families who raised their children on soft drinks because their water wells were polluted by acid mine drainage. Today sodas are an expected part of an everyday meal, and in some areas, they have become *the* major source of dietary calories.

Poor nutrition alone can cause tense muscles, migraines, and worse.

- Muscles that remain shortened or in spasm are weak and must recruit other muscles which are strained by jobs they were never intended to do.

- To avoid the resulting pain, you begin to limit movements and physical activities. Fatigue and depression decrease energy and even the *desire* to stay active.

- Oops! Weight gain! Time to diet! Now come more nutritional deficits which in time may result in severe malnutrition, metabolic diseases, muscle problems, and migraine.

One of the problems is heavily processed food and water.

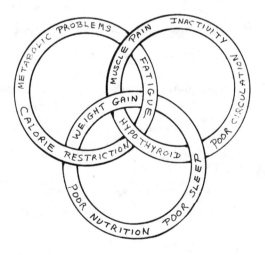

**Figure 85.** THE CYCLE OF MALNUTRITION, STRAIN, AND DYSFUNCTION

# PROCESSED FOODS

"Processed" may need a definition. Almost all food is processed one way or another, but there are extremes.These range from "pick, wash, eat" (for a tomato perhaps), to de-naturing of the original material plus artificial flavoring / coloring / preservatives in addition to pesticide loads. All of these can cause problems, whether they manifest as migraines or something else. They can contribute to the confusion surrounding food sensitivities. It may not be the food itself but what has been done to it.

One example is red meat, which many migraineurs suspect may be a trigger. It may actually be hamburger. Meat from many sources, impossible to track, raised in filthy feed lots, is ground in a very few central processing plants then shipped around the country. Another surprising example is orange juice.

Citrus ranks high on migraine food lists and yet there may be a big difference between a well-peeled orange eaten out of hand and a glass of orange juice out of a carton.In one case you're getting the fruit of an orange. In the other case, say an 8 oz glass of juice, you may be getting the juice of several oranges and many other things as well because of how that orange was processed.

At home, we cut the orange in half and ream out the juice. In industry, whole oranges are pressed like grapes. Skins split and juice comes out with molds, bacteria, and residues from pesticides and/or washing agents left on the skins. And size matters. An 8-oz glass of orange juice is not an orange; it several oranges and will raise blood sugar[1]. And while the juice may have been squeezed from fresh oranges (certainly not *dried* ones!) it isn't necessarily *fresh* as most of us think of that term.

To keep a year-round supply of a seasonal fruit, distributors rely on oranges from Mexico, Brazil, Costa Rica, and other Latin American countries where land and labor is cheaper, environmental regulations almost non-existent, and pesticides illegal in the US can be used. Juice is pasteurized to kill bacteria and molds, then stored in huge tanks from which all air has been extracted. The resulting product poured from your carton of "fresh-squeezed" orange juice may be up to a year old (Hamilton A, 2009).

Most flavor is lost with this treatment, but it can be added back via chemical flavor packs ("not found in nature," says Hamilton) tweaked to fit local taste preferences. If you are bothered by synthetic fragrances at the perfume counter, you might also be bothered by them showing up in your orange juice. Or, it might be something else.

You may notice that home-squeezed orange juice doesn't resemble what comes from the carton. It may be flavorful, but also thinner, less robust. The different mouth feel of commercial juice can be the result of several other chemicals that don't show up on the label possibly including bromylated vegetable oil and propylene glycol[2]. These are standard additives, considered safe for *most* people when used in food (and antifreeze) but they may not be safe for *all* of us.

---

1. There are about 2 oz of juice in a medium orange but this can vary widely.

## WATER

*Migraine can be a symptom of dehydration.*

"But I don't *like* water!" is not an excuse. It is an explanation.

Dehydration is one of the most common causes of headache. In combination with constipation, or body odor requiring ever stronger deodorants, you are almost certain to be dehydrated. If you squeeze your eyelids gently together and see sparkles, it isn't aura. It is dehydration severe enough that the eyeball has begun to deform[1].

Our bodies are approximately 70 per cent water — or should be. Every turn of double-helix DNA requires 500 water molecules. Collagen in our joints and disks is a triple helix requiring even more water. Water is critical for proper cell function, nutrient transport, and removal of waste materials from cells. With dehydration comes fatigue, constipation, impaired muscle function and cramping, slowed metabolism, memory problems, depression — and headaches. Even narrowing of spinal disks is thought to be caused or abetted by dehydration of disks and their collagen fibers. Oddly enough, dehydration can also cause *edema* which may also be involved in migraine[2].

Many migraineurs experience changes in urinary frequency, a symptom which has received little attention[3]. Water retention may be linked with onset of a migraine, its end with sudden "water dumping" and urgent urination. And it isn't ordinary urine, but a clear colorless fluid, suggesting odd behavior in the kidneys. This may involve vasopressin, a hormone secreted by the pituitary by command of the hypothalamus. At low levels vasopressin regulates the amount of water excreted by the kidneys. At higher concentrations it affects other processes, including blood flow.

In studying patients with this symptom, 12 hours after migraine onset, researchers found a significant drop in vasopressin resulting in dumping of water and sodium[4]. Other researchers sampled vasopressin during spontaneous migraine attacks and again after patients had been symptom-free for at least a week. During migraines, vasopressin was consistently raised (the highest levels were seen in the only patient who vomited). Abnormally high vasopressin during migraine attacks may explain

---

2. They need not be listed so long as they make up less than 2% of the juice by weight. Bromylated vegetable oil (containing bromine) prevents separation of citrus oils. Banned in 100 countries, it is still legal in the US.
1. Sparkles in the form of concentric rings or circles can be symptoms of a detaching retina due to age or injury.
2. From (Gr.) *oídema* "swelling" (formerly known as *dropsy* or *hydropsy),* from abnormal accumulation of fluid under skin or in body cavities.
3. If a patient has recently ingested riboflavin (Vitamin B2) pills, urine *should* be bright yellow, but is not (although color returns later).Oliver Sacks mentioned this symptom of oddly clear urine in his book *Migraine,* also mentioning how rarely it is mentioned.
4. Poole CJ and Lightman SL (1988); Hampton KK and others (1991). *Spontaneous migraine* refers to migraines that occur on their own rather than the ones induced by injecting the subject with nitrates or other known triggers. These have been difficult to study due to the prep time required for advanced imaging techniques such as PET scans.

water retention, vomiting, and even changes in peripheral blood flow (cold hands and feet and facial pallor). These symptoms are attributed to hypothalamus problems, but it is also possible that the actual origin may be dehydration which triggers desperate attempts by the hypothalamus to hold on to whatever water it can.

Get enough water for your body to function properly. It's what you're made of. Water requirements vary by weight and activity. There are many formulas, but you need roughly an ounce per pound. That is, 100 pounds, 100 ounces, more with heavy exercise and sweating. The best guide is the "pee test." Urine should be pale yellow. Orange urine signals dehydration[1].

Ideally, *water* should mean *water-colored water*. Not sugar water or Red-Dye-Number 5 colored water. Not tea- or coffee-colored water. We may think we've gotten enough "fluids" during the day by counting up diet sodas or cups of coffee. But many of these (such as caffeine, alcohol, and potassium-rich "diet" drinks) are diuretics which help flush water from the body along with water-soluble vitamins and minerals also needed for good muscle function. The current fad of "vitamin waters" are loaded with sugar, colorings, and preservatives. Stick with *water* water.

On the other hand, electrolytes are lost in sweat and further diluted (with water-soluble vitamins) by constant sipping of water. If you're trying to stay hydrated, what you may really need is *salt*.

## SALT

*Salt* is our common source of *electrolytes*, the electrically charged particles that help run the amazing machines of life. Four of these, calcium, magnesium, sodium, and potassium, are absolutely critical to muscle contraction and relaxation, energy production, nerve conduction, heart function, and water balance.

Mess with electrolyte balance and you may suffer the inconvenience of too many bathroom breaks or the danger of dehydration. You may develop painful muscle cramps, ranging from Restless Leg Syndrome to the ultimate muscle cramp — a heart attack.

"Messing with electrolytes" includes such things as high-potassium "diet" and sport drinks, popping calcium pills, guzzling diuretics (including alcohol and coffee), high-phosphorus soft drinks, and too little or too much actual water. Too much calcium creates deficiencies or imbalances of magnesium, and cramps — muscles that cannot relax. Too much potassium sends water pouring out of the cells, flushing out other electrolytes and water-soluble vitamins.

Sodium allows the body to retain water rather than simply pouring through. Too much raises internal pressures to dangerous levels. Too little and a person may require twice to three times as much water to reach the same degree of hydration as

---

1. Some drugs such as sulfasalazine can cause orange urine.

a person with a good sodium balance. But adding more water can make a bad situation worse, as remaining electrolytes are further diluted or lost. Extremely low levels of sodium in the blood (*hyponatremia* or "low salt blood") results in seizures, coma, and death. It is seen in athletes who consume too much water but too few electrolytes during endurance events, people who fast on juice or water for long periods and people who limit salt intake to an unhealthy degree.

Your grandfather's solution was salt pills but today's salt is not your grandfather's salt. It is nearly pure sodium chloride. There are several reasons for this.

In part, it's aesthetics. Natural salt tends to be gray (often with a swampy tidal zone odor). It is lumpy due to water-absorbing calcium and magnesium chlorides. Taking these out produces a smooth-flowing salt that will run easily through the holes in a salt shaker regardless of the weather ("When it rains, it pours!") When I was a child growing up in the swamps of Southern Maryland, we put rice in the shakers to help shove the salt through the holes. (A friend, who grew up in the deserts of Nevada, thought that was the funniest thing she'd ever seen.) Thanks to refined salt and central air conditioning, I haven't seen rice in a shaker for years.

In part, it's economics. A salt deposit is an *ore*. As with any ore, valuable components are retrieved, the rest is dumped or sold very cheaply. The pure sodium chloride you see at the grocery is a refined waste by-product of the chemical mining industry that sells for pennies a ton while "sea salt" at health food stores sells for $5-$10 a pound. It's the same stuff, right? Maybe. Or maybe not.

When seawater is evaporated, the many different salts precipitate out at different rates. Sodium chloride drops out of solution first. The remaining brine can be piped away to another pond for further drying and separation. This handy chemical fact means that a salt-water refinery can produce a "sea salt" that is not *whole* salt but nearly pure sodium chloride, unadulterated by other electrolytes and minerals. These have been removed (easier to pull them out of salt brine than blast them out of granite) and sold separately on the commodities market. I once bought a box of "Dead Sea Salt," expensive, but said to be "rich in a host of trace minerals." It was a lovely pure white, with perfect cubic crystals completely unaffected by humidity. Apparently what I got was pure sodium chloride of Dead Sea origin.

Natural whole salts have recently appeared in cooking magazines. Taste testers invariably choose them over pure sodium chloride for "*their satisfying depth of flavor.*" It may be that our problems with salt or salt cravings are not because of the salt we get but because of the salts we *don't* get, the 90-some minerals and flavors that are missing and for which our bodies hunger. To satisfy that hunger, consider whole natural sea salt. It may be gray and lumpy in wet weather but contain all the minerals it had when it first left the ocean with the outstanding exception of iodine.

Iodine is critical to thyroid hormone and iodized salt was key to eliminating hypothyroidism across the notorious "Goiter Belt" of the iodine-deficient American Midwest. Iodine is volatile; it is lost during evaporation, during cooking and from any salt that is mishandled or poorly stored, no matter how much you paid for it. Whole sea salt has more natural minerals but *less* iodine than refined commercially iodized salt. If not obtained elsewhere, the current fad of eliminating salt may also eliminate iodine.

"Sports beverages" are touted for replacement of electrolytes lost after illness or sweaty exercise. But electrolytes in these drinks are rarely balanced. A leading brand contains sodium and potassium[1] but no magnesium. You can do it better and more cheaply (and without colorings, preservatives, or artificial flavoring). Stir a bit of sea salt / rock salt into a pitcher of water or fruit or tomato juice diluted with plain water. Add a pinch of Epsom salts (magnesium sulfate).

Whole sea salts are increasingly available and expensive. Personally I ignore the gourmet brands in favor of mined rock salt, *halite*. These deposits are the bones of long-vanished oceans, laid down aeons before oil spills, ocean dumping, and other detritus of modern civilization.

## VITAMINS AND MINERALS

Malnutrition doesn't mean "starvation." Its precise literal meaning is "bad feeding." This can mean perfectly adequate calories but stupid food choices. It can also mean "food that is so downright dangerous that it can and will kill you." All too often it means "failure to get adequate nutrients required for good health and function."

In theory, we get all the nutrients we need from the Standard American Diet. Vitamin and mineral supplements? All you'll get is "expensive urine." Perhaps it all depends on where you want to put your money: expensive urine, expensive migraine drugs, expensive bypass, or expensive hip replacement[2].

Cheery assumptions of nutritional adequacy rarely allow for increased nutritional demands of chronic emotional or physical stress. These may range from Fight Or Flight responses, chemical overloads due to smoking, alcohol, drugs (prescription and recreational), and environmental toxins. Antacids, alcohol, and a long list of prescription drugs destroy vitamins, decrease absorption in the gut, or speed their elimination from the body. Tobacco smoking destroys B vitamins and vitamin C and directly aggravates trigger points while exposing the smoker and those nearby to a host of pathogenic bacteria. (See page 207).

The MDR (Minimum Daily Requirement) is the amount of a substance required to prevent a full-blown deficiency disease. MDR does not address elevated requirements or sub-optimal nutrition. It does not address insufficiencies.

An insufficiency is to a deficiency as a worn tire is to a blow-out. You can travel a long way on balding, suboptimal tires. Nothing terrible will happen and you probably won't

---

1. Electrolyte-balanced Eletewater, mixed with *plain water*, also replaces magnesium. Many athletes swear by its ability to prevent or relieve cramping. See www.eletewater.com.
2. On the other hand, see "The Dark Side of Supplementation" on page 174

die because of them, if everything down the road is optimal. That is, no high speeds, no sudden curves or rough stretches. No speed bumps or potholes. No rain. No sleet. No snow. No stress, no worries.

Similarly, a few days or weeks of quickie burgers and fries will not make you the poster child for scurvy or beriberi. But add some stress, perhaps final exams or a lay-off, tax time, or heavy sweating from heat or hard work. Perhaps you're living on a high carbohydrate / low protein diet from which green vegetables are excluded because "they're too expensive" in favor of Sugar Coated Breakfast Bombs and pizza with the two-liter soft drink special. Add an infection, a series of steroid shots or emergency surgery . . . and you're headed for a blow-out.

There is no ideal one-size-fits-all balanced diet. Ideal for whom? Balanced how?

Nutritional insufficiency may involve multiple issues.

- *High requirements.* Nutrient demand varies by sex, age, environment, physical and emotional stress, genetic background, and even skin color. Genetically dark-skinned persons in Minnesota have radically higher requirements for supplemental Vitamin D than genetically light-skinned persons.

- *Inadequate intake.* This may include unavailability, processing losses, destruction in the body due to antacids, or interactions with foods and drugs and alcohol.

- *Unbalanced intake.* Too much of one nutrient can cause deficiencies of another; for example, high calcium intake can cause magnesium deficiencies and block absorption of thyroid hormone. Too much of one B vitamin causes deficiencies of the others.

- *Poor absorption.* Lack of co-factors or enzymes needed to process nutrients, or high-fat diets that bind calcium and magnesium, low-fat diets that lose fat-soluble vitamins A and D, high intakes of antacids or soy that block iron, calcium, and many other nutrients.

- *Poor utilization.* Includes cellular resistance, auto-immune functions, and other genetic problems such as gluten intolerance.

- *Geologic location.* Local weather, water, soils and even their bacterial populations.

Family history of disease may involve more than genetics. It can also be a factor of where a family has lived. Finland has some of the worst rates of heart disease in the world yet when Finnish families packed up and moved their same genes to Minnesota, their rates of heart disease plummeted. Similarly, in the US it was long observed that people living in the Atlantic Coastal Plain had higher rates of heart disease than those living just a few miles away in hard rock areas or with a different water system (Seelig, Mildred (2003); Rubenowitz-Lundin E and Hiscock KM, 2005).

These are a few of the many observations that led to the field of medical geology: Where you end up living is a bit of a crap shoot — but it has enormous impact on what is in your local food and water, on what you eat, therefore what you are. And what you are in Finland and in the Atlantic Coastal Plain is usually deficient in magnesium.

What we think of as "different" vitamins work together, different minerals work together, and vitamins *and* minerals work together. No matter how many calcium pills you pop for strong bones, if other bone-building materials are missing (such as phosphorus, magnesium, boron, strontium, Vitamin D), you can't build strong bones.

The B vitamins in particular are commonly referred to as a *complex*. Members are synergistic, that is, they "work together" as a team. Supplementing one can produce deficiencies of others. Except in rare circumstances, we should get our nutrients from *food* as we were designed to do.

It was long said that supplemental vitamins and minerals were unnecessary. All that was needed for good health was a balanced diet. I think that is absolutely true, and I also think that today it is increasingly difficult to find Americans who actually eat a balanced diet in any form. Where balance is off, supplements are a great help, but they should be *supplemental*. Don't try to live on pills and potions alone, then wonder why you just don't feel healthy. Also be aware of some of the chicanery that goes on in the vitamin industry. Exempt from supervision by the FDA, the only watchdog organization I know of is www.ConsumerLab.com, an independent laboratory that tests and evaluates supplements for humans and pets. Their queries are simple:

- *Labeled Amount*: Do amounts stated on the label match contents of the bottle?
- *Purity*: Is the material contaminated with lead or other toxins?
- *Ability to Break Apart.* Does material break up for absorption or does it pass through the digestive tract intact?

This is pretty basic stuff. And yet some of their findings include:

- Probiotics containing less than 10% of beneficial bacteria claimed on the label.
- Calcium and magnesium, green tea, ginkgo, and more, contaminated with lead.
- Glucosamine and chondroitin supplements for joint health that contain lead, but no detectable levels of chondroitin.
- Statin levels in red yeast rice that varied 100-fold — as did toxic fungal contaminants.
- Chromium supplements containing *hexavalent chromium*, co-star of the movie *Erin Brockovich*. I have found supplements in my local grocery with Chromium VI clearly listed on the label, from companies that apparently did not know, sold to customers who also did not know, that this is the hexavalent form (*hex* = 6 = VI) and that it is toxic.

## VITAMINS

A *vitamin* is an organic compound that cannot be synthesized by the body in sufficient quantities and must be obtained from the diet. Vitamins are necessary for life itself.

B vitamins, Vitamin C, Vitamin D (and more) are critical to neuromuscular function. They also appear to play an important role in migraine as they are typically low in migraine sufferers. Several OTC remedies include magnesium (involved in platelet clumping and vascular health), feverfew (a blood thinner which would also affect platelet clumping) and riboflavin (B2)[1]. It may be that these compounds work as well as they do (for *some* if not *all*) because they correct underlying nutritional problems.

*Please do not pick a symptom out of the following lists then buy a bottle of that particular nutrient with the notion of treating that symptom. Look at the Big Picture, look at food lists, and look at the difference between living on real food and real meals versus processed imitation foods and pills popped on the run.*

### B Vitamins

The B vitamins *as a group* help metabolize proteins and fat and convert carbohydrates (sugars, starches, alcohol) to glucose. They are critical to proper function of muscles (including heart), the nervous system, liver, GI tract, hair, eyes, and skin. They are important in producing many enzymes and hormones including: insulin, growth and sex hormones, DNA, RNA, amino acids, and stomach acid. All B vitamins are water soluble, lost in urine and perspiration, meaning they must be supplied daily. Overall these are poorly supplied and poorly balanced in processed foods.

**B1 (THIAMINE).** With fatigue, cold, and weight gain there is a tendency to suspect low thyroid, but low temperature can also come from low levels of iron and B1. When hypothyroid patients are treated with B1 first, symptoms may disappear and thyroid function improve *without* thyroid therapy. Starting thyroid hormone before correcting B1 can produce symptoms that mimic thyroid overdose. (Travell and Simons, 1983).

**B2 (RIBOFLAVIN).** Riboflavin is the vitamin that turns urine a bright sunny "yellow" (L. *flavus*). If yours is colorless, it may not be "expensive" enough. Riboflavin is high in dairy products and organ meats. Deficiencies can appear in restricted diets and heavy exercise can double requirements, especially in women of childbearing age.

**B3 (NIACIN).** Folic acid and its relationship with B12 is an outstanding example of why B vitamins should be supplemented as a complex, not individually. High levels of folic acid *increase* requirements for B12. With low levels of B12 (typical of strict vegetarians) popping folic acid supplements can drop B12 levels even lower. The result can be permanent, irreversible neurological damage.

**B12 AND FOLIC ACID.** B12 is some of the best evidence that pure vegetarianism is not the natural human diet. Requirements are tiny but critical: 2 micrograms per day. Humans on strict vegetarian diets can't get even that much without supplementation. The high levels of folic acid found in vegetables ("foliage") *increase* the need for B12 and it simply isn't available in a purely plant-based diet[1]. You would have to eat the land crustaceans (known as insects) that naturally come with the plants and are high in B vitamins. Deficiency symptoms can progress to coma and death, symptoms which qualify as an evolutionary dead end. An intermediary symptom may be migraine as low levels are often found (with other B deficiencies) in migraine sufferers. If you are taking antacids, you may need to take a B12 supplement to achieve healthy levels.

---

1. MigraHealthTM and MigraLief ® are the same product.
1. Claims for B12 from spirulina (an algae) are not supported by the medical literature.

Many individuals do better supplementing with methylcobalamine than with the more common cyanocobalamine, which is cheaper, but must be transformed to the methyl form in the body to be useful. *Methylation* (adding a sulfur group) can be a challenge for some people's individual body chemistries. MSM (Methyl-Sulfonyl-Methane) occurs naturally in the cabbage family (cruciferous vegetables including cabbage, kale, and broccoli), onions, garlic, nuts, seeds, milk, and eggs. MSM in combination with glucosamine can help supply the raw materials if they are lacking in the diet and, for many, help reduce inflammation (Usha PR and others, 2004).

### Vitamin C

Among its many functions, Vitamin C is required for healthy muscles and vascular system, metabolism of thyroid, calcium, and iron. Many athletes and pain sufferers jokingly refer to ibuprofen as "Vitamin I" and down it by the bottle. But one of the side effects of ibuprofen, aspirin, and other painkillers (besides liver and kidney damage) is active destruction of Vitamin C. Using Vitamin C-destroying painkillers to deal with pain (which may have begun with low levels of Vitamin C) can set off a vicious cycle of vitamin deficiency and muscle dysfunction.

### Vitamin D

Vitamin D is known as the "sunshine vitamin" because it is created by Ultra-Violet (UV) light in the oils and cholesterol of the skin. It is critical to an enormous number of body functions. Vitamin D is actually a hormone, interacting with skin, brain, kidneys, intestines, pancreas, heart, and other organs. It is involved in blood clotting, and the nervous system. Some estimate that it regulates up to 2,000 individual genes.

No matter how many calcium pills you pop "to protect bones," calcium can't be absorbed or bone laid down without Vitamin D. Hence deficiency is associated with diseases of faulty calcium metabolism (including osteoporosis, rickets, and bad teeth) but also linked to high blood pressure, depression, fibromyalgia, Type I diabetes, rheumatoid arthritis, Multiple Sclerosis (MS), and some 17 different types of cancer (especially of the colon, but including breast, prostate, and ovaries).

Historically, children born in March in the Northern Hemisphere have tended to develop schizophrenia at higher rates than those born during other months. Over the 9 months from late June through March, sunlight intensity is either falling or (while increasing) the weather is still far too cold for sunbathing in New England.

In 2003, researchers studied 150 patients who had come into a primary care medical clinic in Minneapolis, Minnesota (45° North latitude) between February and June complaining of chronic non-specific musculoskeletal pain that did not respond to standard painkillers. Most had been told that their pain was "all in their heads." An an overwhelming 93 percent proved severely deficient in Vitamin D, including *all* subjects of African, Hispanic, and Native American origin, and *all* subjects under the age of 30. Of these, 55 percent were *severely deficient*; 5 patients (4 of whom were 35 or younger) had *no detectable levels of Vitamin D at all* (Plotnikoff GA and Quigley JM, 2003).

Severity of deficiency was disproportionate by:

- Age for young women,

- Sex for East African patients, and

- Race for African American patients.


The risk of Vitamin D deficiency has long been thought to be greatest for house-bound persons and the elderly. In contrast, this study found most severe deficiencies in the young, especially women of childbearing age. There's little difference between "house-bound" and "office-bound" for many people, regardless of age, who go to work in the dark and return in the dark.

No one's skin can make Vitamin D when sun is blocked by walls, windows, heavy clothing, or ever more effective sunblock. Due to cancer concerns, any exposed skin may be covered with sunblock or UV-inhibiting cosmetics. SPF8 is 95 percent effective at blocking Vitamin D formation; SPF15 inhibits 99 per cent. The long robes traditionally worn by Muslim women, covering all skin, were protective survival gear under the blazing East African sun. Transplanted to Northern climes, they may be too successful at blocking sun to allow good health without Vitamin D supplementation.

The double-whammy of low intake and low exposure to sunlight is bad enough, but genetics, in the form of skin color, can make it worse. In general, dark-skinned persons are more likely to be lactose intolerant and consume less milk, one of the main modern food sources supplemented with Vitamin D. Dark skin *is* a sunblock, an excellent protection against *too much* sun. Pale skin evolved to survive in the weaker light of Northern climes. It may take several hours for dark skin to produce the same amount of Vitamin D that a light-skinned person can produce in a few minutes.

This is why the possibility of deficiency may not even be considered in light-skinned individuals. Checking Vitamin D levels is particularly critical for dark-skinned Northerners, but all *humans* living in the northern latitudes, regardless of skin color, are commonly deficient in D, especially during the winter months.

But what is "Northern"? It is more Southern than you might think.

In general, persons north of central Virginia may fail to get enough year-round sun exposure to make adequate Vitamin D. Winter light in New York is too weak to make Vitamin D at all — it *must* come from foods and supplements. But the problem is not limited to northerners.

In 2009, Dr. Steve Wheeler found Vitamin D deficiency in 42 per cent of patients with chronic migraine headaches studied at Ryan Wheeler Headache Treatment Center in *Miami, Florida* ("the Sunshine State"). Vitamin D deficiency in one of the sunniest areas of the country suggests severe dietary or sunlight deficiencies, serious "sunscreen abuse," high genetic requirements, or all of these combined.

It does not follow that Vitamin D deficiency *causes* migraine. Deficiencies are foudn in many humans; migraineurs are a minority of the total. Nevertheless, this is part of the total nutritional picture.

The recommended intake of Vitamin D set by the National Academy of Sciences has long been based on an age-related scale as follows:

- 19-50 years: 200 International Units (IU)

- 51 to 70 years: 400 IU

- 70 years and older: 600 IU

This list does not consider occupation, skin color, or latitude. It dates from a time when a majority of the population worked in agriculture; a relatively small percentage does so today. We can no longer assume that we automatically get what we need.

What is really important is actual levels, which you can only know by actual testing. Table  shows current recommendations.

| CURRENT RECOMMENDATIONS FOR BLOOD LEVELS OF VITAMIN D | |
|---|---|
| <20 ng/ml | Deficiency |
| 20-30 ng/ml | Insufficiency |
| >30 ng/ml | Sufficiency |
| >40/50-80 ng/ml | Optimal |
| >150+ ng/ml | Toxicity |

Many Vitamin D researchers now believe that intake should be 1,000 IU / day or higher. Vitamin D should be taken separately, not in multivitamins containing the traditional 400 IU. Taking multiple multivitamin pills to reach 1,000+ IU of D exposes you to overdoses of other nutrients.

D2 (ergocalciferol) is a weakly active synthetic version of Vitamin D derived from plants. It is the type most often found in supplements at the old rate of 400 IU.

D3 (cholecalciferol) is the more potent animal-derived version best suited to humans. This is the one you actually want to take, but again, do not exceed 1,000 IUs per day without testing blood levels. Because of its ability to redistribute and deposit calcium, too much D3 leads to tetany and calcification of muscles, liver, kidney, and other body parts not intended to function as bone. Supplements combined with tanning beds can quickly produce toxic levels of Vitamin D. The 25-hydroxy-Vitamin D test costs about $100, much less than trying to identify and treat overdose.

Too much or too little will result in pain that is *not* limited to your head.

## MINERALS

Minerals build bones and teeth, but also provide electrolytes for muscle action, nerve transmission, and many other functions.

### CALCIUM (CA)

Calcium is critical for muscle contraction. It is also involved in blood clotting, nerve transmission, and is a major component of bone and teeth — but not the only one.

Women are constantly encouraged to supplement calcium "to protect bones" but bones are not made of calcium alone. They also contain phosphorus, magnesium, sodium, and potassium. Trace elements include (zinc, manganese, fluoride, and molybdenum, and strontium). Calcium cannot be absorbed without Vitamin D and magnesium (Mg). In addition:

- Too much calcium with no place to go won't inhibit fractures but *will* create kidney stones and other problems.

- More than 2 units of calcium to 1 unit of magnesium induces magnesium deficiency producing muscle cramps, migraines, and other symptoms of magnesium deficiency including cardiac arrest. (See Magnesium on page 149.)

- Excess calcium supplements and antacids neutralize stomach acid making other nutrients, such as iron, unavailable. Iron can only be absorbed in an acid environment.

- Calcium (whether from a pill, yogurt, or milk in your coffee) binds to thyroid making it unavailable. If you take thyroid hormone and calcium, take them several hours apart.

Calcium is bulky stuff. You won't find it in any meaningful quantity in "one daily" formulas unless you're looking at a horse pill. You've got to get it elsewhere, preferably from food.

Calcium in cultured yogurt is more available than in plain milk and may be edible even for the lactose intolerant as the lactose (milk sugar) has already been digested by the bacteria of the yogurt cultures. The standard recommendation is dairy products, but a serving of high-calcium vegetables such as kale or broccoli can provide as much calcium as a glass of milk. And, because magnesium is part of the chlorophyll molecule, intensely green calcium-rich vegetables can also provide a healthy balance of calcium and magnesium.

Calcium must be balanced with magnesium. And no matter how many calcium pills you swallow, calcium cannot be absorbed without Vitamin D or without stomach acid.

## MAGNESIUM (MG)

What condition has been linked to the following symptoms?

- Vasoconstriction and vasospasm,
- Muscle tension, numbness and tingling, and TMJ dysfunction,
- Type A personality traits, anxiety, tension, hyperactivity and restlessness
- PMS, menstrual headache, and endometriosis,
- Disrupted serotonin metabolism, depression and fatigue
- Sleep problems and insomnia,
- Spreading cortical depression,
- Sensitivity to light and noise,
- Sensitivity to MSG,
- Blood platelet clumping, increased risk of stroke, heart attack, and cardiac arrest

Migraine headache? That's just one of the many symptoms.

The answer is *magnesium deficiency.*

Magnesium is a *macro*nutrient meaning that it is needed in "large" quantities. Whether or not it is actually available in macro quantities depends on supply and demand. It is present in the body only if it is put there, and only as long as losses do not outstrip supply. But supplies of this critical nutrient are ever lower in our processed food and water. For example, magnesium is:

- High in wheat, but one of the many nutrients lost when the bran is removed in refining whole wheat into white flour. It is not returned during the "enrichment" process.
- High in some hard waters; lacking in softened, filtered, and bottled water.
- Blocked by high fat diets.

Historically high rates of heart attack in soft water areas compared to lower rates in hardwater areas led to the realization that magnesium deficiency is heavily involved not only in cramps and spasms of skeletal muscles, but also in the muscles lining blood vessels and in the heart itself.

Calcium *contracts* muscles.

Magnesium (a natural calcium blocker) allows muscles to *relax.*

With the rise of processed foods and waters and transportation, the original "hard water advantage" of local geology — soil, rock, and groundwater — has begun to blur and vanish. Water softening replaces calcium and magnesium with sodium. Even when magnesium is present in food and water, absorption is blocked by high fat diets while the need for magnesium is elevated by sugar and stress.

Magnesium is commonly deficient in the Standard American Diet despite its importance in almost every bodily function. Magnesium is directly involved in over 200 enzyme actions, and indirectly in several hundred more. The SAD — white flour, high fat, high sugar — is a recipe for disaster for many reasons. One is magnesium losses.

Magnesium is absolutely critical to cellular function. It is involved in every reaction of ATP, in every heartbeat. Low levels are linked to migraine (especially menstrual migraine), cluster, and post-traumatic headaches. Low levels have also been reported in hemodialysis headaches and fibromyalgia compared to control groups. Problems with muscle function and crashing fatigue might have something to do with the fact that there is magnesium in every molecule of ATP, which is the beginning of every muscle movement, every heart beat.

No magnesium > no ATP > failure of the ATPase system > failure of the sodium pump

Magnesium deficiencies can also lurk behind depression and insomnia, as magnesium is critical for manufacture of serotonin and melatonin. Requirements rise with emotional stress, loud noise, hard physical exercise, sweating, pregnancy and possibly the pre-menstrual part of a woman's cycle. Poor absorption (due to age, high-fat diets, low stomach acid), increased elimination (diarrhea, diuretics, or laxatives), and a host of common medications can make a marginal or bad situation even worse. Some drugs *aid* magnesium retention and happen to be the same ones used in treatment of heart attack (including aspirin, beta-blockers, and ACE inhibitors) and migraine.

**TABLE 6.** DRUGS THAT DEPLETE MAGNESIUM

| | |
|---|---|
| *Allergy* | Adrenalin, aminophyllin, AsthmaNefrin, Epinephrin, EpiPen, isoproterenol, and Isuprel. |
| *Cardiac Care* | For heart attack or irregular heartbeat: amiodarone, Betapace, bretylium, Cordarone, digoxin, Lanoxicaps, Lanoxin, Quinaglute, Quinidex, quinidine, Quin-Release, solalol. *Diuretics for* hypertension or congestive heart failure: Edecrin, ethacrynic acid, furosemide, Lasix, mannitol, thiazides (drugs ending in -*zide*). |
| *Infections* | Aminoglycosides, amphotericin B, carbenicillin, Garamycin, G-Mycin, Geocillin, Geopen, Jenamicin, tetracyclines, Ticar, ticarcillin. |
| *Psych/ Neuro* | Mellaril, Orap, pimozide, thioridazine, Stelazine, trifluoperazine, |
| *Other:* | Cancer, immune, and antifungal drugs: A-hydroCort, chemotherapy drugs and radiation, cisplatin, corticosteroids, cyclosporine, hydrocortisone, Hydrocortone, Nebupent, Pentam, Pentamidine. |

## Magnesium and Stress

Magnesium levels too low to support energy metabolism leave muscles tense and fatigued. In a fight-or-flight state of stress, adrenal glands release the stress hormones adrenaline and cortisone. These increase heart rate, breathing, transmission of nerve impulses, muscle power and response. Magnesium is urgently needed for all of these responses and quickly mobilized from tissues not immediately critical to survival (such as bone surfaces) and dumped into the blood stream for delivery to the rest of the body. When the threat passes, kidneys excrete excess magnesium.

If body stores are adequate, all is well. If stores are low but stress continues, magnesium may be mobilized even from vital tissues — including the heart and the cell membranes of other tissues. This is how stress and subpar nutrition can convert a slight magnesium deficiency into a migraine, a sudden heart attack, or stroke.

Cell membranes are held together with magnesium in a complex dance with other electrolytes. Magnesium deficiency destabilizes membranes allowing other electrolytes to flood in and out of cells inappropriately. For example, a magnesium "leak" can:

- Result in failure of the blood-brain barrier allowing toxins to reach the brain.

- Allow calcium to flood into cells causing swelling and edema (one mechanism behind destruction of brain cells by MSG and aspartame).

- Change the Ca:Mg balance in muscles so that muscles constrict but cannot relax. In skeletal muscle, this result is known as a *cramp*. In the muscles that line veins and arteries, it may be known as *vasospasm or vasoconstriction*. In the muscle of the heart it may be behind angina or *fibrillation*. The end result may range from heart attack or stroke or migraine.

That magnesium might play an important role in migraines was suggested and tested with success in the 1930s. John Myers, M.D., developed what became known as the "Myers' cocktail," an intravenous formula of magnesium, calcium, B vitamins, and vitamin C. It was originally designed to aid wound healing but later found effective in other conditions, especially migraine, but also including acute asthma attacks, fibromyalgia and Chronic Fatigue Syndrome, acute muscle spasm, and cardiovascular disease (Gaby AR, 2002).

With the rise of the pharmaceutical industry, non-patentable magnesium therapy fell out of favor. In the 1980s the concept was revisited for headaches with mixed results. Magnesium helped *some* headaches (but not *all*) in *some* patients (but not *all*). The greatest improvements were seen in migraine and menstrual headaches (compared to those diagnosed as "tension"), but some studies showed no improvement at all and these conditions did not seem to correlate well with blood tests.

## Magnesium and the Heart

Heart failure is a "growth industry" in the US where it is the leading cause of hospitalizations for cardiovascular disease.

—Peggy Peck, *MedPage Today* (May 29, 2010)

Electrolyte levels in blood and serum are carefully regulated within strict limits representing less than one percent of total body stores. They can change within minutes in response to stress and other hormones. As it became clear that much cardiac disease is related to magnesium deficiency, it also became clear that there was poor correlation between magnesium in heart tissue and blood. Many patients dead of cardiac arrest have been found with no detectable levels of magnesium in the damaged areas of the heart, yet perfectly "normal" levels of serum magnesium. Hence low blood levels may reflect a failure of the mobilization system (seen in persons who are severely ill) *or* dangerously low levels of available stores (seen in persons who appear healthy but are about to become severely ill or dead from cardiac arrest).

Historically we have measured *total magnesium* (TMg), all types and combinations of magnesium combined. But total magnesium turns out to be far less important than what is *ionized* (IMg2+) or *free*, unbound to anything else. To help a migraine, magnesium must be *free* and it must have the proper electrical charge[1].

In the 1990s, new techniques developed by Drs. Burton and Bella Altura, made it possible to test magnesium by type, and to test type against headaches. With this powerful new tool, neurologist Alexander Mauskop designed a double-blind study of over 100 patients that revealed the critical relationship between calcium, magnesium and migraine[2]. Both groups had normal levels of *total* magnesium in blood tests, their electrolytes were all "within normal ranges." However:

- 42% of migraineurs had low levels of *free* magnesium with an elevated ratio of calcium to magnesium. That is, there was less of the critically important *free* magnesium (IMg2+), and what there was of it was out of balance with calcium.

- Only about half as many patients (23%) with severe continuous headaches had similar levels of free magnesium and calcium.

- Even among those with total Mg within "normal ranges," levels were "low normal" in those with low IMg2+. Levels weren't low enough to have raised a red flag in standard blood tests, but comparing the two suggested a background pattern of deficiency.

- Magnesium did *not* relieve headaches if IMg2+ was *not* low to start with.

In summary, this study suggests:

---

1. As analogy, in my town, parking meters use quarters only. I may have pockets full of change, it's all "money," but no matter how much *total* money I have, only quarters produce results. All other coins are functionally "inert."
2. Mauskop A, Altura BT, Altura BM (2002). Dr. Mauskop runs the New York Headache Center, New York, NY. See his research papers on-line at: www.nyheadache.com.

- Current ranges for "normal" and "low" total Mg are too broad. IMg2+ should be above 0.54 mmol/L. Patients with lower levels benefited most dramatically from Mg therapy.

- Balance between Ca and Mg is critical. Random supplementation of calcium without considering its relationship with magnesium is unwise.

- Not all migraines are the same. Even when chemical imbalances are involved, they are not necessarily the same chemical imbalances.

### Magnesium Testing

Actual magnesium status has always been difficult (or unacceptably painful) to test as stores are primarily in muscles and bone. Reliable readings required actual tissue, a biopsy, not a popular procedure.

In the 1990s Dr. Burton Silver discovered that magnesium in skin cells scraped from the floor of the mouth matched levels in heart tissue (obtained in the course of bypass surgery) and skeletal muscle (biopsied from members of the NASA space program). Dr. Silver went on to develop the Exatest which sidesteps the need for invasive biopsy samples. Intact sublingual cells are fixed on a slide then bombarded with X-rays. Energy released at wavelengths unique to individual minerals reflect the levels actually present in cellular tissue. And, because these cells are replaced every two to three days, they can track actual changes in tissue rather than misleading minute-to-minute fluctuations possible in blood and serum.

The Exatest is covered by insurance and is available from:

Intracellular Diagnostics, Inc.
945 Town Centre Dr, Suite A
Medford, OR 97504
(541) 245-3212
www. Exatest.com

Magnesium deficiency may also explain the different responses to MSG and aspartame. Some people are not bothered. In others, these popular food additives trigger migraine, GI tract disturbances and diarrhea, racing hearts and possibly even the "restaurant coronary." See Blaylock R (1997) for details. See Seelig M (2003) for a superb review of magnesium, its critical role in health, and its deadly lack in American diets. If you are low, look at your diet. Requirements vary between individuals, but there is no need to be deficient in this readily available mineral.

Most lists of high-magnesium foods feature chocolate, avocados, nuts, and bananas, items which are not only high in calories but also high on migraine food elimination lists. Focus on intensely green vegetables. Magnesium is to chlorophyll in plants as iron is to heme in the blood of animals.

### Magnesium Supplementation

You can also turn to pills and powders but be aware of the critical *balance* of calcium and magnesium. Ideally the ratio of calcium to magnesium 2:1 or even 1:1. This is increasingly rare; food refining removes magnesium from many foods while the current fad of heavy calcium supplementation guarantees imbalance as there is so little attention to magnesium.At the grocery, I find many supplements for calcium alone, none for magnesium alone. I also find:

- One product combining calcium (1,000 mg) / magnesium (400 mg) / zinc (38 mg). Ratio of Ca to Mg: 2.5 to 1. Not perfect, considering calcium from so many other sources, but not severely out of balance.

- "Stress formulas" containing B vitamins with around 200 mg of added *calcium*. None of these contained magnesium despite its intimate involvement in the stress response, which increases magnesium requirements.

- B-6. No magnesium was included although it is a co-factor with B-6, critical to absorption and function. Like the stress formulas, it included 200 mg of calcium (which was not stated on the front label, only in the small print on the back).

The grocery store may not be the best place to buy supplements, but this is where most people see them. Health food stores tend to stock more expensive options, but price is not always a guarantee of quality[1]. The current interest in high levels of Vitamin D supplementation makes it particularly dangerous to overdose on calcium supplements in the absence of magnesium. Excess Vitamin D deposits excess calcium in kidneys (as stones) or in joints and muscles (producing TrPs, fibromyalgia, arthritis symptoms or worse) and has been linked with heart problems in women.

An informational booklet on migraine (funded by a leading pharmaceutical company), dismisses years of magnesium research on the basis that long term benefit from magnesium would require long-term use. Somehow this was different from long-term use of migraine drugs and different from long-term daily requirements for other macronutrients such as calcium, Vitamin C, air and water. None of these critical nutrients can be replaced by triptans.

## POTASSIUM (K)

Potassium is the body's primary positive ion. It helps regulate water balance, acid / alkaline balance, and to stabilize heartbeat and blood pressure. It is critical to the sodium/potassium pump for nutrient transfer to cells, muscle contraction / nerve transmission, and transport of oxygen to the brain. Fruits and vegetables are all high in potassium.

---

1. You can see this clearly at www.ConsumerLab.com, the only organization that tests health supplements for content and toxins. See their report on a popular magnesium powder found to contain lead.

# IRON (FE)

Oh the irony! Iron can make you stronger, healthier, and more energetic, or like other heavy metals, it can kill you. Iron binds to oxygen (the *heme* part of hemoglobin) transporting it to the cell. No iron, no oxygen transport, no energy for body or brain. Iron is also involved in synthesis of collagen, serotonin and dopamine.

Iron-deficiency anemia is common in women of child-bearing age due to monthly losses. Anemia in men or menopausal women is abnormal and may be associated with gluten intolerance and celiac disease, a bleeding ulcer, low stomach acid, or other problems needing attention beyond simple iron supplements.

Age also takes its toll via poor absorbtion. A study of "well-nourished" women 60 and older in the US found that nearly half had iron deficiencies and their production of germ-fighting T-cells were as much as 50 percent below that of women with normal levels of iron (Ahluwalia, N. and others, 2004). You might also be in the 10 percent of the population that stores too much iron. Men and post-menopausal women have no natural way of removing excess iron from the body.

So before dosing yourself with iron, get a blood test to see if iron-deficiency anemia is even a problem. Years ago, iron compounds were regularly advertised for weary, depressed housewives in the belief that most fatigue was due to "iron-poor blood." but anemia has many possible causes. Treat infection or ulcers first. Treat with iron only if there is a true iron deficiency.

Too much iron is toxic. It creates damaging free radicals and suppresses the immune system. In the pancreas it kills insulin-producing cells resulting in diabetes. It also increases the tendency of blood platelets to clump and clot, increasing the risk of heart disease, including arrhythmia, congestive heart failure, stroke, and *migraine*. Iron accumulations in the heart ("iron heart") lead to cardiac arrest.

Persons with genetic *hemochromatosis*, a common genetic disorder in Caucasians, are extremely efficient at absorbing iron[1]. Instead of the 10 per cent that most people absorb, they may absorb 30, storing the excess (as much as 20 times normal levels) in liver, heart and pancreas. Symptoms usually appear between 30 and 50 in men and after menopause in women. At these ages, early symptoms such as joint pain and fatigue, impotence, loss of menstruation, or pain in the upper right abdomen are quickly attributed to many other conditions and may be treated with a host of remedies including additional vitamin and mineral supplements (including iron) for fatigue, but only make things worse.

Too much iron? Give your abundance to the nearest blood donation center. Win+ Win.

---

1. The gene behind the adult condition is HFE. The juvenile version involves a mutation in a gene called *hemojuvelin*.

# Metabolic Problems

*Migraine can be a symptom of hormonal upsets in both men and women.*

What do you get if you eat a low-fat diet, take estrogen hormone replacement, take calcium to prevent osteoporosis, eat plenty of broccoli and other cancer-fighting crucifers (perhaps via juicing), replace red meat and dairy with tofu and soy milk, drink caffeinated beverages to stay alert at work or on the road, and stay hydrated with the help of your plastic bottle of filtered water?

You just might get a thyroid problem with fatigue and low metabolism. And one of the roots of chronic muscle problems and headaches, is low or slow metabolism.

## HYPOTHYROID

If you're suffering from muscular pain and fatigue, are overweight, tired all the time, sluggish, depressed, your face and ankles are puffy, you're missing the outer third of your eyebrows, can't understand how you can weigh as much as you do considering what you actually eat, or have been diagnosed with fibromyalgia, ask your doctor for a thyroid panel *and* a thyroid antibody test. But first, take your temperature regularly over a week or so of normal health.

If you're reading this, you're a mammal. Mammalian processes require certain operating temperatures. If you "freeze to death," that is, if you "die of hypothermia" (which is possible anywhere below around 95° F) it won't be because your blood freezes to ice and solidifies in your veins. You will die because critical enzyme reactions can no longer take place at subnormal temperatures.

Hypothyroid is common throughout the world in areas geologically deficient in iodine. The American Midwest "goiter belt" is famous for its iodine deficient soils, but so is Austria, the Alps, Nepal, Tibet, the Andes, and other areas[1]. Typically these are mountainous inland areas, far from the sea, and yet the original research on thyroid and hypothyroid began in England. A Dr. Ord described and named myxedema in 1877.

---

1. Morton Salt Co. first introduced iodized table salt in 1924.

## ON THYROID AND TSH

Thyroid function is commonly evaluated by checking levels of Thyroid Stimulating Hormone (TSH), a request for production of thyroid hormone down in manufacturing. The results can be confusing for several reasons.

One is that a high TSH indicates *low* thyroid function and a low TSH indicates *high* thyroid function. It might be easier to think of the TSH numbers as individual requisition forms. If levels are low, there will be a lot of requests. If levels are low, we assume that stocks are adequate.

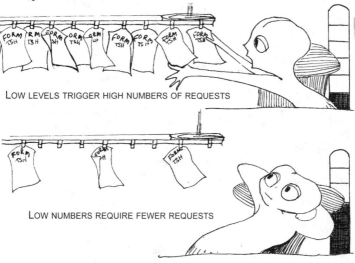

LOW LEVELS TRIGGER HIGH NUMBERS OF REQUESTS

LOW NUMBERS REQUIRE FEWER REQUESTS

**Figure 86.** THYROID REQUISITION FORM TSH

Another problem is that thyroid tests are notorious for a wide range of results interpreted as "normal." As a result, many people drag through years of mental fog and confusion, depression and suboptimal health, weight gain, low libido, and disgust with their "weakness," "lack of discipline and self-control," and failure to function at a higher, hotter level. Ranges have changed since the TSH test was developed back in the 1970s. Then, 6 was high but still "normal." Later it became apparent that the "high normal" end of the bell curve included many people who were actually hypothyroid or would be within a few years. In 2003, the American Academy of Clinical Endocrinologists (AACE) encouraged doctors to treat patients testing outside a range of 0.3 to 3.4 µU/ml. Unfortunately not all labs (or doctors) have heeded this. A report saying that "your TSH is normal" doesn't mean much unless you know the range. Get numbers.

Yet another problem is T4 to T3 conversion. Thyroid hormone comes in several versions, T1, T2, T3, and T4 named for the number of iodine atoms in the molecule. T4 is a relatively inert storage form, while T3 is the short-lived but active form.

De-iodinase enzymes convert T4 to T3. Essentially, these knock an iodine off the 4-iodine molecule (Figure 87) creating the 3-iodine molecule. Currently, most treatment

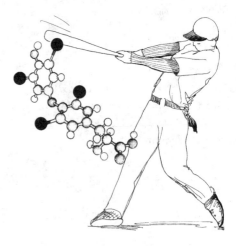

Removing an iodine atom from T4 (the
storage form of thyroid hormone) creates
the active T3 form.
Many drugs block T4-T3 conversion
while TSH tests appear normal.

**Figure 87.** CONVERTING T4 TO T3: DEIODINASE ENZYMES

for hypothyroid involves synthetic thyroid made up of pure T4. The theory is that the body will convert T4 to T3 as needed. This doesn't always happen, yet thyroid tests may appear to be normal.

Thyroid tests are loosely analogous to testing your metabolic fires by calculating the units of oil and air delivered to your furnace. Suppose you tell the janitor that your building is constantly cold. "No way!" he says. "The usual quantity of fuel was delivered this month. According to my calculations *the temperature in your building should be just fine.*" If you feel it isn't fine, a more practical approach is to simply check the temperature in your living unit. If normal building temperature should be 70° but is actually 60°, something is wrong no matter what the calculations may say.

In theory, normal body temperature is 98.6° F. This is not as universal as once believed, but if your temperature stays low by a degree or more something isn't right.

Aside from other symptoms of low thyroid such as heightened cholesterol and blood pressure, increased susceptibility to infections and heart attack, a temperature that regularly runs just one degree low increases your chances of myofascial pain syndromes (including migraine) due to faulty energy metabolism. I have seen apparently healthy bodies riddled with pea- to walnut-sized trigger points despite constant stretching and even dry-needling. What was remarkable in each of these patients was a body temperature of 96-97° F. On getting temperature up to where it should be for a healthy mammal, the trigger points melted away like ice in the warm sun.

Sub-normal temperatures also decrease your chance of correct medical diagnosis. Temperatures above normal are considered to reflect bacterial infection which can be handled by antibiotics. Those below normal are considered to reflect viral infection for which little can be done.

If you are dragging through life at 96.6°, but sick with a temperature of 98.6°, the doctor will only see the "normal" temperature, despite running a temperature equivalent to a fever of 100° in Normals.

Oddly enough, body temperature one or two degrees low is often dismissed as being of no importance. "Well, my dear, maybe your temperature just *naturally* runs low." Maybe it does — and needs correction. It is common after head injury and trauma to the hypothalamus.

*Hypothalamic obesity* is intractable weight gain after damage to the hypothalamus and nervous system, often after a head inury. It is not unusual for victims to gain weight even on severely restricted diets. Hypothyroid symptoms such as low temperature and severe fatigue may appear, making it extremely difficult to exercise. Meanwhile, the vagus nerve stimulates insulin secretion and fat storage. Attempts to treat the condition with drugs and bariatric surgeries (such as stomach stapling and bands) have been largely unsuccessful (Lustig RH, 2008).

The health consequences of subnormal temperatures can be painful and damaging. Low temperature is abnormal. Get it checked. Take your healthy-day temperature. Go from there.

Temperature measurements are just one part of a complex picture. They don't consider your age, antibodies, stress levels, exercise, or diet. The temperature test reveals only that something may be wrong — but that is a great starting point.

Low temperatures can occur for reasons other than hypothyroid. One is iron-deficiency anemia. A deficiency of thiamine (B1) alone can result in low basal temperature or, if thyroid supplements are given, can produce symptoms that may be interpreted as the thyroid supplementation being "poorly tolerated."

Adrenal function must also be considered. Supplementing thyroid when adrenals are exhausted from stress, a regimen of cortisone shots, or poor nutrition can bring on a full-fledged condition of adrenal failure.

Be aware that thyroid may not be the problem, and a prescription for thyroid hormone may not be the answer. Healthy thyroid function is part of a hugely complex ring of relationships that may be severely unbalanced by nutritional problems, brain injury, and environmental toxins. Thyroid levels may be disrupted by nutritional deficits, sedentary lifestyle, a head injury, or even your anti-depressant and shampoo.

## MODERN PLAGUE, MODERN REASONS

One reason for the plague of hypothyroidism and related ills is a world awash in a sea of modern chemicals that disrupt thyroid and normal endocrine function.

Americans now eat large quantities of soy, heavily marketed as part of a healthful cancer-preventing diet, pointing to low rates of breast cancer in Japan. But this ignores the high rate of stomach cancer in Japan as well as other dietary customs that have little to do with soy and much to do with a diet high in seafood and vegetables.

One reason why hypothyroidism is so common in women is that estrogen binds thyroid. But its effects are not limited to women. Just as females produce and have receptors for testosterone, male bodies produce and have receptors for estrogen. Both males and females can suffer further disruptions from estrogens from outside sources.

### Estrogens, Phytoestrogens, and Xenoestrogens

*Xeno-estrogens* ("foreign-estrogens") and *phyto-estrogens* ("plant"-estrogens) are chemicals similar enough to human estrogen to fool the body, but not close enough to actually do the work required of them. They are found in foods, cosmetics, spermicides, plastics and other household/industrial chemicals. Sources include *paraben* (common in lotions and moisturizers), and the ubiquitous *bisphenol-A*, a plastic used for water and food containers, baby bottles, coatings on cash register receipts, and countless other materials.

Another problem is *phytates*. Found in the bran or hulls of all seeds, soy has them in large quantities. As weapons of chemical warfare against plant-eating predators, phytates block uptake of essential minerals including calcium, magnesium, copper, iron, and zinc.

These chemicals are not destroyed by cooking. In its long history of cultivation, soy was considered a valuable green fertilizer (it is a nitrogen-fixing legume) but not food for humans until the Chinese learned to ferment the beans. Fermentation breaks down many of the damaging compounds but these remain intact in unfermented American tofu, soy milk, yogurt, ice cream, infant formula, and soy oil, now used in nearly all processed foods. But there's more.

Today's soybeans are not your grandfather's soybeans. Genetically modified soybeans now make up over 90 per cent of the US crop. The soybeans were modified to resist a dose of herbicide high enough to kill any other plant. In theory, this would reduce the time and expense of tilling and cultivation while increasing yields. What it seems to have done is to create superweeds that are now resistant to many times the recommended dose of weed killer. Some researchers suspect that many problems attributed to soy use in the US are actually side effects of the burgeoning levels of weedkiller and toxic by-products on crops, some concentrated in the oil of the beans themselves.

## Foods and Food Handling

- *Goitrogens.* These "goiter-makers" are found in cabbage, kohlrabi, broccoli, cauliflower, kale, rutabagas, turnips, and millet. To actually block thyroid function requires large quantities, but juicing helps. By reducing an entire cabbage to the contents of a teacup, one may ingest goitrogens in quantities impossible in their solid vegetable state.

- *Soy, Phytates and Phytoestrogens.* They inhibit enzymes, disrupt natural hormones, and block iodine needed to make thyroid hormone.

- *Out-of-Season Fruits and Vegetables.* DDT and other endocrine-disrupting pesticides may be banned here, but sprayed on crops imported from tropical areas outside our growing season. This includes coffee which (outside of Hawaii), is not a US crop.

- *Calcium Supplements.* Calcium binds thyroid and besides imbalance with magnesium, often found in migraineurs, overdose is linked to heart problems and kidney stones.

- *Plastic Bottled Water.* A source of xenoestrogens from plastics especially bisphenol-A.

- *Fluorine (F), Chlorine (Cl), and Bromine (Br).* Halogens ("salt-makers") are highly reactive elements that can substitute for each other. In the game of chemical musical chairs, they can replace iodine (I) but the end molecule is not thyroid. Fluorine is specifically used to depress an overactive thyroid. Fluorine in anti-depressants may explain why they often decrease thyroid function, in turn a common *cause* of depression.

- *PFCs (Per-Fluorinated Compounds.* These compounds (from Teflon to Scotch Guard) provide stain, oil, and water resistance. They persist in the environment as organic pollutants due to the strength of the bond between carbon and fluorine.

- *Low Salt and No Salt.* If iodine is not obtained from other sources, current emphasis on eliminating iodized salt may also eliminate iodine.

- *Severe Dieting.* The body, interpreting this as famine and risk of death, slows metabolism as a survival mechanism.

## Medications that Block or Bind Thyroid

Many drugs interfere with thyroid, in part, by interfering with conversion of T4 (the relatively inert storage form) to T3 (the active form of thyroid hormone). These include anti-inflammatories (glucocorticoids), anti-convulsants and cholesterol-lowering drugs. Some anti-cholesterol drugs bind thyroid so effectively that several hours should be allowed between taking them and any thyroid medications. Salicylates (aspirin and aspirin-like compounds) and nicotine have also been implicated. Anti-depressants can cause hypothyroid even though low thyroid can cause depression. Some specific examples are listed below.

- *Hypertensives.* Blood pressure medications such as propranolol and beta-blockers cause weight and energy problems by interfering with T3-T4 conversion.

- *Anti-Depressants.* SSRI medications such as Prozac (fluoxetine), Paxil (paroxetine), and others) can cause problems possibly because fluorine replaces iodine in the thyroid molecule; the result is not real thyroid. Lithium actively blocks T4 and T3 production.

- *Anti-Cholesterol Drugs.* Cholestyramine, Colestipol (Colestrol, Questran, and Colestid)

- *Corticosteroids.* Believed to block T4 to T3 conversion.

- *Anti-Convulsants.* Phenytoin (Dilantin) and Carbamazepine (Tegretol) can speed metabolism of levothyroxine (synthetic T4); tests may show decreased levels of T4.

- *Anti-Tuberculins.* Rifampin speeds metabolism of levothyroxine (synthetic T4); tests may show decreased levels of total T4.

- *Heart Medications.* Amiodarone HCL (Cordarone) can cause both *hypo-* and *hyper*thyroidism. Patients should be monitored on a regular basis.

### Medications Impacted by Thyroid

The following medications can have different effects in the presence of thyroid supplements. Be sure your doctor knows you are on thyroid *before* starting the following medications.

- *Anticoagulants.* In the presence of thyroid hormone, blood thinners (such as Warfarin, Coumadin, Heparin) can become *more* effective.

- *Insulin.* Thyroid hormones can reduce the effectiveness of insulin.

- *Asthma Medications.* Theophylline, an asthma drug, metabolizes more slowly in hypothyroid patients, more quickly as metabolism rises. Be aware of dosages.

### Cosmetics and Personal Care Products

Many personal care and beauty products contain thyroid and endocrine disrupters, carcinogens, and neurotoxins that can be absorbed through the skin. Individually or in concert these are linked to allergies and asthma, birth defects, early puberty, brain disorders and more. Cosmetic companies are now required to list some ingredients on labels with two outstanding loopholes:

- *Fragrances* are exempt on their own *and* when combined with other products, as in lotions or soaps because fragrance formulas (including perfumes and colognes) are considered trade secrets.

- *Unintended materials or by-products* include compounds created during the combination of other chemicals in the course of creating the product. This category can include metals from the pipes and processing vats[1].

In the US, Cosmetics are not tested or controlled by the FDA, nor, apparently, by anyone else. Supposedly, safety concerns are met by the Cosmetic Ingredient Review (CIR) founded in 1976 as an arm of the cosmetics industry trade association. Over the last 30 years, the CIR has managed to safety test about 10 per cent of common cosmetic ingredients and identify just 10 as *objectionable*. In contrast, the European Union has banned 1,300 known or suspected of causing cancer.

The Environmental Working Group (EWG) began a campaign for safer cosmetics and developed a database of ingredients. When it became clear that there was more in the

---

1. Can include chemical reactions claimed to be unintentional. For example, sodium hydroxy-methyl-glycinate releases formaldehyde which need not be listed on the theory that it was *unintended*. This is like listing hydrogen and oxygen, but failing to mention the water that results when they combine. This might explain an oddity with carpet fumes (see page 212). Formaldehyde is a poison and can be a powerful migraine trigger.

bottle than on the label, EWG sent samples off to a laboratory for chemical analysis. Tests of 17 name brand fragrances revealed an average of 14 chemicals in the bottles that were not listed on the labels. Mystery ingredients included hormone disrupters, allergens, and other chemicals never tested for safety. For details, see Malkan S (2007) and www.cosmeticsdatabase.com.

EWG recommends avoiding the following.

- *Alpha- and Beta-Hydroxy Acids.* Skin irritation, possibly to the point of scarring.

- *DEA (diethanolamine).* Skin irritation, inhibition of choline (an important brain nutrient).

- *Lipstick containing lead.* Over 60% of name-brand lipsticks tested by EWG.

- *Skin lighteners.* Some contain mercury and cadmium. Hydroquinone, a possible carcinogen, endocrine and immune disrupter, has been banned in the EU since 1976.

- *Nano-technology.* Heavily advertised, completely unregulated.

- *PABA (Para-Amino-Benzoic Acid).* Photo-allergic reactions including blisters.

- *Phthalates.* Linked to endocrine disruptions, birth defects, and sperm damage.

- *Sodium Laurel Sulfate / Sodium Lauril Sulfate (SLS) / Sodium Dodecyl Sulfate (SDS).* Skin and eye irritation. In toothpastes, linked to canker sores.

The following chemicals may be particularly dangerous for migraineurs.

- *Fragrances, synthetic.* leading cause of cosmetic-related allergies and sensitivities, from skin and eye irritation to nausea, fatigue, depression, and headaches.

- *Hair dyes and p-phenylenediamine diaminobenzene (PPD).* PPD is found in almost every hair dye on the market, the darker the dye the more PPD it contains, including dark dyes claiming to be "henna". PPD may be a carcinogen, but definitely an allergen. In 2006, the American Contact Dermatitis Society voted PPD "Allergen of the Year."

- *Hair straightener and conditioners containing placenta.* From sex organs of butchered pregnant livestock, placenta is a super source of estrogen, producing breasts and pubic hair in toddlers, and thyroid problems in adults.

- *"Antibacterial" soaps with triclosan.* Triclosan mimics thyroid hormone binding to the hormone receptor sites and blocking normal thyroid hormone.

- *Formaldehyde.* In nail polish, soap, shampoo, carpets, and building materials.

- *Parabens.* Used as a preservatives in various cosmetics and toothpastes. They are endocrine disrupters, can cause skin eruptions, and have been found in breast cancers.

# Menstrual Headaches

*Migraine can be a symptom of hormonal disruptions.*

A woman's monthly cycle is an ever-changing fluctuation of hormones punctuated by ovulation and menstruation. Migraine tends to accompany both events.

For many women, menstruation is famously painful. If you suffer that, you don't need a migraine as well. Even less do you need to be told that your pain is "psychosomatic" or "an excuse to avoid responsibility." Chances are excellent that it is something else entirely: *prostaglandins*. These are hormone-like substances involved in inflammation, contraction and relaxation of smooth muscles including the muscular lining of blood vessels (affecting blood pressure), intestines, and uterus. Contraction and relaxation depends on the ratio between different groups of prostaglandins[1]; different types are used to stall or to induce labor.

Prostaglandin levels rise with ovulation. In some women, they rise so high that they escape the uterus and enter the blood stream, affecting other smooth muscles. Intestines move food along too quickly, causing diarrhea. Blood vessels expand or constrict too suddenly, causing surges of heat or feelings of cold. The uterus may contract so strongly that it compresses blood vessels, cutting off its own blood supply. The result is cramping and pain. Despite the traditional claims of psychiatric causes, despite the snickers and sneers, the pain is very real. Functionally, it is remarkably similar to (and about as funny as) the crushing pain of angina and heart attack, that is, pain arising from decreased blood supply to the muscle of the heart.

The pain that many women endure is truly phenomenal. The late Dr. Penny Wise Budoff (1980) told of a young woman whose doctor dismissed her injuries as "bruises." When she was still walking oddly after two weeks, her father demanded more tests. Subsequent X-rays revealed that she had broken her back and coccyx, yet for two weeks she had followed her usual schedule, working and walking with a broken back and no pain relief. How? Compared to her monthly cramps, it was business as usual.

One client, a competition dancer, weight lifter, and scuba diver (hardly a wimpy neurotic looking for excuses "to avoid effort or responsibility") had landed in the ER with pain so severe that only morphine could relieve it. Said another athlete, "compared to the monthly cramps, recovering from surgery from my C-section was a cake-walk."

"Have a baby!" has often been recommended as a cure for migraine. Not only is this untrue, but many women report that their labor pains were never as bad as their menstrual cramps which returned after delivery. Many women report that, when told to head for the hospital only when the labor pains became worse than normal cramps, they "nearly had the baby in the living room; at no time were my labor pains as bad as what I experienced every month!"

---

1. First found in seminal fluid, named for the "prostate," but later found throughout the body.

---

## PAIN AND PROSTAGLANDINS

Psychogenic causes are the most common and the most important in cases of primary dysmenorrhea. . . Most reaction could be obviated by proper counseling prior to puberty. The individual who does the counseling under ordinary circumstances, should not be the mother, older friends, or girls of her own age, but should be a physician. Additional necessary help might be obtained by the use of trained psychologists.

— Brewer, *Textbook of Gynecology* (1962)

We have come to consider it as a psychosomatic illness. . . Many reports suggest that psychotherapy is the sole answer to the problem.

— Parsons and Sommers, *Gynecology* (1978)

The men who wrote and read these textbooks trained me and every other physician, and it is difficult for any physician to reject ideas that have been so deeply ingrained.

— Penny Wise Budoff, M. D (1980)

In 1976, Dr. Penny Wise Budoff was asked to speak on health problems of "Women in Industry." To prepare, she researched the causes of menstrual cramps and found *nearly nothing.* "In 1974," she reported, "in the entire world's medical literature, there were just 8 articles dealing with the pain of dysmenorrhea." Budoff began to wonder why there was so little real scientific data on menstrual cramps and why the scant material that existed invariably blamed the pain on women's psyches.

I had had menstrual pain since I was sixteen, and I was pretty confident that I was not neurotic. Menstrual cramps often awakened me from a sound sleep at 4 A.M. Certainly, if I were as hysterical as all the literature postulated, I could have picked a more convenient time for my cramps, such as the middle of a busy afternoon with all my phones ringing and all my patients complaining of long waits in the reception room.

There were tantalizing hints that prostaglandins might be involved. Women who get severe cramps produce up to five times the levels of prostaglandin compared to women who don't, but researchers had never followed up on this lead. Budoff set up the first double-blind study to test this observation, proving the link and the effectiveness of Ponstel®, a prescription prostaglandin inhibitor[1].

Thirty-some years later, there seems to be only limited awareness of the cramping / prostaglandin connection. Menstrual pain is still treated with birth-control pills which offer relief to many women, but involve 21 days of hormone treatments for just 3-7 days of pain. Meanwhile, standard OTC remedies specifically marketed for menstrual pain rarely address prostaglandins.

One well-known brand lists the following ingredients.

---

1. Strangely, Budoff was criticized because, although Ponstel® had been on the market for many years for relief of arthritis pain, it had not been approved by the FDA specifically relief of *menstrual* pain.

- *Acetaminophen*: Not an NSAID and less effective than aspirin (a mild prostaglandin inhibitor). Actual NSAIDs appear in only 2 out of 4 members of the product line.

- *Pyrilamine maleate:* Usually listed as "diuretic" but actually an antihistamine "to reduce irritability." An antihistamine can make you too sleepy to be snappish, but as it also blocks and binds acetylcholine, it can help block smooth muscle contractions.

- *Pamabrom*: For "muscle cramping," but primarily a gentle, electrolyte-sparing diuretic. It may help block increased pressure on blood vessels and nerves, thus preventing restricted blood and nutrient supply to muscles with resulting cramping.

- *Caffeine:* For fatigue or to counteract drowsiness from the antihistamine. One formula contains 60 mg of caffeine, roughly equivalent to 2 cups of coffee. Caffeine *increases* prostaglandins but is standard in migraine remedies as a gentle vasoconstrictor.

- *Diphenhydramine*: Better known as an antihistamine and sleep aid by its trade names, Benadryl and Sominex. Included in some *night time* formulas (see formula 5).

**TABLE 7.** INGREDIENTS THAT DO AND DO NOT INHIBIT PROSTAGLANDINS

| | Prostaglandin Inhibiting | | Prostaglandin *Non*-Inhibiting | | | | |
|---|---|---|---|---|---|---|---|
| | Ibuprof.[a] | Naprox.[b] | Acetamin.[c] | Pamabr.[d] | Pyrilam.[e] | Diphen.[f] | Caffeine[g] |
| 1 | | | 500 mg | 25 mg | | | |
| 2 | | | 500 mg | | | | |
| 3 | | | 500 mg | | 15 mg | | 60 mg |
| 4 | | 200 mg | | | | | |
| 5 | | | 500 mg | | | 38 mg | |
| 6 | 200 mg | | | | | | |

a. Ibuprofen (Trade names: Advil, Motrin, Nuprin). Formula 6 is ibuprofen only, 20 pills for $8. One aisle away, 300 pills are offered for the same dose and price.
b. Sodium Naproxen (Aleve, Naprosyn, Anaprox, Naprelan)
c. Acetaminophen (Trade name: Tylenol)
d. Pamabrom = diuretic (Trade name: Aqua Ban)
e. Pyrilamine maleate or mepyramine= antihistamine
f. Diphenhydramine = antihistamine (Benadryl and Sominex)
g. Caffeine. See page 234.

⁀n I was a teenager, it felt like someone was punching me in the stomach. Later I
⁀ that two naproxen sodium at the onset of my period, and maybe one the next
vas enough to keep real pain at bay. A rheumatologist friend recommends
⁀en over ibuprofen, due to lower dosing frequency (8-12 versus 4-6 hours) which
⁀ less stomach irritation and possibly less damage to filtering organs (liver and
⁀). Of course some people tolerate one or the other better, and should go with
rks for them.

—Emily Dolan-Gordon

Best to ignore the "feminine products" aisle where pills for PMS and menstrual cramps are the same as or less effective than generic NSAIDs at huge markup. Used correctly, NSAIDs will treat cramps from prostaglandins at the source. For an NSAID such as Motrin, Budoff advised:

1. Take 1-2 400 mg capsules after a meal or with milk immediately after the first sign of spotting or cramping. If cramps don't normally appear until the second day, you may wait and take it then.

2. Follow with one capsule every 3-4 hours, but no more than needed (limit: 6 per day). Do *not* tough it out, do *not* wait until the cramps get bad. You must *block* prostaglandin formation, not try to play catch-up once it has risen to painful levels.

   More recently, researchers found that a single table combining sumatriptan and naproxen was effective against both cramping and menstrual migrain, effectively blocking formation of prostaglandin that causes uterine contractions (Durham and others, 2010).


## MENSTRUAL MIGRAINE AND MAGNESIUM

Recent research implicates other issues in pre-menstrual syndrome and menstrual migraine. At the New York Headache Center in Brooklyn, NY, A Mauskop and others (2002) found that magnesium deficiency and / or levels out of balance with calcium played an important role in menstrual migraine. Testing 61 women with menstrual migraine for levels of ionized calcium ($ICa2+$), ionized magnesium ($IMg2+$), and total magnesium, showed consistent deficiency and/or imbalances of these electrolytes.

- Magnesium deficiency was found in 45% of women suffering menstrual migraines but dropped to 15% between menstrual periods.

- In menstrual migraines, calcium *levels* were within norms, but *balance* with magnesium was off, typically with calcium far too high.


Chemical imbalances that trigger migraine are brought on not only by poor nutrition or advice to overdose on calcium pills. They can also be triggered simply by *breathing*, especially in women.

# The Chemistry of Breathing

*Migraine can be a symptom of inadequate air supply, whether from sleep apnea, tight clothing, or energy over-efficiency at home or office and poor air exchange. If you always get a headache at the ski resort or yawn more than anyone else at closed-room staff meetings, you may have found a clue to your migraines.*

Lack of oxygen (as in sleep apnea) or low-oxygen environments (part of Sick Building Syndrome) is a powerful factor in migraine and other conditions.

Oxygen ($O_2$) is our most critical nutrient and we need a constant supply of it. Oxygen feeds cell function, improves mind / body coordination, increases energy, enhances confidence. Healthy breathing:

- Allows balanced intake of $O_2$ and excretion of $CO_2$. But $CO_2$ also has an important role in the body and must be balanced with $O_2$.

- Assists in mechanical circulation of fluids including blood and lymph.

- Improves cell and organ function, critical to higher brain function.

- Controls blood flow through the brain and therefore its metabolism, neuronal activity, and seizure thresholds (Fried R, 1993).

- Helps prevent hypoxia of depression and hyperventilation behind panic disorders.

- Assists mobility and health of the spine and the intervertebral discs through regular movement of the ribs.

- May be responsible for greatly improved health and well-being documented in regular church-goers. Besides increased social, emotional, and spiritual support, services that involve singing or chanting promote effective breathing.

- Can be used for relaxation, auto-suggestion, to form or modify habits and behaviors, improve learning, and sleep.

- Serves as a bridge between the conscious, subconscious, and unconscious levels of mind, linking concepts and sensations developed during various physical disciplines.

Poor health due to poor breathing is common and thoroughly documented in the medical literature. Symptoms of bad breathing range from dizziness, depression, anxiety and panic attacks, back and chest and arm pain (angina), numb or tingling or cold fingers, potentially deadly heart arrhythmias, high blood pressure, and tight crampy muscles — all of which are related, involved with, or linked to migraine headaches.

How is this possible? Via disruptions, biochemical and muscular, to the respiratory system, hence to the entire body, of which migraine is just another symptom.

## OXYGEN (O₂) AND CARBON DIOXIDE (CO₂)

> All physiology textbooks point to . . . the vasoconstrictive effects of sympathetic stimulation. But they fail to emphasize that low arterial blood $CO_2$ (low $PaCO_2$) is as powerful a peripheral vasoconstrictor as sympathetic stimulation.
> — Robert Fried, Ph.D. (1993), *The Psychology and Physiology of Breathing*

We tend to think of oxygen as "good" and carbon dioxide as "bad," a mere waste product to be expelled, but this is not so. The balance between the two controls the body's critical acid-alkaline (pH) balance. Ideally, blood is very slightly alkaline (a pH of 7.4).

*Too much $CO_2$ in the blood*[1] shifts pH below 7.4 (more acid). This is seen in upper chest breathing due to emotional stress, restrictive clothing, or poor posture. It can happen at high altitude and high humidity (less available oxygen) and in disease conditions that produce metabolic acidosis[2]. The result is vaso*dilation*, the hallmark of migraine.

*Too little $CO_2$ in the blood* shifts pH above 7.4 (more alkaline). This occurs during hyperventilation, especially with rapid, shallow "chest" breathing. When $CO_2$ is lost faster than the body produces it, blood vessels constrict (vaso*constriction*); less *oxygen* reaches brain and extremities, often a first stage of a migraine attack) and nerves become more sensitive. Numbness or tingling around the mouth is a common first symptom. Hyperventilation is so effective in constricting blood vessels that victims of acute head trauma are purposely hyperventilated to constrict swollen blood vessels which could cause deadly brain swelling.

Deep *diaphragmatic breathing* best maintains the $O_2$ - $CO_2$ balance but usually requires slower breaths. *Exception*: the heavily obese, heavy smokers, or those with metabolic acidosis. When $O_2$ supply and exchange are already low (*hypoxia*), or $CO_2$ is metabolically high (*hypercapnia*), slowing breath further can be deadly. Gas exchange is worsened by hot and humid weather, chronic pain or stress, and changes in elevation or the equivalent in the form of incoming weather fronts.

*Paradoxical breathing* is breathing with the upper chest while blocking the action of diaphragm, abdomen, and lower chest, forcing the muscles of abdomen and chest to work *against* each other while altering the $O_2$ - $CO_2$ balance. Paradoxical breathing:

- Centers expansion at mid-lung where gas exchange is less efficient.

- Moves air mostly between the upper and lower chest but little air *in and out* of the lungs causing air starvation in body and brain.

- Produces chronic muscle tension in respiratory muscles of abdomen, chest, and neck.

- Invokes the fight-or-flight response of the sympathetic nervous system.

---

1. *Hyper*capnia (too much) and *hypo*capnia (too little) $CO_2$ from (Gr.) *kapnos*, smoke.
2. Chronic anemia, diabetes, liver / kidney failure, cancer, shock, heart failure, dehydration, lactic acid from exercise or diet (milk products) can trigger hyperventilation as the body attempts to reduce acid levels by eliminating excess $CO_2$. See Chaitow L (2002); Fried R (1993).

Strained respiratory muscles (and the neurovascular tissues they entrap) can produce a wide range of pain and bizarre neurological symptoms ranging from headache and back pain to thoracic outlet and carpal tunnel syndromes. These commonly include:

- Rectus abdominis (associated with abdominal, stomach, and back pain), especially in persons who lock down abs to "suck in" a waistline,

- Diaphragm (which causes "stitches" in the ribs and shoulder pain),

- Intercostals (responsible for "stitches" in the ribs during active exercise),

- SCM (a common origin of frontal headache and nausea; see diagram on page 49).

- SCALENES (the neck muscle behind arm, back, and chest pain; see diagram on page 62).

Women are at special risk because progesterone stimulates respiration[1]. Pregnancy not only means eating for two, it also means breathing for two. Shifting into this state when *pre*-pregnant (pre-menstrual) sets the stage for hyperventilation and may be responsible for some PMS symptoms. During the luteal phase (day 22 on), $CO_2$ may drop by 25 per cent. Hyperventilation when $CO_2$ levels are already low can cause chest pain and panic attacks. This is worsened by Western cultural ideals of the heaving bosom and slender waistline[2] (or in men, flat abs). If breathing seems an unlikely trigger, remember that migraines are strongly linked with:

- Asthma or Chronic Obstructive Airways Disease (COAD).

- Hyperventilation (also associated with asthma and COAD).

- Depression: Decreased oxygen in brain decreases production of serotonin and other neurotransmitters.

- Menstrual cycle: $CO_2$ is lower in the later part of the cycle.

- Thoracic Outlet Syndrome: migraine may be a first symptom.

- Hypertension, stroke, and heart disease.

---

1. Men with identical symptoms are usually tested for heart attack (Chaitow L, 2002, p. 44).
2. This is perpetuated even in biofeedback breath trainers. A well-known brand instructs *men* to fasten the belt around the *diaphragm*. *Women* are told to fasten it around the *upper chest*.

# Specific Biochemical Issues

## INSOMNIA AND DEPRESSION

Today it seems that nearly every problem is attributed to serotonin and should be treated with anti-depressant Selective Serotonin Re-Uptake Inhibitors (SSRIs). Depressed? You need SSRIs. Fatigued? SSRIs. Sleeping too much or too little? SSRIs! "Because," we are told, "serotonin is the key neurotransmitter." OK, but if serotonin is key, what is the key to serotonin? Amino acid L-tryptophan in combination with Vitamin B6, magnesium, and Vitamin D. The Standard American Diet is typically low in all three. Levels in migraineurs are often extremely low.

Ideally, serotonin produces the sleep hormone *melatonin*, but, if the body is deficient in B6 and magnesium, it cannot make melatonin. Now we have sleep disruptions plus the deficiency symptoms of those individual nutrients: depression, disturbed sleep, disturbed neurological and muscular function, platelet clumping, poor resistance to stress, and more. If you don't provide your body with the raw materials, your body can't make the snazzy neurotransmitters needed to function. Sorry, but there it is.

For proper function, a body must be properly fed, watered, and exercised. Over a dozen basic nutrients have *depression*, sleep disorders, and muscle problems as their first presenting symptoms of deficiency[1]. These symptoms are commonly associated with migraine and commonly treated with antidepressants (because "depression hurts!") but they are also common symptoms of sub-optimal nutrition.

Imagine that it is your custom to make a piece of toasted home-made bread and jelly as a bedtime snack. It improves your mood and helps you sleep. Making the bread for the toast requires flour and water, yeast and eggs, butter and sugar. If you don't have those ingredients, you can't make the bread. No problem! I will give you a prescription for toast and jelly. And in theory, since you no longer need to make your own bread, you no longer need to be concerned about keeping those ingredients on hand in the house. But in fact *there is a problem* because those same raw materials are needed for other household products and activities, from making waffles and omelets to doing laundry and waste disposal.

Some products require other inputs. Obviously you can't make chocolate-chip cookies without chocolate chips. But you also can't make them without the fundamental basics of flour and sugar, and the minerals — iron, copper and zinc — that make up the oven, or without functioning wires and pipes from the utility stations.

Much of our health system is now based on prescriptions for toast or chocolate chip cookies while ignoring the raw materials.

---

1. One psychopharmacologist will not accept insurance because the companies refuse to pay for blood tests to check nutritional status of his depressed patients. Their rationale: if his patients are depressed, he should put them on anti-depressants for which they *will* pay.

## THE CHEMISTRY OF SLEEP

Insomnia is often interpreted as a symptom of depression because both conditions are intimately involved with serotonin. Melatonin, the sleep hormone, is produced in the pineal gland from serotonin (the "feel-good" hormone) in response to light.

Serotonin > Melatonin

We all suffer short-term depression and difficulty sleeping at some time. A bad day at work, noisy neighbors, a bed partner who snores, bad news and sad memories will do the job. These stresses produce stress hormones (such as cortisol and adrenaline) which block serotonin production, hence they also block melatonin.

Stress > stress hormones (cortisol / adrenaline)

No matter how cozy the bed or dark the room, melatonin cannot be produced without serotonin. Normally, melatonin is produced in the pineal gland from serotonin which in turn is produced from the amino acid tryptophan, that is:

Tryptophan > Serotonin > Melatonin

But biochemistry is rarely that simple. To make serotonin from tryptophan requires other raw materials including Vitamin B6, magnesium, and Vitamin D (the sunshine vitamin). To make melatonin from serotonin requires still more B6 and magnesium. No serotonin, no melatonin. So the pathway is actually:

Sunlight and Vitamin D

v

Tryptophan > Serotonin > Melatonin

^

B6 and Magnesium

The B6 we get from food and supplements must be converted to the biologically active form (known as P5P) before the body can use it. This requires an enzyme (pyridoxine kinase) which in turn requires zinc. So the pathway is really more like this: ,

Sunlight and Vitamin D

v

Tryptophan > Serotonin > Melatonin

^

(B6 + Zinc) > P5P + Magnesium

No zinc > no B6 conversion > no serotonin > no melatonin. And this will be true no matter how many calcium pills or yoga classes you take. It is especially true if you live in an area deficient in zinc[1].

Absorption of zinc (and other minerals) requires picolinic acid, an isomer of niacin[1]. Niacin is so critical to the body that if it is low, the body will try to make its own from the amino acid tryptophan. But this process is so extremely inefficient that it must be seen as a biochemical act of desperation, a last ditch survival strategy. Tryptophan is hijacked for niacin production at the rate of 60 to 1, that is, 60 units of tryptophan are needed to produce one unit of niacin. If there is no tryptophan left over to make serotonin, you are going to be short on serotonin and melatonin as well. But the body doesn't much care about that. The body sees this as a choice between happy and *dead* versus depressed but *alive*.

This is why niacin alone can correct depression and insomnia in *some* people (but not *all*). It is why depression and sleep disorders can arise from many seemingly different things: low levels of B vitamins, minerals, a low-protein diet, and a basement office. Even if protein and B vitamins are well supplied, all these chemical reactions require "energy packs" in the form of ATP (Adenosine Tri-Phosphate, from the Krebs cycle). Magnesium makes and breaks those energy bonds with every heartbeat and every muscle action.

Normally, as light increases in the morning, serotonin rises and melatonin falls. As light levels fall in the evening, melatonin rises. Artificial lighting has its place of course, but don't be surprised if you cannot go from a brilliantly lit room or TV to bed and sleep if melatonin never had a chance to develop. This is especially true if your late-night light (or computer screen) is *blue*.

Early morning light is shifted towards high energy blue frequencies. This is the light that told early humans that it was time to wake up and safe to come out of the cave. Towards nightfall, light gradually decreases shifting towards slower frequencies, the sunset colors of yellows and oranges and reds. Besides computer screens, blue LED lights have been showing up in many electronics along with complaints of sleeplessness. Avoid bright lights, especially blue ones, before going to bed.

Inappropriate levels of adrenaline at night when you're trying to sleep can cause insomnia and nightmares. This can occur in abusive or traumatic situations. You can also produce adrenaline by watching scary TV programs (such as the news) before bedtime, a good reason to keep TV out of children's bedrooms and perhaps your own

Sleep-disrupting adrenaline can also come from hypoglycemia. The brain lives on glucose and when it gets hungry it sends a message to the adrenal glands which produce adrenaline. Adrenaline converts glycogen (the storage form of glucose) back into glucose to feed the brain. Meanwhile, that hungry brain blocks production of serotonin. (*If Brain doesn't feel good, why should you?*) and melatonin (*Sleep? You want sleep? Not until you feed me!*)

---

1. Hedaya (personal communication, 2004) notes that his patients from Pennsylvania rarely have zinc deficiencies; those from the Washington D.C. area often do. It's the difference between a hard water limestone area and the soft water of the Atlantic Coastal Plain.
1. *Isomers* are chemicals with the "same-parts" but usually different properties.

This can be a problem with diets that strictly forbid any food after 6 pm. It can also be a problem with foods that spike blood sugar leading to an insulin crash and hypoglycemia during the night. A *light* bed-time snack, a balance of protein, carbohydrate and fat, can help to stabilize blood sugar and avoid being awakened by a hungry brain screaming for food.

## THE DARK SIDE OF SUPPLEMENTATION

Today it is often said that it is impossible to get adequate nutrients from food. That can be true, but it is certain to be true if you don't eat real food, if you try to live on heavily processed, "fun" foods, sugar or soft drinks as your major source of calories, or if you don't eat at all because your life is too sedentary to allow normal weight without drastic calorie restriction.

On the other hand, many of us have higher requirements than others due to many factors including genetics and geology. Yet vitamin and mineral supplements were long dismissed as unnecessary to anyone eating a balanced diet. All you would get, it was said, was "expensive urine." That claim can also be true, but it first requires that a balanced diet actually be eaten.

Problems may be less an issue of *expensive* urine than of frankly *toxic* urine. Yes, you can overdose on vitamins and minerals. Problems arise when:

- You don't know your actual nutritional status.

- Nutrients are out of balance.

- Supplementation is based on inaccurate information.

It can be foolish and dangerous to supplement with no idea of where or how you are. Many researchers now recommend levels well above the traditional 400 IU, but I've also heard of vitamin salesmen recommending 10,000 units per day. Vitamin D overdose is particularly nasty and may result in calcification of soft tissues . There is also evidence that too much Vitamin D with too little Vitamin A suppresses immune function. Before taking high ongoing doses of Vitamin D, get your blood levels tested. What you need depends your status, which you can't know without testing.

Read labels and notice what's really in the bottle[1]. I recently realized that what I thought was B-complex *only* was actually B vitamins *and* A, C, D, E, iron, selenium, copper, *and* chromium all in wildly different levels ranging from 25 per cent up to 5,000 per cent of the recommended daily value. Did I really need that? Not likely.

Beyond the MDR and the RDR there is the UL, the Upper Level of Tolerable Intake, the highest level of daily intake beyond which adverse health effects may begin to appear.

---

1. Don't confuse *milli*grams (mg) with *micro*grams (mcg or µg, 1/1000th of a milligram, or one millionth of a gram. Convert mcg to mg by moving the decimal three places to the left.

Like everything else, ULs vary by age and sex (and sometimes by race, as for Vitamin D). Do not exceed the UL without close medical supervision[1]. Manufacturers are not required to indicate whether their products exceed ULs and many do.

Lately there has been much emphasis on selenium "to protect against cancer." The upper limit of selenium intake verging on toxic is considered to be 400 *micrograms* per day. Just one ounce of Brazil nuts (about 6) can supply that and more. Adding pills can push a reasonable intake to toxic levels, especially in the Dakotas or eastern Montana where selenium in soils and crops reaches toxic levels (Muth OH and Allaway WH, 1963). On logging my food intake, I see that I am averaging over 200 per cent per day from food alone. Do I need to supplement with more? Probably not.

In contrast, my thiamine intake is consistently low. Supplement? Seems reasonable, but I hold in my hand a bottle of B1 (thiamine) containing 300 mg (20,000 per cent) of the daily value. It that sensible? Because B Vitamins are water soluble, they are generally believed to be safe at any dose. This is incorrect.

First, B vitamins work so closely together that consistent overdose of *one* is the best possible way to produce deficiency symptoms of *others*. Second, some B overdoses cause serious symptoms all their own. Toxic overdoses have been documented from supplements, not from food, although both contribute to the UL. There is no UL for B1 (thiamine), B2 (riboflavin), or B12 (cobalamin), yet keeping a reasonable balance seems more rational to me. Other Bs have revealed problems.

- *B6.* The UL is assumed to be 1 gram per day but overdose (with painful neurological symptoms and skin lesions) has been reported at levels as low as 200 mg per day.
- *Niacin.* High doses have caused dangerous liver inflammation.
- *Folic acid.* UL for adults is 1.0 mg. Excessive intake from supplements and fortified foods has been linked to symptoms including kidney damage and a doubled risk of prostate cancer. In a large study of diabetics with kidney disease, patients dosed daily with 2.5 mg folate (over double the UL — *why*?) with high-dose B6 and B12, developed *worse* kidney function with increased risk of heart attack, stroke, and death compared to the placebo group (House AA, 2010).
  Folic acid is the most sensitive of the B vitamins, destroyed by heat and air. If what was in the bottle is damaged in shipping or storage, the balance is broken.

Know what you actually need, and know what you're getting — or not. Keep a food and migraine diary, and for supplement safety see: www.ConsumerLab.com.

---

1. "Close medical supervision" does not mean, "Come back in 3 months and we'll see how you are doing." It means daily or weekly monitoring of status and potential side effects.

## PELLAGRA: THE "CORN DISEASE"

Pellagra is a deficiency disease caused by inadequate niacin. It spread with the introduction of native American corn (*maize*) to other populations; *pellagra* is an Italian word, describing the "rough-skin" typical of the disease that swept Europe after the introduction of the wonderful new grain from the New World. It was rampant throughout the American Deep South throughout the 1930s, in company with a diet of corn, fatback, and molasses.

Pellagra is another reason why you can't expect to live well on popcorn and bourbon[1]. Without special processing niacin is unavailable from corn. The body can make it from tryptophan, but this is metabolically expensive and impossible on a low-protein diet.

Native Americans boiled corn in alkali or lye. Known as *nixtamalization*[2], this process unbinds niacin, makes tryptophan more available, improves balance of amino acids, and destroys molds and bacteria. This is the process behind *hominy* corn, which, dried and ground, is known as *grits*.

The technique failed to transfer completely to Europeans who saw no point to the extra time and expense of extra processing[3]. The resulting "corn plague" caused centuries of disability and death in Europe and the US.

Today we just grind the corn, as the Italians did. Despite our heavily corn-based diet, we expect people to have other sources of niacin, from supplements or other foods, so pellagra is associated with poverty, alcoholism, and disease especially where other foods may be unavailable.

Pellagra is easy to treat, but easy to miss if one assumes that it is no longer an issue. It should be suspected in patients with any of the Three A's: Anorexia, Alcoholism, and AIDS, conditions which are very much with us today. In 2008, L. Delgado-Sanchez and others described a patient with the Three D's of "Diarrhea, Dermatitis, and Dementia" in Brooklyn, New York. Fortunately, her condition was recognized and treated before appearance of the fourth classic D: "Death."

Milder niacin deficiency may fail to raise alarm bells. Today, the early symptoms (slowed metabolism and decreased cold tolerance with irritability and anxiety, poor concentration, fatigue, apathy, insomnia and depression) are most likely to be treated with anti-depressants and sleeping pills. Women may be at higher risk; historically, their deaths from niacin deficiency have been double that of men. Like thyroid, niacin may be impacted by estrogen (Brenton BP, 2000).

---

1. Bourbon is made from corn mash.
2. From the original Aztec language (Nahuatl) from *nextli*, "ashes" (the source of lye) and *tamal*, "corn dough" familiar in Spanish / English as *tamale*, a corn-based food.
3. Modern Westerners fail to appreciate traditional fermentation techniques used by Eastern cultures to render soybeans edible.

## NON-PHARMACEUTICAL SOURCES OF SEROTONIN

There are at least four ways to increase serotonin levels without pharmaceutical drugs: meditation, bright light, exercise, and food.

PET scans[1] have measured synthesis of serotonin in the brain while subject thought about positive things or depressing things (Perreau-Linck E and others, 2007). Up moods? Higher serotonin. Down moods? Lower serotonin. The findings suggest a two-way flow, with serotonin influencing mood and mood influencing serotonin (Young SN, 2007). This can explain why Cognitive Therapy can be as effective for depression as drugs (DeRubeis RJ, 2005). It matters what you think about, where you dwell.

Bright light has long been used to treat Seasonal Affect Disorder (SAD) and has also helped women with Premenstrual Dysphoric Disorder (PMDD), an extremely severe form of PMS (Lam RW and others, 2005). Bright light is involved in serotonin production in the brain and autopsies have revealed lower levels in persons who died in winter than in summer (Carlsson A and others, 1980). This finding was verified in live human. Overall, serotonin levels were lower in winter, but varied with hours of sunlight exposure on the day samples were taken, regardless of season (Lambert GW and others, 2002). Attempts to depress healthy women by depleting tryptophan were successful in dim light, but completely blocked in bright light (aan het Rot M and others, 2007).

Like bright light, exercise increases serotonin levels and has worked as well or better than anti-depressant drugs. Exercise in bright light is even better, but increasingly rare. Many of us drive to work and come home again in the dark. Relatively few engage in the outdoor work labor of our ancestors. Even on cloudy days, outside light is almost always lighter than indoor light.

Aerobic exercise for depression and insomnia has been found to be just as effective as SSRI antidepressants for *some* people (but not *all*) because if the actual root problem is magnesium or related deficiencies, the exercise program wonderfully beneficial to one may offer little more than fatigue and muscle pain to another.

Why can't we just take serotonin pills? Because serotonin itself does not cross the blood-brain barrier. How about gobbling down a precursor such as tryptophan, said to be high in turkey? Sure, but there are many foods higher in tryptophan than turkey. Milk for example. Lactalbumin, in milk and whey protein, contains more tryptophan than most other proteins (and certainly more than a diet of soda pop and crackers). Chick peas, a Middle Eastern staple, are another source. Domesticated peas have tryptophan contents almost *double* that of wild varieties and almost two-thirds of it is free, unbound to the protein. Researchers suspect that seeds were selected for higher tryptophan content (Kerem Z and others, 2007).

So consider the possibilities: meditate, eat right, and dance and play in the sunshine, even when there are clouds in the way.

---

1. Positron Emission Tomography (PET) reveals changes in metabolic activity.

# Chapter 6

# Triggers and Thresholds

*Migraine can be a symptom of nutritional, structural, and emotional stress. It can also come from clothing, furniture, computers and car seats, trades and hobbies, even musical instruments.*

Some triggers are painfully obvious and well-known but there's much more to migraine than red wine, cheese, chocolate, and tyramines. These are the clichés of migraine. The problem with clichés isn't that they are untrue. It is that they tend to be accepted in place of further investigation. Many a migraineur has found that no matter how faithfully they eliminate these foods they *still* get migraines. Tyramines may be a factor, but not the only cause.

## Headaches of X Origin: Where Systems Collide

So, are your headaches myofascial? vascular? neurological? chemical?

Imagine that a bundle of nerves, fascia, and blood vessels arise through a hole in a granite counter top then spread out to supply distant muscles and organs. Drop a hammer on top of these delicate structures so they are caught between two hard, unyielding surfaces.

Would problems be vascular, neurological, muscular, or organic?

When tissue is sufficiently irritated to fire off alarms and protective responses throughout the entire system, the only good answer is "all of the above." The body is a *system*. *All* systems would be impacted.

Like Borromean rings (page 19), migraine triggers can interlock and collapse in very similar ways. You may be unaffected by any *one* thing, but put combine several triggers and you will have a migraine. Remove one and maybe, just maybe, you *won't*. Remove more, and your chances of losing your migraines are even better. The best migraine drugs can't work well if the source of the migraine pain is actually structural: strained muscles, distorted structure, or nerve involvement. The Rectus Capitis Posterior Minor, the smallest of the Suboccipitals, can strain the dura mater and neurovascular tissue in the brain, causing severe headache in addition to proprioception / balance problems, inflammation, and chronic neck pain (McPartland JM and Brodeur RR, 1999). It's hard to track the problem back to the source if one simply stops at the diagnosis of *migraine.*

Case in point, 9-year-old Andrew" suffered 6 months of relentless headaches. These were diagnosed as *migraines,* apparently on the basis of their severity only, because no matter how carefully questioned, he gave no description of the vascular pulsing and pounding typical of true migraine. Eventually the pain became so severe that Andrew could no longer engage in physical activities. He spent a month out of school, mostly sitting on the couch watching hours of TV and playing computer games. He spent days in the hospital on an amitryptaline drip with no relief.

As a last resort he was brought for biofeedback treatments but on intake he was found to have extremely tight neck and shoulder muscles. Gentle pressure on TRAPEZIUS and SCM immediately fired off a series of vagal responses.

Two events occurred before the headaches began.

- *Carrying a heavy load of school books.* On noticing this, father weighed the backpack and found that it weighed almost 30 pounds.

- *Orthodontic work.* Right before the headaches, a palate spreader had been removed.

On discovering the muscular and cranial issues, Andrew was referred out to Eduardo Cortina, a Washington, D.C. body worker. Cortina is not a physician or neurologist. He is a licensed massage therapist specializing in Upledger's craniosacral work and an instructor of Alexander Technique. A few sessions of cranial and postural work reduced Andrew's relentless headaches to one per week, controlled by 2 Advil.

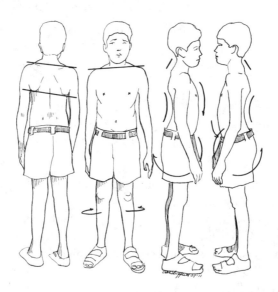

**Figure 88.** POSTURAL DISTORTIONS AND MIGRAINE

# Bones, Joints, and the Occasional Odd Wiring

*Migraines can be a symptom of malformed or misaligned bones, from feet to head. If you have a callus at the base of the second toe, a swayback, and you carry your head forward of your shoulders, you have found a clue to your migraines.*

Bones provide our solid framework. They also create the restricted spaces which allow pressures to build, compressing nerves and blood vessels. These distortions strain muscles and fascia. A less familiar concept is that bones can hurt too. Pain sensitive structures include the *periosteum*, the nerve-rich layer of tissue surrounding bone.

One of the best ways to trigger hysterical warning messages from neurovascular and myofascial tissues is by hitting them over and over and over . . . *with a bone.*

## TEMPORO-MANDIBULAR JOINT DYSFUNCTION

The Temporo-Mandibular Joint (TMJ) is the jaw joint between the temple and the the lower jaw (mandible). This structure is usually diagrammed from the outsidebut Figure 89 shows what's going on inside. Everything there is a branch of or supplied by the trigeminal nerve, from the muscles and ligaments, to the teeth and the nerve-rich, pain sensitive periosteum surrounding the bone, right down to the joint capsule itself. Here, muscular, vascular, neurological and structural interactions combine with potentially dire consequences.

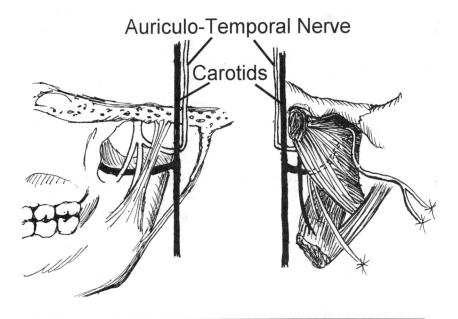

**Figure 89.** TMJD AND NEUROVASCULAR STRUCTURES

TMJD is not usually thought of as a neurological condition, but it can have devastating neurological impact on trigeminal, facial, and vagus nerves, triggering the trigeminal alarm system with other neurovascular symptoms we call "migraine."

Several jaw muscles are entrappers. MEDIAL PTERYGOID can entrap the chorda tympani nerve (a branch of the facial nerve) as it runs through the ear on its way to supply salivary glands and taste sensation to the tongue. LATERAL PTERYGOID can entrap the buccal nerve (a branch of the trigeminal nerve). A tight MASSETER can entrap the maxillary vein causing fluid backups in the network of vessels that drain the face. These three jaw muscles alone may be responsible for toothache, sinus pain, odd taste sensations, migraines, and more[1].

Some still sneer at the "laundry lists" of symptoms attributed to TMJD, partly because they are so *long*. But their length is the natural result of so many neurovascular impacts. Bones, teeth, nerves, and vascular supply all came into play, eventually firing off the trigemino-vascular alarm system. TMJD is specifically linked with migraine (Gonçalves DA and others, 2011).

All of this activity can start with muscle strain, whether from gummy bears and tough meat or clenched teeth and anxiety. Very often it starts with *malocclusion* (a "bad " bite or "closing").

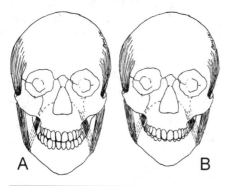

**Figure 90.** TMJD AND MALOCCLUSION

Upper teeth should fit on top of their lower counterparts (Figure 90-A). Teeth that do not fit properly require the jaw to shift eventually overworking jaw muscles.

Imbalances elsewhere in the body can also distort and unbalance the jaw stressing the joint and the teeth.

Results can range from *facets*, (shiny worn areas on teeth) or a lower jaw that appears oddly short, to severe neurological symptoms including migraine.

A jaw that must shift backwards in order to chew, producing an overbite (Figure 90-B), is especially damaging. With every bite, every chew, the condyle of the jaw slams into the joint and all its associated fascia, sensors, nerves and blood vessels.

---

1. The dentist will also look for infected, impacted, or otherwise damaged — or damaging — teeth. A former migraineur reported wisdom teeth growing in sideways and intermingling with and crushing nerves. Removing them removed the migraines.

There is a simple Ear Test for this:

1. Stick your little fingers in your ears and push them forward,
2. Move jaw normally as if chewing.
   You should feel *no* significant movement within the ear canal. If you feel the jaw slamming against your fingers,
3. Shift jaw slowly forward until you find the *first* position where pressure on fingers disappears. This is the point where your jaw needs to rest in order to relieve stress on muscles and nerves.

The Hat Test allows you to see and feel the strain of TMJD on the muscles of jaw and head. You can see this in any eatery where men wear their hats. You can feel it yourself with an inflexible and snug-fitting hat or headband.

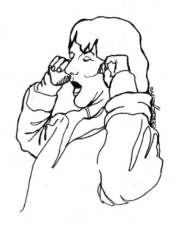

**Figure 91.** TMJD EAR TEST

1. Put on hat.
2. Eat something crunchy.
   If the hatband is sufficiently inflexible, you will feel every move of your jaw as muscles shorten and bulge. As in the TMJD Ear Test,
3. While chewing, shift jaw forward until you reach the first position where you no longer feel the bulging and pressure against the hatband.

If there is significant movement, you may have found a significant migraine trigger. It is even possible that some food sensitivities are not a problem of ingesting those foods, but a problem with *chewing* those foods. Chewing activates the FRONTALIS muscles of the forehead, another source of pain commonly diagnosed as migraine.

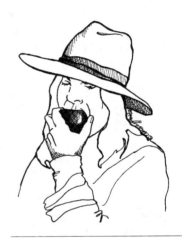

**Figure 92.** TMJD HAT TEST

Figure 93 is an sEMG trace of a patient with TMJD. The lower graph shows imbalance between right and left MASSETERS. The upper graph shows the FRONTALIS muscles firing in time with the MASSETERS

What is actually happening here? An interplay between muscles, nerves (both facial and trigeminal), bones and joints. Most problems originate not with the joint but with the muscles that should control it but cannot, allowing the jaw to move in ways that were never part of the original design. When the jaw slams against the joint capsule and muscles tighten around nerves that signal their distress, the trigeminal nerve sounds the usual alarm.

When TMJD became popular in the media, I scoffed at the latest fashionable ailment. (Earlier, all problems had been due to *hypoglycemia*). Later I was stunned to discover

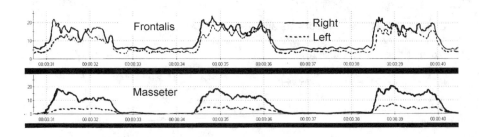

**Figure 93.** sEMG:MASSETER AND FRONTALIS MUSCLES

that a big part of my problem was simply that my teeth didn't fit. In such a situation, a properly designed splint can eliminate the daily grind on the trigeminal nerves and can make radical changes in migraine attacks. Mine dropped by approximately 50 per cent in frequency and severity.

.IRelief can manifest in other forms. A fellow student in a physical fitness program fell while rock-climbing, later suffering migraines and radical deterioration of physical condition. Rock-climbing requires excellent upper-body strength, but during almost two years in the program, I had never seen her manage more than two or three very shaky pushups, followed by total collapse. Noticing that her jaw seemed odd, I urged her to see my dentist. The results were striking. In his office, with splint in place, she went to the floor and did a dozen pushups.

Is TMJD an issue for you? See for yourself if there is any difference between how many push-ups you can do:

1. With teeth clenched and jaw shoved into the joint capsule versus
2. Jaw open, muscles stretched and relaxed.

Or, swing your partner! I loved contra dancing, but could never survive more than two or three "swings" without severe dizziness. An unexpected side effect of a good TMJ splint was the sudden overnight ability to outlast nearly everyone else in a dance consisting almost *entirely* of swings.

You may see a big difference. Or not. It may be enormously helpful to relieve a TMJD, or it may be a small part of the problem, just one of many neurological stresses that can add up to a migraine or severe tension headache.

Problems can even come from other sources. You can create an overbite with a Head-Forward posture alone. Sometimes proper jaw mechanics have been lost to childhood orthodontics that resulted in lovely, even teeth but life-long headaches. There's nothing for it but go back and do it right. See "Dentists" on page 236.

# NECK (CERVICAL) BONES

> By one of those unconscious divisions which assign the medical specialties according to certain anatomic landmarks, the cervical spine has become the province of the orthopedic surgeon. As a consequence, anatomic studies of the cervical spine, with its delicate and complex nerves and blood vessels usually emphasize the skeletal structures. Some very important organs are not given enough attention, and others are completely ignored, because of their seeming structural unimportance; but these are the very elements that, as the result of some disorder or injury, give rise to most headaches of extracranial origin. To the neurologist and the neurosurgeon, the spinal skeleton is important only as the support and viaduct of nerves and vessels which may suffer from encroachment due to any slight dislocation.
>
> —Emil Seletz, MD (1958)

Neck bones can be heavily involved in headaches. A first step in any head or neck pain is to check bones of the neck and spine for proper alignment.

Misaligned vertebrae can press on blood vessels and sensitive nerves. Every bone, every joint is surrounded by *periosteum* (the stuff "around the bone"). Periosteum (just another version of fascia) is richly supplied with nerves and capillaries. When two bones press together in ways they shouldn't, they hurt. Whether by accident or design, the professions most likely to help most simple causes of head pain are marginalized as "alternative."

## C1-C3

The *atlas* vertebra (C1) is the first vertebra of the cervical spine, the interface between spine and skull. Unlike other cervical bones, it is relatively free-moving, neither impeded nor reinforced by interlocking surfaces. It is secured only by muscles and ligaments. This allows great flexibility of head and neck, but also allows the atlas to slip out of alignment with relative ease.

Displacement is usually unrecognized and untreated despite serious consequences. Correcting the displacement reduced hypertension in a double-blind, placebo-controlled pilot study at the University of Chicago. Researchers reduced systolic blood pressure by 17 points and diastolic by 10. In adults, hypertension is defined as systolic pressure of 140 or higher and diastolic pressure of 90 or higher. Subjects beginning the study had a mean blood pressure of 147 / 92.5 which fell to 129.8 / 82.3 after treatment— well below the level requiring medication (Bakris and others, 2007).

Atlas vertebrae were rotated out of alignment by an average of just one degree. Returning them to their proper position (0 degrees rotation) produced the remarkable improvements in blood pressure.

C1 gives rise to (and can entrap) the suboccipital nerve which supplies SUBOCCIPITAL muscles. C2-C3 give rise to the greater occipital nerve. Distortions in this area may strain nerves and fascia, specifically the dura from brain and spinal cord which attach to the first 3 vertebrae.

## SKULL BONES

*Eppur si muove*!
"And yet it moves!"

—[Attributed to] Galileo

We tend to think of the skull as a sort of bowling ball with a couple of holes and a mouth, perhaps a movie screen behind the eyes, but otherwise, solid.

In fact, the skull is an amazingly complex structure made up of 8 major cranial bones and 14 facial bones. There are 22 skull bones in all, with holes for nerves and blood vessles, with joints in between. Joints? Do cranial bones move?

According to Western medical tradition they *do not*.

According to Eastern medical tradition *they do*.

That group East of here includes Italian physicians who traditionally considered fixed skull bones to be pathological. The case is strengthened by the presence of skull sutures that look remarkably like gliding joints — with intricate crenulations, like sliding dove-tail joints — joined by flexible fibrocartilage.

Belief that skull bones *do not* move in normal skulls beyond adolescence comes from some very old and very flawed research combined with a tradition of dissection involving preserved remains. (There is good reason why bodies pickled in formaldehyde are referred to as "stiffs.") Schools that emphasized fresh dissection, as the Italians, believed otherwise. Many modern studies clearly show that skull bones *do* move, apparently as part of a pressure relief system in brain and spinal cord.

In the 1980s, studies under the electron microscope revealed that suture surfaces are richly supplied by blood vessels and nerves. Which nerves? *Trigeminal* nerves. Thus movement of cranial bones (or lack of it) explains yet another migraine trigger and another issue in barometer headaches.

In the mid-1990s, these heretics were joined by NASA and Soviet space agencies for whom the physiology of pressure changes are critically important. They dismissed the notion of the skull as a rigid container of constant volume (Ueno and others, 1993, 1996).

In 2009, scientists at Lawrence Livermore Laboratories discovered that part of the mechanism of brain injury from surprisingly small explosions was because "direct action of the blast wave on the head causes skull flexure, producing mechanical forces in brain tissue comparable to those in an injury-inducing impact, even at non-lethal blast pressures." Skulls rippled along the sutures.

*Cranial-sacral rhythm* (CSR) is said by osteopaths and cranio-sacral therapists to be a regular involuntary movement of the skull unrelated to blood circulation. Others dismiss the existence of a separate CSR, and yet CSR or something like it is monitored in hospitals by means of a screw drilled through the skull to serve as a pressure gauge.

What *is* unusual is the idea that its tiny pulses can be detected by sensitive human hands. Not everyone can feel them. I can't, but there is no doubt about what a good craniosacral therapist or an osteopath with manual manipulative skills can do. For my clients and myself, they have repeatedly eliminated or greatly reduced barometer migraines. Lack of movement appears to be strongly related to severe headaches including painful and frightening neurological symptoms.

Skull movements are believed by osteopaths to regulate and relieve intra-cranial pressures (Upledger JE, 1983; Gard G, 2009). Pressure variations in cerebrospinal fluid control how much blood drains into veins. This beautifully fluid system can be changed in response to atmospheric pressure, injury and disease, or as we have seen, by lying down and sitting up. It can also be impaired by myofascial constriction.

The osteopathic tradition strove to recognize and correct relationships between all body parts, including skull bones. Their movement out of alignment and back in again via manual manipulation has been measured and documented. Oleski and others (2002) found angles of change averaging 2.5° for the sphenoid bone and atlas.

The sphenoid bone is considered to be the "keystone" of the skull. Correcting a mis-alignment of the sphenoid often improves other pain, especially barometer headaches. Skull-bone movements appear to be another pressure-release mechanism; if bones are locked in place due to birth injury or other trauma, internal volume is also locked in place. Pressure applied to bones in craniosacral therapy is intended to shift or release strain on the fascia of the brain.

These movements, or a pathological lack of them, can be affected by skilled hands. They can also be affected by feet.

## FEET

The "bio-imploded" (or collapsed — as in rounded, dropped shoulders, head forward, lower back flattened, off balance) posture resulting from long-standing hyper-pronation is a major (if not *the* major) perpetuating factor in this chronic condition. In my experience, this postural abnormality is present in most patients with chronic [myofascial pain syndrome] and must be corrected for treatment to be successful in the long term.

— Bernard E. Filner, M. D.

The base of the body is *feet*. Problems at the base can cause knee, hip, back, and head pain due to changes in posture, torque, and gait. You may have noticed all-over aches and pains beginning with something as simple as a blister on your heel.

The origin of many ills is in the bones of the feet, specifically those of the second toe and a condition with the wonderful name of "Dudley J. Morton Foot" or "long second toe[1]." But there's more to it than toe length; the real problem is enlargement of the *base*

---

1. Named for its description by Dr. Morton in 1934. Also known as "Classic Greek Foot" for its common appearance in Greek statuary where this configuration was apparently thought to be extremely elegant—at least as feet go.

of the second toe (second metatarsal head). This configuration is so common that it is difficult to class as "abnormal." It may be a simple artifact of footwear.

We tend to think of "foot-binding" strictly in terms of classic Chinese foot binding. In constrast, consider the hard leather shoes worn "for support" by Western children beginning as toddlers and on through adulthood. "In shoeless areas of the world," says an anthropologist, "feet look like Fred Flintstone feet, broad and blobby with widely spread metatarsals. Any problems with enlarged metatarsal heads simply vanish." If you have Western-style feet, you may need to understand why and how to make adjustments to avoid Western-style aches and pains.

The "balls of the feet" are the two rounded bumps at the base of the big and little toes (formally known as the metatarsal heads). Ideally, a tripod of support forms between these and the heel. The Morton foot lacks that stable tripod configuration. There may be no *balls* on which to balance; there may be only *a ball* in the middle of the foot, at the base of the second toe. Trying to balance on that is like trying to balance on a marble or a knife-edge, and that can be a tough balancing act indeed. It makes standing, walking, and many athletics far more difficult than they should be.

You can see the problems by doing a half-squat while standing in front of a mirror. Properly supportive feet and muscles should allow ankles to simply flex forward and back. With an unstable foot, arches, ankles and knees tend to collapse inward; attempts to maintain balance cause a cascade of muscle strain. Hammer toes form when toes constantly grip the floor. You may notice an odd bulge a few inches above the outside of the ankle, an overdeveloped peroneal muscle overworked by attempting to stabilize foot and ankle. When overworked muscles can no longer stabilize an unstable foot, the result is "weak" ankles and repeated sprains, knee, hip, and back pain that spreads upward to cause shoulder pain, jaw problems, and headaches.

The real clue is not the length of the toe, but the size of the metatarsal head.[1] Bending toes back may reveal a prominent mound at the base of the second toe that rises above the heads of all the other toes. If the head is large enough, a callus forms here. There may also be calluses on the outside of the big toe and in other areas as shown to protect against abrasion when the foot rocks inside the shoe. The base of the second toe can become painful. But padding the callus "to relieve pressure" (as directed on packages of commercial foot pads) will make the problem *worse*. Placing the pad below the base of the big toe re-establishes the stable configuration.

You can check your feet or check existing orthotics which may not be doing the job despite their expense. See instructions for "The $3 Test Orthotic" for testing only. *See a podiatrist for professional corrections.*

---

1. This is also true among fashionable women who are now having long second toes surgically shortened to look good in sandals, a process which brings its own set of problems.

## THE $3.00 TEST ORTHOTIC

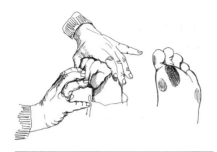

**Figure 94.** SECOND TOE AND CALLUS

Correcting imbalances caused by the Morton foot can be key to treating dysfunction elsewhere in the body. A podiatrist can make a good set of permanent orthotics but a temporary set for testing or emergency use can be made of Molefoam/Moleskin, duct tape, corrugated cardboard, and Dr. Scholl's Air Pillow insoles. Women use men's sizes; men use 2 sizes larger than normal shoe size. Trim as needed. Use no more than 2 layers of cardboard or padding. If you need more, you need to see a podiatrist for *immediate* professional attention. With a partner or mirror,

1. Stand comfortably with feet shoulder-width apart on a pair of shoe inserts; mark around feet and toes and cut to fit.

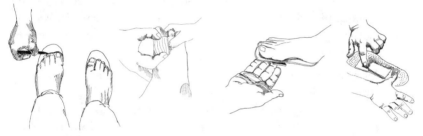

**Figure 95.** MEASURING AND PLACING PADS

2. Do a half squat (knee bend) *keeping heels on floor.*
3. Watch for any medial collapse of ankle and knee.
4. That is, do ankles or knees move in towards the centerline?
5. If ankles stay where they should and the knee does not deviate, you're OK. not . . . .
6. Apply a square of Molefoam sized to cover the bump at base of the big toe.
7. The foam should not touch the base of the second toe nor extend into the are of the arch.
8. Slip foam into position under insert. Squat again to test correction; increase layers until ankles neither collapse to the in-(medial) side nor deviate to the outside (overcorrection).
9. A knee that still deviates after ankles are stabilized needs arch support. For each one,
10. Cut 2 strips of Molefoam/moleskin or corrugated cardboard to reach between ball of the big toe to just in front of heel.
11. Test by squatting as above and add layers until the knee no longer deviates.
12. Tape the corrective pads into position on the underside of the insoles.

Dancers and others who practice barefoot may tape the pad to the ball of the big toe and wrap with athletic tape. End tape on top of the foot so that it will not pull loose.

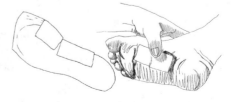

**Figure 96.** PLACING ARCH SUPPORTS

## HEADACHES FROM THE HIPS

Head and neck pain also arise due to pelvic distortions and one of the most common causes of the Head-Forward posture is a pelvis that is out of balance.

The pelvis is the structural center of the body. It may look and feel like one big bone, but is actually three separate bones joined by fibrocartilage. The sacrum fits like a wedge between the two rear "wings" forming the sacroiliac (SI) joints and supporting the lower (lumbar) vertebrae of the back. Traditionally, the joints between the three pelvic bones have been considered to be as fixed and immovable as the cranial bones, a notion coming from centuries of studies on cadavers. There is good reason why dead remains pickled in formaldehyde are referred to as "stiffs" but in live folk, the situation is very different.

The three pelvic bones can be torqued, twisted and tilted up, down and sideways. This can happen from shocks and blows, or through muscle strain. The pubic bone (actually two branches of bone "joined together" at the *symphysis*) can shift and move during childbirth or a bad fall and fail to return to proper position afterwards. Because the pelvis is a three-part structure, it is impossible for any one piece to be misaligned without distorting the other two. .

Even a perfectly shaped pelvis can be rotated too far forward at the hip sockets by muscles in front of the thigh (such as tight quads) or rotated too far backwards by muscles in back of the thigh (such as tight hamstrings). Think of the pelvis as a wheel or pulley seen from the side; the spine is perched on the rim, so any rotation shifts the base of the spine along with the wheel as it turns or tilts forward or back. In the normal

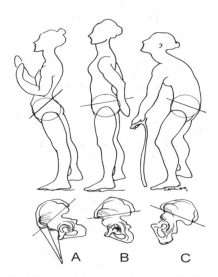

**Figure 95.** PELVIC ROTATION: FRONT, NORMAL, AND BACK

position (Figure 95 B) the "hip bone" (the Anterior Superior Iliac Spine or ASIS) is approximately aligned with the pubic bone.

*Posterior* pelvic rotation places the ASIS *behind* the pubic bone flattening the back and causing a hunched-over posture. *Anterior* rotation places the ASIS *forward* of the pubic bone with swayback and protruding buttocks. It gives the odd appearance that legs are following along behind the rest of the body. "Big Butt" can certainly be due to generous padding, or genetic variations in the position of the sacrum. It can also be a severe anterior pelvic rotation.

With "Big Butt" comes "Big Gut." Normally the viscera are cradled in the bowl of the pelvis. When the pelvis rotates too far forward, the abdominal contents spill forward over the pelvic rim, straining against the abdominal muscles. So what looks like "fat" isn't necessarily. For a quick test,

1. Lie on your back on the floor or other solid surface.
   Soft tissue should shift and adapt to the surface; bones will not. In this position,
2. Check for a swayback by reaching a hand between back and floor.
   If a hand or arm fits easily between your back and the floor, chances are excellent that at least part of the problem is anterior pelvic rotation.

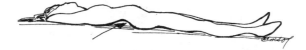

Therapists measure pelvic tilt by finding the Anterior Superior Iliac Spine (ASIS) and Posterior Superior Iliac Spine (PSIS) and comparing their angle to a horizontal line. The proper angle of pelvic tilt in males is considered to be 0-5°, in females 0-10°.

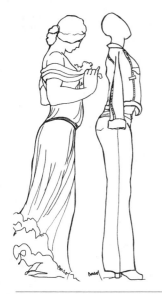

**Figure 96.** THE FASHION PELVIS

An anterior tilt of 40° or more (producing a swayback or "bubble-butt"), is often seen in gymnasts and dancers. A posterior tilt is commonly seen in persons with shortened hamstrings, especially the elderly. The result of either posture can be head, knee, and back pain because when the pelvis is wrong, everything is wrong. The body must strain to adapt to body mechanics that are completely outside of design specs.

Through the 1920s until recently, women's fashion emphasized *posterior* pelvic rotation with hips thrust forward and buttocks flattened or tucked under. Mannikins for trendy young female fashions are now being made with a swaybacked posture that hasn't been seen since the early 1900's. Then it was known as "the fine figure" and controlled with corsets and stays. Weak or shortened muscles will also do the job.

## ARMS AND LEGS

In most ethnic groups, elbows normally reach almost to the waist. In others they do not. This structural condition is primarily a problem when *sitting*.

Belief in "short leg" is common, but a genuinely short leg is rare; the diagnosis should always be verified by X-ray and precise measurements. The real culprit is usually muscular, especially the QUADRATUS LUMBORUM (QL) muscle of the lower back. This unfamiliar muscle is one of the most common causes of short leg and persistent lower back pain. QL hikes up the hip; if short and tight, one leg appears shorter than the other. Simply inserting a heel lift under the apparently shorter leg perpetuates the problem by encouraging the muscle to shorten even more, worsening the problem. Walking casts do the same; a half-inch of cast under one foot means a short leg on the *other* side.

A leg may also appear short due to a short hemi-pelvis, a congenital condition in which the pelvis or one of the sitz-bones is actually smaller or shorter on one side. Sitting creates a tilt to the shorter side. Everything above must shift to compensate. This produces a functional scoliosis as the body tries to keep head and eyes level, eventually straining muscles throughout the body.

# Postural Strain

One individual may experience his losing fight with gravity as a sharp pain in the back, another as the unflattering contour of his body, another as constant fatigue, and yet another as an unrelenting threatening environment. Those over forty may call it old age; yet all these signals may be pointing to a single problem so prominent in their own structures and the structures of others that it has been ignored; they are off-balance; they are at war with gravity.

— Dr. Ida P. Rolf

### THE HEAD-FORWARD POSTURE

The Head-Forward posture has been seen as elegant and glamorous since the days of Nefertiti, at least in women. Strangely, it is never as attractive in men, who are labeled as "mouth breathers" and "knuckle-draggers" when muscle strain begins to take its toll.

In men, what *is* admired is a "military" or "regal" bearing often developed by necessity. The importance of good body mechanics becomes painfully clear when wearing a heavy crown, a 5-pound medieval helm, or heavy equipment on a long march. Attempting to support weight with muscle rather than bone is a terrible strain.

And yet, the ramrod-straight military posture is more form than function, more for display than actual application. You will see it at Buckingham Palace and the Tomb of the Unknown Soldier. You won't see it in war zones where the goal is to be low and small, to be less of a target, possibly while heavily loaded. WWII infantryman (such as Bill Mauldin's ever-weary riflemen, Willy and Joe), carried about 80 pounds of equipment. Today the load averages more than 100 pounds.

"Depending on the soldier's job," notes Army veteran Chuck Gordon, "it may run as high as 200 pounds. The average load for an infantry rifleman includes up to 60 pounds of body armor, a 3-4 lb Kevlar helmet (K-pot), primary weapon and ammo that can range from 5-6 pounds up to 15-20 pounds for a machine gunner. A mortar troop

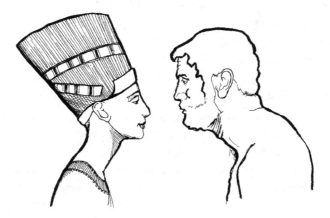

**Figure 97.** THE ELEGANT HEAD-FORWARD POSTURE

may carry an additional 15-20 pounds of mortar gear and ammo. Add rucksack, personal items, food and water, and a foot soldier may be carry anywhere from 30-105 per cent of his or her body weight into combat.

In combat zones, troops are on duty 24 hours a day, 7 days a week, catching sleep when they can. Even in "rear" areas troops will likely be required to wear body armor and carry primary weapons round the clock, working 12-16 hours a day, 7 days a week."

Members of the military are fighting a war on two fronts: with hostile forces and with their own equipment and enormous physical wear and tear. Overt damage includes traumatic brain injury (TBI) and amputations from explosions, but a more insidious damage is muscular and structural. Many vets see civilian physicians with no military experience of their own, and no idea of what combatants have been through or why they might have terrible back pain and headaches.

Monsters and devils are typically portrayed with Head-Forward posture. Perhaps they snarl and behave so badly because they *hurt*. The Head-Forward posture strains muscles of back and neck. It also strains jaw muscles (Figure 98).

The more forward the head, the greater the pull to open the jaw. Attempting to keep the jaw closed keeps jaw-*closing* muscles under constant strain. These include MASSETER, TEMPORALIS, and PTERYGOIDS, all involved in TMJD. All can cause brutal pain on their own, and all can trigger the trigeminal alarm system so heavily involved in migraine.

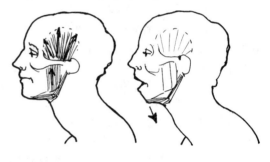

**Figure 98.** HEAD-FORWARD MUSCLE STRAINS

The Head-Forward posture also shortens chest muscles, rotating shoulders and arms (and knuckles) forward, impeding proper breathing and reducing oxygen supply.

It also deforms the neck. Ideally, the weight of the head rests on the neck bones which are separated by discs that act like springs. The further the head moves forward, the harder muscles must strain to keep it from falling down. Stress on bony attachments produces bone spurs. Aging bones may even develop stress fractures and remodel into the classic dowager's hump which is not at all elegant. Other problems arise.

When the neck tilts forward, face and eyes are tilted down. To see forward, head and chin must tilt up. This is the job of the SUBOCCIPITAL muscles. One of these (RECTUS CAPITIS SUPERIOR MINOR) connects directly to the dura of the brain and spinal cord. Strain on the dura means strain on the meninges and its complex network of nerves and fascia and blood vessels. The result may be migraine of "mysterious" origin.

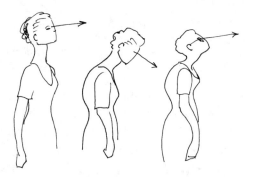

**Figure 99.** HEAD-FORWARD POSTURE AND SUBOCCIPITALS

Another problem is the straight neck that has lost its curve (also known as "Military Neck"; see Figure 108 on page 243). A normal curve acts as a spring. Normally, discs and vertebrae compress and rebound vertically and obliquely forward. In a straight neck, they are vertically compressed with every step, which can lead to disc narrowing and stress fractures.

Head-Forward posture and abnormal spinal curves are strongly associated with TMJD which is also associated with bad bite, but you can change your bite simply by changing your posture.

While standing up straight, ears over ankles (have a friend help you with this),

1. Relax your jaw completely then tap your teeth together. Note position.
2. Move your head strongly forward (into a classic "mouth-breather" pose) and notice how your bite changes.

# Foods and Additives

> She had never forgotten that, if you drink much from a bottle marked "poison," it is almost certain to disagree with you, sooner or later.
> —Lewis Carroll, *Alice's Adventures in Wonderland*

We tend to think of food sensitivies as problems with the food itself. But problems can originate in contamination and breakdown products, additives, and processing side effects that are blatantly toxic. Food sensitivity is a common migraine trigger, often disguised so effectively by a 2-3 day delay, that we may fail to recognize a problem.

If you suffer migraines, you have probably been given a list of common "trigger foods" usually consisting of foods high in tyramines. You may find that faithfully following the list makes absolutely no difference in your headaches. There are at several reasons for this. Besides common triggers like red wine, chocolate, liver and onions:

1.  Tyramines do not reliably cause migraine. Standard tyramine-containing food lists have little in common with foods actually found to trigger migraine under laboratory conditions, including injection of tyramines into the body (Jansen SC and others, 2003).
2.  Your headaches are not triggered by food intake, but by other food-related factors such as chewing. Or,
3.  Your headaches are triggered by almost all the foods you eat, because the triggers are the additives and preservatives present in almost all processed foods.

The problem may also be the condition of the food, processed or not. In some people, any decay — mold, pathogenic bacteria, toxins, or breakdown products — may trigger an alarm which triggers the trigeminal system which triggers a migraine.

Nerve fibers that respond to or secrete catecholamines[1] are in the pain-sensitive dura mater surrounding the brain. When brain is exposed to formaldehyde vapors, catecholamines are detected. More catecholaminergic nerve fibers were found in the dura at the base of the brain than in the upper regions and more were found *surrounding* blood vessels than in the areas *between* blood vessels (Cavallotti D, and others, 1998).

Unfortunately, tests for food sensitivity are still uniformly unreliable. The best route is to eliminate obvious triggers and take sensible steps to avoid the not-so-obvious ones. Buy fresh food, store it in the coldest part of the refrigerator (the door is the warmest). Eat it fresh and don't even think of using the week-old casserole.

Our automated food supply system increases opportunities for bacterial infection while decreasing traceability. Meat from many sources, impossible to track, is ground in a very few central processing plants then shipped around the country. Enjoy your hamburger but have it ground at the butcher's and enjoy it *thoroughly* cooked. Save "medium" and "rare" for meat from a known source or ground in-house[2].

---

1.  Catecholamines (from the adrenal glands) are also known as "stress hormones," more familiar as neurotransmitters epinephrine (adrenaline), norepinephrine (noradrenaline) and dopamine.
2.  The documentary movie *Food, Inc.* makes the reasons for this vividly clear.

## ALLERGENS AND SENSITIVITIES

Many have been identified as migraine triggers. These include, some say, all the ones worth eating. Some are highly variable, perhaps due to variability in the food itself. For example, while citrus is a common trigger, I could safely eat an orange but not commercial orange juice (see page 137).

Buy locally and buy in season. It is your best chance for peak nutritional quality and avoids an unfortunate legal loophole: Is a pesticide banned in the US? No problem! It is simply sold across the border and applied to foreign crops that are sold right back to us as raspberries in January.

Observe your asthmatic friends and when something fires them off, take notice. Apples are not on the standard migraine food lists but they almost always gave me a migraine. Then I learned that an asthmatic friend risked anaphylactic shock if she bit into an unpeeled apple. No peel, no asthma, no shock. And for me, when I followed her example, no migraine.

Some of this is variability in the person, for example, those who recommend a banana diet as a sure cure for migraine. Individual successes may reflect individual issues such as low potassium. For me, bananas have always been a no-fail migraine trigger. Something in me does not like bananas. I, in turn, do not like Honeydew melon or Delicious apples; to me they produce a nasty metallic aftertaste, noticed by other migrainous friends over the years, although too few to draw any sweeping conclusions. Perhaps it is genetic. If your family hates the taste of a popular food or has a tradition that "onions are poison" it is best to pay attention.

On the other hand, some food sensitivities have nothing to do with the food itself, everything to do with what has been added to it.

## MSG AND OTHER EXCITOTOXINS

*Excitotoxins* are added to food to block the "tinny" and "stale" flavors of canned, packaged, and over-processed foods. They create wonderful taste sensations ("You can't eat just one!") They allow manufacturers to use lower quality ingredients by fooling the brain into thinking that the food tastes much better than it does. They do this by exciting the brain cells to death. Hence the term.

The most familiar excitotoxins are free glutamates in the form of Mono-Sodium Glutamate (MSG) and aspartame (found in various artificial sweeteners). Both are powerful migraine triggers, a statement for which many food companies swear there is "no evidence." There is plenty of evidence by researchers not funded by food companies. You may disagree with it, but the claim that there is *no* evidence is just plain wrong[1]. How then, can the conclusions be so different?

The food industry specializes in many short studies lasting no more than an hour or two, but as migraineurs and asthmatics know all too well, symptoms of a trigger may appear hours or days later. Some double-blind trials failed to show significant reactions compared to placebo, or, subjects taking the placebo had reactions that were strangely worse than those in the "challenge" group — because aspartame and/or MSG were used in both the challenge samples *and* the placebos. Other creative approaches have been used. For example, of all test animals:

- Human brains are the *most* sensitive to glutamates.

- Monkeys aren't much bothered.

- Mice are closest to humans in sensitivity (although less sensitive than humans). Therefore, *if you are looking for real results,* the best test animals are mice.

In vivid contrast, a widely quoted safety study:

- Used monkeys and fed MSG at rates known to induce vomiting.
  At a professional conference, the investigator is said to have admitted that the monkeys had vomited (which would invalidate the test) then denied it later in print.

- Sedated the animals with the most powerful glutamate antagonist known.

- Presented results showing "no damage" based on a sample taken from the wrong part of the brain (Blaylock RL, 1997).

- Conclusion: MSG is safe for the real test animal, *you.*

Glutamate is one of the building blocks of protein. Hence, *free* glutamate is formed by hydrolysis, breaking protein back down to its basic components. This is why the phrases "protein isolate" and "protein concentrate" appear on labels rather than the relatively rare "MSG" which so many people are now trying to avoid despite protests by the food industry that MSG is *natural.*

Free glutamate is harmful precisely because it *is* natural. Areas with the most glutamate receptors are most vulnerable to glutamate damage. One of these areas is the heart. Another is the hypothalamus, the control center for such diverse functions as appetite, endocrine glands, thyroid and sex hormones, sleep-wake cycles, immunity, and emotional balance.

It has been known for decades that excitotoxins actively destroy brain cells. When magnesium (a natural channel blocker) is low, calcium floods into the neuron, changing osmotic balance and attracting water. The neuron balloons to several times normal size and dies within an hour or two, along with the neurons attached to it. Many researchers link excitotoxins to neuro-degenerative diseases such as Parkinson's, Alzheimer's, Amyotrophic Lateral Sclerosis (ALS, "Lou Gehrig's disease") and such diverse conditions as sudden cardiac death and Irritable Bowel Syndrome (IBS), even "restaurant coronary."

---

1. Blaylock RL (1997) includes an extensive bibliography with explanatory comments on the research. Read it for yourself.

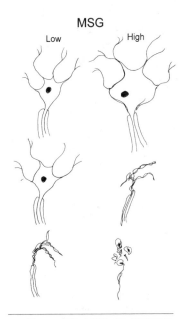

**MSG**

Low      High

**Figure 100.** MSG AND NEURONS

(After Blaylock R (1996)

In concussion and stroke, injured cells release a flood of free glutamates that cause damage for hours or days after the initial trauma. In 12 severely brain injured patients, levels rose high enough to destroy neurons within 24 hours of the injury, reaching their highest point 48 to 72 hours after the injury (Baker AJ and others, 1993).

You can't recover from brain injury if you re-injure your brain on a daily basis. You can't overcome migraines by living on additives considered to be a serious migraine trigger by every headache clinic in the country[1].

Excitotoxins can be absorbed through the skin, a possible explanation for reports of adverse reactions to many personal care products containing "hydrolyzed protein."

Glutamates cross the blood-brain barrier and the placental barrier from mother to unborn child. In the US, MSG was banned from baby food in the 1970's. *In theory*, babies no longer swallow MSG with their strained carrots, but you will still find these ingredients in food for toddlers. Feeding your child from the table? The amount of MSG added to adult foods in the US has doubled in every decade since the 1940's. They are now almost impossible to avoid and especially damaging if you are actually hungry. Excitotoxins are absorbed more easily on an empty stomach and from liquids (such as soups, juices, and diet sodas) than from solids. And glutamate damage is greatest when magnesium is deficient and blood sugar is low.

If you choose to eat these products that is your choice, but it should be *your choice*, not something that you are fooled into, *especially if they trigger asthma or migraines*. The issue is what is good for *you*, not how many other people are *not* bothered. If it causes you problems, don't eat it. Onions are generally recognized as safe, but for me, a single bite of raw onion once meant a nasty three-day migraine.

The best defense is cooking from scratch. If that is not possible, read labels with an eagle eye. In the following lists the suffixes *-lyze* and *-lys* indicate a "breaking." *Hydrolyzed* protein is "broken" into its component amino acids; one is glutamic acid.

---

1. Aspartame was once included in Merk's Maxalt-ML; some patients got worse after taking it (Newman LC and Lipton RB, 2001). It was later removed, and Maxalt is now considered one of the better migraine drugs.

Free glutamates destroy brain cells regardless of the source, whether combined (or not) with sodium or potassium (or their equivalent in Latin), whether they arrive via meat or vegetarian cuisine, and whether or not the label claims "no MSG added" as the actual MSG content is so often disguised behind other words.

---

**TABLE 8.** ADDITIVES WHICH ALWAYS CONTAIN FREE GLUTAMATES

- Autolyzed yeast

- Gelatin, powdered or capsules

- Hydrolyzed gelatin, protein, or plant protein

- Hydrolyzed oat / soy / wheat / corn flour

- Hydrolyzed vegetable protein (HVP) (Typically contains 10-30% MSG).

- Monosodium Glutamate (MSG) and Natrium Glutamate (*natrium* is simply Latin for "sodium")

- Monopotassium Glutamate (MPG) is glutamate bound to potassium.

- Plant protein extract; this includes wheat protein isolate, soy protein isolate or concentrate. May also appear as protein from peas, beans, corn, etc.

- Sodium / calcium caseinate (casein is milk protein)

- Textured protein

- Whey protein concentrate (from milk)

- Yeast: autolyzed, extract or as yeast food

---

**TABLE 9.** ADDITIVES WHICH COMMONLY CONTAIN OR ARE FOUND WITH MSG

- Bouillon cubes, broth, and stock

- Disodium guanylate and disodium inosinate. These costly food additives work in combination with low-cost MSG. If they are on the ingredient list, MSG is almost certainly in the food even if not stated on the label[a].

- "Flavoring" and "Natural flavoring": may contain 20%-60% MSG.

- Malt extract, malt flavoring

- "Natural beef / chicken / pork (etc.) flavoring": may contain 20%-60% MSG.

- "Seasoning" and "Spices"

---

a. Inosinate is said to increase the flavoring power of MSG "by fifteen-fold" (K Lopez-Art, 2010). In theory, if present, there may be *less* MSG, but there's no way of knowing.

**TABLE 10.** ADDITIVES WHICH MAY CONTAIN MSG OR ASPARTAME

- Carrageenan

- Croutons (extremely high)

- Diet foods and diet / Diet / sugar-free sodas (aspartame)

- Low-fat and fat-free foods (removing the fat removes much of the flavor; MSG enhances what's left)

- Enzymes (especially *protease* enzymes, used to break down proteins)

- Salad dressings (extremely high)

- Soy protein concentrate and isolate

- Sugarless gum (aspartame)

- Ultra-pasteurized dairy products especially those containing carrageenan

## RECIPES

Crackers and salad dressings are some of the worst offenders. Can't live without them? You can make your own in less time than it takes to run to the store.

### Basic Crackers

Preheat oven to 400 degrees F, bake 12-15 minutes.

1 cup flour
1/2 tsp baking powder
1/4 tsp salt
1/3 cup water
3 Tablespoons vegetable oil
1 egg white + 2 Tablespoons water
Toppings: Seeds (sesame or poppy), herbs and spices (thyme, oregano, hot pepper flakes) your choice.

1. Preheat oven and lightly grease a cookie sheet.
2. Combine flour, baking powder and salt. Combine water and oil.
3. Mix wet and dry ingredients together and stir into a smooth dough.
4. Roll out dough thin and flat on sheet. Prick with fork and score with a pizza cutter.
5. Beat together egg white and 2T water. Brush mixture onto top of dough and sprinkle with desired topping. Bake, cool, and enjoy!

### Salad Dressings

Simple, inexpensive, and safer to make at home. You'll find the basics in any general cookbook (such as the venerable Joy of Cooking), hundreds more on the Internet. For these and other recipes, with user ratings, see:www.allrecipes.com .

### Sausage

Trying to avoid flavorings and preservatives but miss your breakfast sausage? You can make that too. *Sausage* is an ancient meat preservation technique involving chopped or ground meat that has been "salted," spiced, and flavored, often with garlic, sage, rosemary or wine, all of which have anti-bacterial properties.

For example, Andouille sausage is made of ground pork, salt, garlic, black and red peppers, mace, allspice, thyme, sage, and red wine. Bratwurst contains pork, salt, sugar, coriander, sage, paprike, cayenne, rosemary, mustard, pepper, and nutmeg.

Casings are available at most grocery stores but spiced meat packed in a box is still sausage. Hundreds of recipes are available on the Internet. Even if you don't them, it's good to know what's in a product beyond the "spices" listed on commercial labels. Some people are allergic to allspice[1]. Knowing that an ingredient is used in one sausage (but not others) can be valuable information.

See: www.thespicysausage.com.

---

1. Allspice was known to produce seizures in Brian Othmer, who apparently died from a slice of spice cake. See his story at www.EEGInfo.com.

## SULFITES

*Sulfites* are sulfur-based antioxidants that prevent wilting and discoloration in foods, especially light-colored ones that tend to brown when exposed to air, such as lettuce, guacamole, apples, coconut. In shrimp, lobster, and crab they prevent *melanosis* ("black" spot), a harmless but unappetizing discoloration. Sulfites develop naturally in wine and beer during fermentation but are also added to kill wild yeasts and fungi on grapes, and added to finished wines (especially whites) to kill bacteria and preserve color. They condition bread dough, bleach flour and cornstarch, and stabilize drugs. They work so very well that they were banned from use in meats not because of sulfite safety but because of *meat* safety. Sulfites preserve a fresh pink color in meats that might be days or weeks old (while destroying thiamine and other B Vitamins).

Sulfites have been in common use since at least the 1600s and approved for use in the US since the 1800s. So many uses over so many years earned them GRAS status, which indicates a substance is Generally Recognized As Safe, so safe that it is exempt from FDA restrictions. If added to a food it need not be listed on the label. But for some sensitive people (especially asthmatics) sulfites are extremely *un*safe. Reactions can range from asthma attacks, hives and swelling, to nausea, stomach cramps, diarrhea, and headaches, anaphylactic shock, and death.

In 1982, after many reports of severe reactions, including deaths, the Center for Science in the Public Interest (CSPI) petitioned the FDA to rescind GRAS designation for sulfites but little happened. Sulfites, after all, were safe for *most* people, but 10-year-old Medaya McPike, an asthmatic, wasn't one of them.

In 1985, at a local restaurant, Medaya ordered her "usual," a guacamole tostada. At home, half an hour after finishing the sulfite-laced meal, Medaya went into cardiac arrest. She was resuscitated at the emergency room but with brain damage so severe that she died 5 days later. Her death prompted Congressional hearings leading to a 1987 FDA ban on sulfites on *fresh* fruits and vegetables in salad bars and supermarket produce, and required warning labels on all sulfite-containing prescription drugs.

In 1990, after thousands of reports of reactions and several deaths from canned and frozen potatoes, the FDA revoked GRAS status of sulfites on fresh and frozen potatoes that would be served unlabeled to consumers. In announcing the ban, the FDA again emphasized that sulfites are harmless to *most* people, estimating that about one person in 100 is sensitive. But levels in foods vary widely. While they rarely exceed several hundred ppm they may approach 1,000 ppm.

Companies are now required to list sulfites or chemical combinations that give rise to sulfites of at least 10 ppm or higher[1]. They must also list any sulfates with "functional effect" in the food regardless, of the amount present. Ronald A. Simon of the Scripps Clinic Research Institute, notes that severe reactions can be triggered by trace

---

1. The equivalent "ink concentration" would be 40 drops in a 55-gallon barrel of water.

amounts as low as 5 ppm and even today, the FDA continues to recall foods due to illegal or undeclared sulfites (Grotheer and others, 2005).Asthmatics are at greatest risk. Sulfite reactions in nonasthmatics are *said* to be rare but they happen, typically within 15-30 minutes of eating. The reason for sensitivity is uncertain, but it can develop at any time, sometimes not appearing until middle age.

Migraineurs may fail to notice sulfite headaches because headaches are business as usual. One day after lunch at a salad bar I returned to my office with yet another migraine. "Oh!" said a co-worker from across the room, "You have a migraine." Yes, but how could she *see* that? We often complain that migraine is invisible; we don't break out in spots. But apparently I did. "When you have a migraine," she said, "your neck turns red." Apparently this happened every time I went to the salad bar. Lettuce sprayed with sulfites was giving me headaches I could easily have avoided.

Sulfites appear on labels as *sodium* or *potassium sulfite, bisulfite, metabisulfite*, or as *sulfur dioxide gas*. Even bulk foods at the deli or restaurant must list this information; ask the clerk. If you know you react to sulfites, carry an antihistamine.

### TABLE 11. SULFITE-CONTAINING FOODS

| | |
|---|---|
| Alcoholic Beverages | Beer, cider, wine and wine coolers, drink mixes. |
| Baked goods with dough conditioners | Cookies, crackers, crusts for pie / pizza / quiche; flour tortillas. |
| Condiments | Dried and glacéed fruit and jams, horseradish, cocktail onions, pickles and pickle relishes, olives, salad dressing mixes, and wine vinegar. |
| Dairy Products | Filled milk (skimmed milk with added vegetable oil) |
| Fruit | Trail mix, maraschino cherries, fillings and pectin jelling agents; juices (lemon, lime, apple, grape), shredded coconut. |
| Gelatin | Flavored and unflavored, in puddings and fillings |
| Grain products | Cornstarch, modified food starch, spinach pasta, hominy, breading and batters, noodle/rice mixes, tempura. |
| Meat products | Gravies and sausages. |
| Molasses | Sulphur is added to immature sugarcane. *Un*sulphured molasses is from mature sugarcane and of higher quality. |
| Seafood | Clams, shrimp, lobster, scallops, crab, fresh or in soup mix. |
| Sugar and syrups | Brown, raw, powdered, or white sugar, corn (high fructose), maple syrup, and fruit toppings. |
| Soups | Dried soup mixes. |
| Teas | Instant and liquid concentrates. |
| Vegetables | Pickled / canned vegetables. A popular vegetable juice lists "natural flavors"; the low-sodium version lists "natural flavors" *plus* disodium guanylate, disodium inosinate *plus* sulfites. Prepared guacamole may also be extremely high as Medaya Piked learned to her sorrow. |

# Sleep and Sleep Disruptions

*Sleep deprivation can make you sick and crazy. It's a classic technique of abusers, and linked to increased risk of serious diseases ranging from diabetes to cancer.*

> Within everyone there is a battle between "Morning Guy" and "Night Guy." Night Guy doesn't care that Morning Guy has to get up, sober-minded and alert, to go to work; Night Guy wants to party all night, and Morning Guy hates him for it!
>
> —Jerry Seinfield

Exposure to light when it should be dark has a powerful impact on a body's internal clock, hormones, and metabolism, leading to stress, weight gain, migraine and more.

Our biological clock controls sleep, wakefulness, and myriad other biological processes, but the clock is controlled by cycles of light and dark. Through millions of years of evolution, daily and seasonal patterns of light and dark were the one constant and reliable trigger for eating, sleeping, mating, and migrating. Disrupt those signals — easy to do with artificial lights, shift work, and the absurd notion that we should all be available 24/7 — and you disrupt everything else.

The part of the hypothalamus responsible for sleep/wake cycles is the SCN nucleus. Its cells are sensitive to light. For sleep, keep the room as dark as possible. If you must have a nightlight, stick to red. Red light is slow wave, low energy wave. The red glow of coals in a stone-age fire pit would have done little to disrupt sleep; late-night surfing with a blue computer screen, or blue LED on a bedside radio *will.*

Your body works best when it is exposed to regular cycles of light and darkness. Thanks to electric lighting, late night TV, and computer exposure, there may be *no pattern at all.* To correct this, *make* a pattern.

- Get some outdoor sunlight exposure during the day, every day.

- At evening, reduce brightness and wavelength of artificial light. Avoid fluorescent lights (which tend towards the high energy blue end of the spectrum) in favor of the more golden glow of incandescents.

- Avoid eating heavy meals within 4 hours of bedtime. Do have a light bedtime snack which includes some fat, protein, and carbohydrate.

- Go to bed at a regular time as soon as possible after natural dark — turn off the phone and other potentially disruptive devices.

- Keep the bedroom as dark and quiet as possible or wear a sleep mask. Limit night lights, including clock radios, to red.

- Get up at a regular time. Get a sunrise clock to wake more naturally.

# Infections and Antacids

*Helicobacter pylori* is a bacteria now firmly linked to ulcers. But, whether or not you have ulcers, one symptom of infection can be migraines. Migraineurs found to be infected with *H. pylori* had significantly more migraines (without aura) with no differences in GI symptoms. Nevertheless, when the bacteria was treated, headaches completely disappeared in 17 per cent of patients. In 69 per cent of the remaining patients, intensity, duration, and frequency were significantly reduced (A Gasbarrini and others, 1998).

*H. pylori* colonizes our stomachs where other bacteria cannot normally live because of the extremely acid environment[1]. Once established, it also works to reduce acidity in the areas it has colonized, rather like intrepid pioneers who, having staked a claim on the wild frontier, send home for oriental rugs and china tea sets to make things more comfy and home-like. But lower acid makes the stomach more comfy and home-like for other bacteria and far worse for us. Food can't be digested; it just sits there and rots. This is great food for opportunistic putrifying bacteria, but for us, many nutrients are unavailable leading to lowered immunity, metabolic problems, and frank deficiency diseases. There are three basic types of antacids.

- *Calcium carbonate and other alkalies.* Used to neutralize stomach acid. These include OTC brands such as Maalox, Mylanta, Rolaids, Tums.

- *H2 blockers.* Histamine triggers acid production so H2 drugs work by blocking histamine receptors in the stomach's acid producing cells. They begin working within an hour; effects may last for up to 12 hours. Brands include Zantac, Pepcid, and Tagamet.

- *Proton pump Inhibitors (PPIs).* These inhibit creation and secretion of stomach acid. Effects may last for 24-72 hours. Brands include Nexium, Prilosec, and Prevacid.

In 2009, US sales figures for PPI drugs alone surpassed $300 billion, better for the drug companies than for the patients. Read the small print on the patient information sheets and you will find warnings to limit use to no more than two weeks *because of severe side effects if taken longer.* These include include fatigue, depression, constipation, diarrhea, increased risk of osteoporosis and hip fractures, and *headaches.* There are interactions with cardiovascular, epilepsy, and antifungal drugs and increased risk of infection with pneumonia, salmonella, and *Clostridium difficile* ("C diff", a bacteria that causes diarrhea and other intestinal upsets). PPIs can also create dependency; if the drugs are discontinued, former users may suffer through a one-to-two-week rebound period of *increased* acid secretion This is a high price to pay for an initial condition that may have been due to stress and bad food in the first place.

The war against stomach acid may also be associated, in part, with the increase of migraines in women since the 1980s.

---

1. Normally, the acidity (pH) of stomach acid ranges between 1.5 and 3.5. Vinegar usually measures around 2.5. Acid in the stomach and acid in the pickle jar both inhibit bacteria.

# ALCOHOL

> Alcohol is a very dirty drug in that it does not interact with just one system.
> — Scott Swartzwelder, MD

Alcohol may be a pleasure, but it's also a poison. It damages brain neurotransmitters including dopamine, serotonin, GABA, and glutamate. It destroys B vitamins including thiamine (B1), a cofactor of enzymes involved in cardiac and vascular / microvascular function. Besides being hard on your liver (which must break down the toxin), alcohol interferes with deep REM sleep. If we ignore all that, there's still the problem of wanting to avoid headache, for migraineurs, an iffy issue when alcohol is involved.

One of the problems is *congeners*. These develop during fermentation and, like their buddy ethanol, they are extremely poisonous. While your liver works to break down the alcohol, congeners contribute to the upcoming hangover. In general, the more expensive and lighter-colored alcohols contain fewer congeners. In theory, the darker the drink, the worse the hangover. Whiskey, brandy, rum bourbon and red wine have more congeners than high quality vodka, gin and white wine (but watch for the sulfites that keep it white). Bourbon is said to be the worst of all. That said, if you have a hangover, taking Tylenol or NSAIDS for the pain, risks liver and kidney damage.

# TOBACCO

Tobacco sets the stage for migraine in several ways. Nicotine constricts blood vessels reducing oxygen to tissues. It is also an outstanding source of toxins.

Tobacco products contain over 40 known carcinogens with hundreds of other toxins. Besides nicotine, tar, and carbon monoxide, there is also formaldehyde, ammonia, hydrogen cyanide, arsenic, pesticides, and radioactive radon products. In the short term, smoking is associated with high blood pressure, coughing, and breathing disruptions, which can cause headaches all by themselves. Migraine has been linked to infections, and smoking (whether first- or second-hand) definitely causes infections.

It has long been thought that high rates of lung infections in smokers was due to decreased lung function and immune response thanks to destruction of Vitamin C and other effects. Now it turns out that tobacco itself provides a broad range of pathogenic bacteria.

In 90 per cent of samples, researchers found pathogenic bacteria that cause food poisoning, fever, diarrhea and cramps, botulism, pneumonia, urinary tract infections, ulcers and skin infections, periodontitis, meningitis, endocarditis, destroy red blood cells, and produce endotoxins and carcinogenic nitrosamines (Sapkota and others, 2010). *Pseudomonas aeruginosa,* found in *all* the cigarette samples tested, is the leading cause of all hospital-acquired infections in Europe and the US.

# Barometric Changes

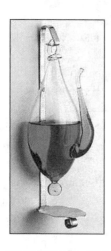

**Figure 101.** WEATHER GLASS

When I was a child, my father kept an empty but sealed half-gallon metal gas can in the jumble of tools on the floor of his car. There was always an entertaining pop as he sped up and down a steep hill on the road home. The empty metal can was serving as an aneroid barometer[1]. You may have had a similar experience while driving through hilly country with a plastic water or soda bottle. And so, perhaps, has your brain.

Pressure changes cause many physiological changes. Many who once questioned the reality of migraine have experienced the vivid reality of Altitude Sickness.

Pressure rises regularly with decrease in altitude and falls with rise in altitude, up to about 10,000 feet where rate of change shifts markedly. Many have problems at high altitude, or at their normal altitude when exposed to the pressure equivalent in the form of stormy weather.

You can see this effect most vividly with a "weather glass," the original water-based barometer. It looks like a distorted glass teapot, half-filled with water. The narrow spout rises from below water level to above the water level. Air is easily compressed but water is not. Water in the spout seals in air but rises and falls with air pressure changes. When air pressure is lower than when the body was sealed, water rises up the spout; when pressure is lower, the water in the spout drops. The change is more striking than a small dial on the wall, and helps to make the effects of pressure change more visible to others.

## WEATHER AND STORMS

At sea level, barometric pressure normally ranges between 28 and 31 inches of mercury, falling in stormy weather and rising in fair. Tissues expand and contract, often with painful results. This is the physiology behind the weather-predicting bunion or arthritic knee. For many migraineurs, pressure changes are a game of atmospheric Whack-a-Mole, the source of many headaches.

In March of 1993, the Atlantic Seaboard was hit by a "thundersnow," a *snow hurricane* complete with thunder and lightning and one of the lowest barometer readings ever recorded in Virginia. What was especially notable (besides swirling snow lit by bolts

---

1. In contrast to the original water barometer, an *aneroid* barometer has "no fluid." It is a made of a flexible metal box or cell from which most of the air has been removed. An internal spring prevents the box from collapsing but small changes in external air pressure cause the box to expand or contract, in turn driving a dial that indicates air pressure.

of lightning) was the headaches. I wasn't bothered much out of the ordinary, but after the storm, many Normals commented on the terrible headaches they had suffered, *the worst they had ever had.*

One of the greatest fears and frustrations of chronic migraineurs is never knowing when the next attack will strike. www.Accuweather.com provides several health indices including Aches & Pains, Allergy, and Respiratory, with a US map of pollen (grass, tree, ragweed, and mold). Changes in temperature, humidity, and pressure are presented as visual charts and numeric values ranging from Beneficial or Neutral up to Extreme Risk. Watch the reports to see how well they correspond to your headaches, or if they correspond at all.

These maps may not be ideal, but they reveal useful trends, especially if you track all three; the Migraine Index alone does not appear to cover all the bases. At the end of August, I was surprised by a week of relentless headaches. They correlated poorly with the Migraine Index of 1-2 (Beneficial), better with the Arthritis Index of 4-5 (neutral to mildly risky), all too well with high levels of Mold and Ragweed Pollen (6). As I write this on a September morning, severe storms are moving in. Although weather is not the trigger it used to be, my head is slightly achy and body a bit puffy. Migraine Risk is said to be low (2) but weather-related Arthritis Pain index is High (8). I do not suffer arthritis but the pressure changes, which cause joint pain in arthritics, can also cause pain in migraine brains and bodies.

## ALTITUDE AND HYPOXIA

The percentage of $O_2$ in air remains at approximately 21 per cent, but air pressure (and number of $O_2$ molecules per unit of air) drops as altitude increases. Bodies accustomed to low altitudes try to adapt by producing more oxygen-transporting red blood cells. This makes blood thicker, a situation worsened by dehydration. The painful or fatal results are called "mountain sickness."

Sensitivity varies. For some healthy people, symptoms of acute altitude sickness can begin to appear around 6,500 feet (2000 meters). It is very common above 8,000 feet (2,400 meters). At 10,000 feet (3,050 m) most low-landers find it difficult to breathe.

The primary symptom of altitude sickness is *headache*, but this is also a first symptom of *dehydration*, common at high altitude because water vapor from the lungs is lost more easily in the thinner air. Altitude sickness is diagnosed based on headache plus:

- Lack of appetite, nausea, vomiting,
- Fatigue, weakness, drowsiness, but also insomnia,
- Shortness of breath on exertion, dizziness or light-headedness,
- Peripheral edema (swelling of hands, feet, and face),
- Persistently rapid pulse.

Similarities between altitude sickness and migraine inspired tests of sumatriptan in treating altitude sickness. Success was limited and fleeting, suggesting that some underlying pathophysiology of migraine is missing (Utiger D and others, 2002).

The best treatment is prevention. Altitude acclimatization is the process of adjusting to decreasing oxygen levels at higher elevations by producing oxygen-binding red blood cells. Experienced mountaineers emphasize "climb high, sleep low." The idea is to never sleep more than 1,000 feet (300 meters) higher than the point where you have acclimated. This is why a high-altitude climb such as Mt. Everest takes many weeks. It isn't trudging up to the peak that takes so much time (or these days, waiting in line). It is the repeated ascending and descending from one base camp to another and back again trying to acclimate. This process is necessary even with supplemental oxygen. Acute mountain sickness can progress to life-threatening High Altitude Pulmonary Edema (HAPE) or High Altitude Cerebral Edema (HACE)..

**TABLE 12.** LOCATIONS AND ELEVATIONS

| Location | Feet | Meters |
|---|---|---|
| Washington, DC, USA | 0-409 | 0-125 |
| Pittsburgh, Pennsylvania, USA | 1,223 | 373 |
| Salt Lake City, UT | 4,226 | 1288 |
| Denver, Colorado, USA | 5,281 | 1,609 M |
| Glacier National Park, Wyoming, USA | 6,280 | 1,914 |
| Machu Pichu, Peru | 7,710 | 2,350 |
| Park City Ski Resort, Park City, UT (max) | 10,000 | 3,049 |
| Cuzco, Peru | 11,152 | 3,399 |
| Snowmass Ski Resort, Snowmass, CO (max) | 12,510 ft | 3,813 |
| Mt. Everest, Himalayas, Nepal | 29,035 | 8,850 |

If you're not a mountain climber, why do you care? Because barometric changes also apply to incoming weather fronts and to the stresses and strains of travel.

Passenger airliners climb to altitudes of around 30,000-40,000 feet, but cabins are pressurized to between 5,000 and 8,000 feet. Some passengers may suffer symptoms of altitude sickness just as they would if they were on the ground in Denver or Machu Pichu. On long-haul intercontinental flights, take all possible precautions. Even "Normal" passengers may suffer the symptoms of altitude sickness. Dehydration and alcohol will add to any problems.

En route to high-altitude destinations,

- If flying, schedule an intermediate-altitude stopover. In keeping with "climb high, sleep low," spending the night at an intermediate elevation may save pain and discomfort. For example, if flying from Los Angeles to Denver, consider a stop-over in Salt Lake City. On the other hand, avoid "puddle jumpers" with repeated take-offs and landings.

- Drink plenty of water for several days before leaving to avoid dehydration; supplement to avoid electrolyte depletion. See "Water" on page 138.

- Avoid alcohol / coffee / diuretics on the plane and for 24 hours after arrival at altitude. This may require pre-flight preparation as a sudden halt to caffeine can trigger painful withdrawal headaches.

- Avoid strenuous activity for the first 24 hours at altitude.

- On the ground, take the slowest routes or travel in stages. Problems may occur after a too-rapid ascent or descent. Take the scenic route, take breaks, take pictures.

- Avoid crossing the 10,000 foot boundary.

There are two commonly cited examples of recent and rapid human evolution. One is the spread of lactose *tolerance* in adults among Europeans about 7,500 years ago with domestication of goats, sheep, and cattle. The ability to digest milk in adulthood opened up a vast new food resource, renewable daily.

The other is adaptation to high altitudes as seen in Tibetans, a shift that opened up new pastures and water supplies. Some 3,000 to 7,000 years ago, Han Chinese moved up to the Tibetan plateau at altitudes of 13,000 feet and higher. The thin air has 40 per cent less oxygen than is available at sea level, yet Tibetans rarely suffer mountain sickness. When biologists compared genomes between Tibetans living at 14,000 feet and Han Chinese living just above sea level, they found some 30 genes rare in the Han but now common in Tibetans. The most outstanding example was gene HIF2a found in a mere 9 per cent of the Han but 87 per cent of Tibetans (Wade N, 2010).

Tibetans with this gene have fewer red blood cells and less hemoglobin. The mystery: How is it possible to compensate for a low oxygen environment by making even *fewer* red blood cells? Whatever the mechanism, it is a textbook example of natural selection: Han Chinese living in Tibet suffer infant mortality triple that of native Tibetans.

But hypoxia and its damage can occur for many reasons other than altitude.

# Other Environmental Stressors

In my family, migraines are said to be genetic.

Uncle Billy suffered severe migraines all through his life until, one day while plowing, a rock shot up and smashed him in the forehead. After the injury was repaired with a metal plate, he took great glee in triggering metal detectors, but he never had another migraine. "So here's what you do," he would say. "Take a rock. . . ."

Alas! It didn't work for me. Despite being hit in the head with rocks, mats, concrete and curbs (and even an elbow while contra dancing) they only got worse. They became hellishly worse —in a building where chemists and geologists worked with toluene, bromoform, and hydrofluoric acid. I rarely used these, but shared an office with an ammonia-based blueprint machine and a photographic dark room. Air intake was over the loading dock where truckers would idle their engines on rainy days.

Every Tuesday morning, like clockwork, I woke with a screaming migraine, regularly landing in the emergency room (Normals with contacts complained of itchy eyes). Since I was well enough on weekends to play soccer, backpack, and do other fun things, I was obviously just lazy, and it nearly cost me my job. Some 10 years later, long after I had resigned, a former co-worker, now the Safety Officer, called to report that all that time the safety hoods in the chemical labs had dumped fumes *not* to the outside, but back into the inside air, apparently a hideously misguided attempt at energy efficiency. I may have a genetic tendency for migraine, but I was also poisoned.

"Sick Building Syndrome" includes obvious stressors such as toxic molds and bacterial infections. Low levels of air exchange and oxygen supply can cause severe problems for persons whose oxygen supply is already compromised, especially when this is combined with off-gassing from carpet, building materials, and cooking.

## CARPETS AND LAMINATES

Many construction materials are toxic, offgassing formaldehyde and other fumes. But one of the worst is carpet, which may be treated with formaldehyde and pesticides, offgassing a host of other toxic chemicals. Industry spokesmen have claimed that formaldehyde, benzene, and toluene (all carcinogens) are no longer used in manufacture of synthetic carpet. Oddly enough, emissions of all three of these chemicals have been found in new carpet samples by several investigators. In a study by the US Consumer Product Safety Commission (CPSC), formaldehyde was found to be one of the top eight emissions (Duehring C, 1993), odd behavior for a chemical that isn't even there.

Carpet alone isn't the only offender. Rubber backings and glues may be a large part of the problem. If you must have carpet, opt for woven natural fibers (avoiding mothproofing pesticides) and secure with carpet tacks rather than glue. For more information,see the following article from the *Townsend Letter for Doctors and Patients* (August 2001) available on-line at:

http://findarticles.com/p/articles/mi_m0ISW/is_2001_August/ai_78177235/

For reports from the carpet installers themselves, including a list of the over 1,000 chemicals used in synthetic carpet see: www.holisticmed.com/carpet/tc2.txt

## CARS

Even that new car smell is toxic. Cars contain or produce dozens of chemical toxins ranging from bromine, chlorine, heavy metals and allergens to frank carcinogens. The worst offenders are vinyl (PVC or polyvinyl chloride), flame retardants, and break-down products created when these materials are exposed to heat and sunlight. Among the worst: Chevy Aveo, the Mitsubishi Eclipse, and the Honda Tucson. See more at: www.healthystuff.org/departments/cars/product.using.php

## NON-STICK COOKWARE

Over-heated, non-stick coatings break down and give off toxic fumes that kill birds. If you don't keep birds why should you care? Because these same fumes sicken and injure humans. It's just that the birds get sick and die *first*. If you are a migraineur, spring-loaded to respond to toxins, *you* are the canary in the coal mine kitchen. Non-stick coatings are everywhere: on broiler pans, drip pans, cookie sheets and entire oven interiors. Combined with a high-temperature self-cleaning feature, these can be deadly to pets and maybe to you.

Some reports claim there is no danger below 600 °F, said to be "well above normal cooking ranges." Not so, according to tests commissioned by the Environmental Working Group (J Houlihan and others, 2003). They found that drip pans *under* the burners (the cool spot) may reach 1,000°F, but problems begin long before that.

Birds are reported to have died in the vicinity of biscuits baking at low temperatures (325° F) in a coated oven. At 446°F (after just 2-3 minutes heating), toxic particulates are released. At 680°F (easily reached on a burner on "high") coatings release at least 6 toxic gases, and MFA, poisonous to humans at even low doses. At 1,000°F, non-stick coatings break down to PFIB, a chemical warfare agent, that causes severe lung edema in humans, similar to the lung edema seen in dead birds.

In humans, symptoms of "polymer fume fever," go largely unrecognized, appearing 4 to 8 hours after exposure and easily mistaken for symptoms of the common flu: chills, fever, chest tightness, perhaps a mild cough, and *headaches*.

Consider cookware of stainless steel, cast iron, ceramic, and glass. If you use non-stick pans, save them for *low*-temperature cooking such as delicate sauces and eggs. Never use them for frying or browning meat (which they don't do very well anyway). And if birds are dropping dead in your kitchen, it can't be a very healthy place for you either.

## CELL PHONES AND OTHER EMF SOURCES

We are increasingly awash in a sea of electronic signals. Much of this electronic fog now comes from cell phones and their towers. The biological stress is believed to come from the signals that resonate with biological systems. We are all unshielded antennas, as anyone will know who remembers being required to stand in a particular spot to improve TV reception during the "rabbit ears" years of television.

Many people and many studies report problems including fatigue, sleep disruptions, memory, and headaches. Larger better-funded studies find no problems and conclude that the various complaints should be attributed to other causes including imagination. Others retort that the funding comes from special interest groups more concerned about profits than public health.

Again the problem may be the trigeminal nerve. Cutting the nerve in homing pigeons eliminated their ability to detect magnetic fields (Mora CV and others, 2004). Perhaps for some humans, the problem is they also detect those fields, all too well.

In working with LENS, a stim neurofeedback system (page 260), extremely sensitive migraineous clients have been quite aware of tiny signals. These are said to be below the level of human awareness. And yet, "I see *blue*," they will say. These tend to be the same clients who get headaches if they talk too long on a cell phone. (See Kramarenko AV and Tan U, 2002).

Why this is, we don't yet know. At least the jury is still out. Cell phones and microwave towers are *supposed* to be safe, and we hope they are, but wishful thinking does not make it so. Err on the side of caution. See a map of cell-phone towers in your area at:www.antennasearch.com.

Meters and test equipment (and yes, even tin-foil hats!) are available from: www.LessEMF.com.

See safety rankings of cell phones at: www.ewg.org/cellphone-radiation

## AIR QUALITY

Air and fumes can trigger headaches just as surely as food, water, and muscle strain.

### *Pollen*

If you have two weeks of migraines on the same two weeks each May, find out what's blooming (and where it's *not*). Get tested for your local allergens. Before making any major moves elsewhere, get tested for *those* local allergens.

An Eastern migraineur triggered by mold thought that a move to the Western desert would be just the thing, only to discover that she is allergic to sagebrush. In contrast, a woman from central Texas, violently allergic to Juniper pollen (which blows during the winter, triggering life-threatening bronchitis and pneumonia) found relief by moving East to humid mildewy Maryland.

## Air Pollutants

Headaches from air pollution are many and varied. In Norway, nitroglycerine ("dynamite") headaches, from local soapstone mines, were frequently found (Sjaastad O and Bakketeig LS (2006). Mining and processing of oil and gas, can produce hydrogen sulfide ($H_2S$) a poisonous natural gas which also arises from more natural sources. HS affects the body much like cyanide; headaches are just one of its many nasty effects.

Normal air levels are less than 1 part per billion (ppb) but heavier than air, it accumulates in low-lying areas. It can reach concentrations of thousands of parts per billion (Skrtic L, 2006). Common sources include pulp mills and wastewater treatment plants, high sulfur oil and gas fields, including poorly plugged wells, refineries, flares, and compressor stations, volcanic vents, and decaying organic material including swamps, marshlands, and animal feed lots.

High risk days for various allergens are tracked at: www.Accuweather.com.

The EPA Air quality index for ozone and particulates is available at: www.airnow.gov.

# The Fashion Migraine

*Migraines can be symptoms of ill-fitting clothing and accessories. Why your migraines may be coming from shoes, bags, wallets, and even glasses frames.*

## UNDERWEAR

The days of whalebone corsets may be gone, but modern versions of steel and Spandex can damage circulation, nerves, and muscles as efficiently as their predecessors.

### BRASSIERES

Brassieres with narrow straps combined with heavy breasts can directly traumatize TRAPEZIUS. Underwires and side stays can also cause damage. Look for *wide* straps and proper fit. Anything tight enough to leave a red mark is too tight or too narrow.

### GIRDLES

The corset has reappeared as a desperate remedy for the thickening waistlines of aging Baby Boomers. Known today as "body shapers" these offer the same side effects as their historical forebears by compressing nerves and blocking circulation. But pressing belly fat into the aorta or vena cava can trigger heart attack or stroke. The same is true of the man's too-tight belt.

### KNEE BRACES

Eastic braces are often worn to treat swelling, but should never be worn to support an unstable joint and never worn tighter than intended. They should always have a cut-out space at the back of the knee to allow normal circulation through the popliteal artery in the back of the knee. Blocking this artery can lead to continued or even worse swelling and Deep Vein Thrombosis (DVT), in which case, headaches may be the least of your problems. If a knee is actually unstable, see your doctor for prescription braces that to support the joint rather than merely compressing its blood supply.

## OUTERWEAR

Heavy coats that hang from the shoulders can strain TRAPEZIUS and other muscles, while tight compressive clothing can strain everything else.

### TIGHT JEANS AND PANTS

The 1980's introduced an affliction popularly known as "Designer Jeans Syndrome." Compressed nerves and blood supply caused symptoms ranging from pelvic pain, tingly thighs, and calf cramps, to panic attacks due to impaired breathing. In the medical literature it appears as "Tight Pants Syndrome." Few men wear jeans as tight as some women, but the same problems appear in men via tight belts and Neoprene "warm pants" worn to prevent muscular injury. All of these can impede circulation to and from the legs. Not only do they block microcirculation, they can even set the stage for deep vein thrombosis (DVT) and risk of pulmonary embolism even in the young and fit (Jowett NI, Robinson CG, 1996).

## FABRIC FINISHES

Fabric finishes can be powerful triggers, even in clothing that made of all natural fibers or harmless synthetics. Some are used to ease the weaving process. Some are anti-microbial chemicals, designed to reduce bacterial growth. The short list includes a wide range of toxic chemicals.

- Benzimidazol derivatives,
- Copper naphthenate, copper-8-quinolinate,
- Dichlorophene,
- Formaldehyde,
- Mercury compounds,
- Triclosan (2,4,4'-trichloro-2'-hydroxydiphenyl ether).

## SHOES

Shoes are a prime offender, especially pointed high-heel shoes that risk sprained ankles, broken bones and even death[1].

High heels shift weight forward. Weight that should spread over the entire foot is concentrated onto the base of the big toe. Pointed toe boxes cram bones together narrowing space for nerve and blood supply (Csapo R and others, 2010). The painful results include bunions and corns, hammertoes, "pump bump" (Haglund's Deformity), bursitis, Achilles tendonitis, bone spurs, varicose veins, Morton's neuroma, and distortions of posture and gait resulting in osteoarthritis of knees and spine. Problems don't stop there of course, but continue upwards to produce the Head-Forward posture and eventually a dowager's hump, but in the meantime, *headaches*.

Calf muscles and Achilles tendons can shorten to the point that women who have worn them too long cannot tolerate flats and must tiptoe when barefoot. Some may even wear high-heeled bedroom slippers, seeing this as a sign of femininity rather than the pathological condition it truly is. Oddly enough, "sensible shoes" with low, wide heels and stiff soles also cause problems by blocking the natural motions of foot and ankle and straining the knees (Kerrigan CD, 1998).

Look for proper fit, toe room and *flexibility*. Soles should *bend*. And they should provide secure traction. Smooth-soled shoes keep the body in a constant state of tension guarding against slipping.

---

1. Survivors of the New York World Trade Center disaster reported piles of women's shoes in the emergency stairwells, abandoned when their owners were attacked not only by terrorists but by their own footwear (Ripley A, 2008).

## ACCESSORIES

### Totes and Bags

A heavy weight carried on one side of the body is a strain to anyone's posture. This is true for both adults and for children whose bones are still forming, and whether it is a fashionably huge designer purse or a knapsack of school books.

Lighten up! Use small purses or empty the large ones. Use rolling luggage, get carts, get help. If heavy loads can't be avoided (as in backpacking) use a hip strap to distribute the weight. Even if weight is properly distributed, experienced backpackers recommend carrying no more than 1/3 of body weight; 1/4 is considered ideal. Thus a fit 170-lb man might carry 40-50 lbs, a 100-pounder should be limited to 25-30.

*No child should be required to haul around a 30-lb backpack.* Figure 88 on page 180 depicts a 9-year old boy who suffered 6 months of relentless headaches, diagnosed as "migraine," that seem to have been triggered in part by a 30-pound bag of schoolbooks.

Problems can start at 5 per cent of body weight with a Head-Forward posture, but in children, loads at 15 per cent of body weight have been found to change *all* postural angles (Ramprasad M and others, 2009). MRI scans, performed on children while standing and loaded with backpacks, have also documented disc compression and lumbar assymetry resulting in back pain (Neuschwander TB and others, 2010). Back pain quickly propagates upward into neck and head pain.

### Ties and Collars

Tight collars and neckties can traumatize the STERNOCLEIDOMASTOID and arteries of the neck. Men may suffer referred muscular and autonomic pain from this source with problems ranging from sinus headache to nausea and dizziness. Again, anything that leaves a red mark is too tight.

### Wallets

Men may laugh at women's body-straining purses and tote bags, but fall victim to "Back-Pocket Sciatica" or "Wallet Butt"). Sitting on a wallet simulates a short hemipelvis on the opposite side resulting in posturally induced scoliosis. A wallet that rides too high in the pocket to sit *down* on, may still cause problems if sat *back on*. A thick wallet between hip and chair back requires a sideways position in the chair or, worse, torquing of hips and torso in an attempt to sit straight. If these results are mistakenly diagnosed as "short leg" a heel lift may initially relieve then perpetuate or worsen the problem. Consider carrying a (thin) wallet in a side pocket. It will be safer from light-fingered persons and you will be safer from back pain and headaches.

### Headwear

Tight hats, hair, wigs, or helmets can ruin a Big Day in many painful ways. A bride with tightly pulled hair, or wearing a tight headband to support a heavy veil, may spend the reception with a head that aches right down to her teeth. She will be in good historical company.

King George IV of England didn't have much fun on his Big Day either. The foppish "Prinny"[1] appeared at his coronation on a hot July day in full (winter) Tudor regalia, including a heavy wig and a 27-foot ermine- and gold-embroidered train. The heavy gem-encrusted crown had to fit tightly enough to stay on a head that had to bow before the Archibishop of Canterbury. Apparently strain and heat triggered a tooth-ache so severe that proceedings were halted to pull a molar. Muscles or tooth? We can't know at this late date, but see the TEMPORALIS pain pattern on page 51.

### Eyewear

A common first step in headaches is an eye exam, "but how often," I asked, "do you find problems relating to headaches?" "Almost never," said the doctor. "We are often the first to find hypertension or tumors because people come to us rather than their physicians. But the eye is rarely the problem."

The usual concern is incorrect prescriptions but the problem may be the lenses themselves. Lenses in small frames (especially progressives) have a small point of focus. Bifocals and trifocals require the wearer to hold the head in a fixed position order to focus at all. Fixing the head *up* to look *down* strains SUBOCCIPITALS at the base of the skull and can cause pain in the back of the head, the temple and eye, and strain on the dura, possibly with vertigo and balance problems. But any lens that is reflective or scratched can force the wearer to hold head and eyes in a fixed position in order to see. Always get non-reflective scratch-proof lenses.

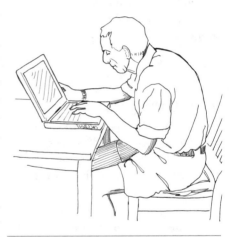

**Figure 102.** SEEING AND C-ING

Focal length should be appropriate to the job. Rather than bifocals, consider reading glasses, computer glasses, even card-playing glasses. Otherwise, the problem may be less of *seeing* than "C-ing," curving into a slouching head-forward C-shape with all its associated myofascial strain.

---

1. "Prinny" was the Prince Regent who took over from the mad King George III lending his title to "Regency" romance novels.

Even frames can be damaging. Glasses must be wide enough and ear pieces must fit properly. The auriculo-temporal nerve arises forward of the ear. If compressed, it can trigger a migraine just like other trigeminal nerve branches. Compressing the local artery starves the TEMPORALIS muscle. If earpieces on your glasses have dug a ditch into the side of your head, you may have found another clue to your migraines.

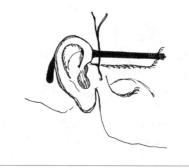

**Figure 103.** NERVES AND FRAMES

## MUSICAL INSTRUMENTS

Musical instruments can be occupational hazards that contribute to migraines and other headaches. Be aware of how they affect your body. sEMG can show the problems in minutes. Many musicians use the Alexander Technique to discover ways to play even more beautiful music without hurting. In all caes, the starting point is a good teacher and good posture.

### Piano and Keyboard

Keyboard players (including computer users) commonly suffer from overstretched TRAPEZIUS and shortened PECTORALIS muscles which can cause headaches, TMJD and more. They also set the stage for debilitating "piano cramp" associated with tendinitis due to tightening of forearm muscles. As always, posture is critical. Ensure that eyes or corrective lenses have the proper focal length to read without hunching forward or falling into a Head-Foward posture.

### Violin and Strings

For violinists, poor posture can result in severe damage and pain. A good teacher will work on posture and form for weeks before the student is allowed to pick up a bow.

The violin rests on the clavicle and the jaw rests on the violin. And it must *rest*. If it is slippy or the player has a particularly long neck, the space can be evened out with a non-slip rubber-coated shoulder rest. Attempting to keep the violin in position by hunching the shoulder and pressing with neck and head causes TRAPEZIUS and SCALENE strain, Thoracic Outlet and Carpal Tunnel Syndromes in many violinists. Symptoms include hellish pain running down the upper back and chest, into arms and fingers, or extending up the neck into the temple, back of eye, and possibly jaw and teeth. The *first* symptom may be migraines. (See "Thoracic Outlet Syndrome" on page 97.)

Shoulder muscles can be remarkably unbalanced in string musicians. Dr. Fishman, who has treated shoulder problems in more than 700 patients using yoga techniques, says it has helped about 90 per cent of them, with the exception of string musicians, "whose shoulder muscles are overtrained" (Brody JE, 2010; see page 265).

*Wind Instruments and Voice*

Wind instruments strain respiratory muscles. Reed instruments, such as clarinet and sax, can strain muscles of the jaw. The musician must retrude the jaw, . breathing through the corners of lips while holding the correct mouth position (*embouchure*) on the instrument. Keeping lips pulled back into the slight smile of a proper embouchure can strain muscles of face and jaw.

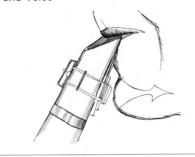

**Figure 104.** CLARINET JAW POSITION

*All* wind instruments (including *voice*) require breath control and diaphragmatic breathing. Chest breathing strains accessory muscles of breathing which includes the SCALENES and other pain-producing neck muscles. You can see and hear this on TV in the tense necks, heaving chests, and breathy voices of many starlets.

## FURNITURE AND OTHER EQUIPMENT

> Every day I go and I sit in a booth like a veal.
> —Lucy (*While You Were Sleeping*)

Another source of pain is planting a body in one position and leaving it there for hours, that is, repetitive *non-motion injuries*. Chairs, computers, and other items offer many opportunities for strain.

Many companies now offer ergonomic equipment. Others make up for it by wildly unnatural working conditions. For example, operators at one well-known telephone company are allowed a 30-minute lunch break. Other breaks are permitted provided they don't exceed 11 minutes total in the course of an 8-hour day. "Airline Thrombosis" gets all the press, but you're far more likely to die from problems developed while confined to desk and chairs, especially those that do not offer proper support.

How different the impact on muscles can be is shown in Figure 105. This is an sEMG tracing of a fibromyalgia patient who could no longer work due to severe pain while sitting at her station. The pattern at left shows wildly firin,painful thigh muscles. The . huge improvement at right came from simply putting a stool under her feet.

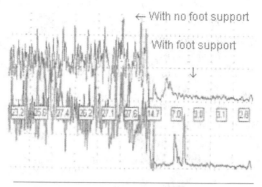

← With no foot support

With foot support

↓

**Figure 105.** Dangling Feet and Muscle Strain

## Chairs

The more time you spend seated, the more damage you can do. Arm-rests too low and seats too high strain many muscles. Pad armrests, use cushions and footstools.

- *Arm-rests.* If too low to provide support for short arms, they force the sitter to lean into them, then to actively hold the head level, straining the neck muscles. If too high, they shorten Trapezius, SCM, and other muscles of shoulder girdle and neck.

- *Seats.* If too high, the sitter cannot place feet firmly on the floor keeping calves in a shortened position. Sharp edges can cut off blood circulation at thigh or knee.

- *Back supports.* Lumbar supports help maintain proper lumbar curve. Loss of this curve, rounding of the back, contributes to Head-Forward posture.

- *Cars.* Bucket seats in cars shorten psoas and other hip flexors, possibly for hours. Too often we select vehicles based on radio and paint. Choose what fits your body.

- *Computers and Workstations.* Work-related injuries often come down to poor posture. Check posture, raise the monitor, lower the chair, use a foot-rest.

## Beds and Mattresses.

If you awaken every morning with a headache, look at your sleeping arrangments.

- Beds that slope towards the head (even due to a carpet at the foot) shift shoulders towards head shortening Scalenes. Can contribute to acid reflux and sleep apnea.

- Pillows that flex the neck strongly forward shorten SCM in front of neck and overstretch muscles (including Trapezius) in back of neck. Hard pillows used by side sleepers may compress the carotid arteries decreasing blood supply.

- Toes weighted down with heavy blankets shorten Gastrocnemius and Soleus muscles impairing circulation, causing calf cramps and possibly headaches.

- Sleeping too cold, chilling all muscles and encouraging a fetal position.

- Fetal position shortens Psoas in hips, and overstretches Trapezius in back.

- Blockage of blood vessels. See "Extreme Sleeping" on page 101.

# The Emotional Component

*Migraine can be a symptom of abuse and brain injury.*

The one enduring symptom common to both Post Traumatic Stress Syndrome (PTSD) and Traumatic Brain Injury (TBI) is headache. In migraineurs, both child and adult, a history of abuse and emotional trauma is higher than in Normals.

Abuse changes the brain in many ways. Stress changes the hypothalamus and even alters DNA[1]. While stress is not the only cause of migraines, or even the major cause, it is far from trivial. Migraine is exhausting and stressful all on its own, but emotional its emotional stress may show up in unexpected ways.

One is an apparently odd reluctance, even stonewalling and refusal, to try new treatments, especially ones requiring more money, more energy, and more organizational skills than you have left or can imagine ever having again.

Another is a strange *disappointment* on learning that there is no tumor or other deadly disease. Hypochondria? Not necessarily. No matter how frightening it may be, a "real" condition such as a tumor provides an acceptable reason for the pain and offers the hope that something can be done about it. Otherwise, "nothing is wrong" is interpreted as "nothing can be done."

Both responses may seem odd to outsiders, but make perfect sense to sufferers who long ago stopped hoping and now aim for mere survival.

Sometimes available survival skills are not the best or the ones most needed.

---

1. Gabor Maté (2010) documented the uniformly abusive backgrounds of chronic drug addicts and radical changes in neurotransmitters. See also the National Geographic film *Stress: Portrait of a Killer.* It documents health changes in primates, found to be identical between a troup of baboons and employees of the British Civil Service.

## LIFE SKILLS

While writing this book I needed to make a short trip out of town for research. With a week of lead time I worried about what to pack, whether the bills were all paid, what projects and promises needed to be re-scheduled, an oil change for the car, how my business would survive without me (for just 3-4 days), and so forth. On noticing my stress over this short trip, it dawned on me: *this is what life was always like before.*

For chronic migraine sufferers, headaches that last two to four days or even a week or more are not unusual. Their lives are nothing like normal lives. As mentioned in Chapter 1, they are more like tales of UFO abductees[1]. You don't get to plan the trip, you won't be functional while it is happening, and you will be disoriented for a couple days after you get back. When you do return to Normal Life, you must do what needs to be done *and* catch up with everything else.

At such a time, laundry and menu planning may be the last thing on your mind, but a sure way to bring on another headache is to miss meals, starve your brain, and make it even more difficult to function. Of all people, migraineurs need regular habits, but many tend to live in ways that drive Normals wild with frustration.

Well-meaning suggestions to reduce the stress of such a lifestyle range from the inane to the superficial: "Enjoy a bubble-bath by candle-light" and "Massage the temples with circular motions." These can be useful to relax tense muscles while feeling for trigger points (and assuming no sensitivity to scented candles or bubble soap). But they do not address the root problem which is often no clue how to run a household or a life. This is almost always true for adult children of alcoholics. It is also true in children of families whose dysfunction did not necessarily come in a bottle.

---

1. A favorite fictional example is Buffy the Vampire Slayer, a super-hero sadly lacking in real-life skills, who slowly goes mad from scheduling issues. After her mother's death she lives on burgers and sugar cereals, wonders why she is depresed, and is eventually reduced to asking Spike the vampire for financial advice. There are many real-life examples like her.

## THE LEGACIES OF ABUSE

> I broke my ankle at school. The office called my father at noon. He showed up at 3 PM. I begged to be taken to the hospital. He said no and took me home. Helped me hobble to my bedroom. Made me get back in the car at 5 PM because he wanted to go out to eat. He backed his seat onto my foot before putting the car in gear. I begged for crutches. He wouldn't get them because they cost money.
>
> —T. B.

Abusive families do not place a high emphasis on growing functional adults. After the screams and the blows, did the victims get proper medical care? Or do they still carry injuries that lead to fear, fogginess, ADD, and learning disabilities? Is there a sense of time and place to provide structure and predictability? —or is everything awash in a swirling sea of uncertainty and unreliability? Do such families practice or teach responsible financial management, or how to plan and prepare nutritious meals? Do they even know or care why these things are important?

The opposite situation is also damaging. Well-intentioned parents may handle every life detail leaving their treasured children as unprepared as abused ones for life on their own. They may have no clue how to deal with laundry ("Just buy more!") and eat all their meals at fast-food restaurants ("Free 30-oz soft drink special!) seemingly unaware that food is more than pain-relief for the symptoms of hunger.

The result is a house and body that is a stress rather than a refuge, a sink of anxiety, depression, and migraine triggers ranging from dust and mildew to unstable blood sugar, nutritional deficiencies, and an overwhelming sense of helplessness and confusion. Relentless CHAOS ("Can't Have Anyone Over Syndrome") feeds isolation, shame, and desperation.

When you can't find the other shoe, can't find the bills or remember to pay them and haven't changed the sheets for months, the house, the desk, the life is such a mess that it becomes too embarassing to even ask for help until things are Better.

But how can Better happen when you don't know how to make it happen?

The A&E TV series *Hoarders* revealed the problems of people who suffer compulsive hoarding. For Normals, the show is extremely stressful[1]. Imagine your life spinning so badly out of control that you actually had to live like that. Hoarding and clutter can be symptoms of the same injuries or abuse that set the stage for migraines in the first place, and migraineurs are even less able than Normals to recognize items in a cluttered environment (Vincent MB, 2007). This suggests brain injury which may be adding to the stress and strain.

One option is to call in professional cleaners and organizers, but can be expensive and improvements temporary if the root problem remains unchanged.

---

1. My Normal brother reports that every 5 minutes of *Hoarders* inspires an hour of housework.

# Chapter 7

# Getting Help

*The many things you can do on your own — and where to get professional help.*

Perhaps you will agree by now that migraine is not a random act of the universe or a life sentence due to bad genes. It can be a symptom of many conditions and life choices that are under our control. Some are not, but start with the ones that are.

## Helping Yourself

> A slave is one who waits for someone to come and free him.
> —Ezra Pound

The causes and symptoms of migraine can interweave and intermingle in gruesomely complex ways that simply cannot be untangled and resolved in the course of a 5 or even 15-minute appointment. Fortunately, you can do a lot of the basic investigation yourself, and you have more than 15 minutes in which to do it.

Start by keeping a headache diary with pain diagrams (Chapter 1). Write down your symptoms, their dates and times. Write down what you've been doing, what you've been eating, and how you've been sleeping. Write down your dreams which may offer clues and insights.

Too much trouble? Not if you really want to get better and not when you realize that no doctor is going to do this for you. Make the process easier with good tools.

### TOOLS AND EQUIPMENT

#### NUTRITION TRACKERS

A first step towards helping yourself out of migraine is striving for regular schedules, and regular healthful meals. It matters what you eat and when you eat. It even matters who you eat it with. Start by getting nutritional status under control. That alone can improve sleep, fatigue, and confusion. There are many diet and calorie trackers on the market, from Weight Watchers to various phone apps.

My personal favorite is www.DietPower.com. This program tracks 30+ nutrients plus weight, water intake, and calories burned through exercise (from Aerobic Dance to Zither Playing) and calculates your metabolic rate. It is based on the USDA nutrition database including many chain restaurant foods. You can add your personal recipes, vitamins, and supplements, track and graph changes in weight, blood pressure, girth, and more. Enter height, weight, and goals, and you're on your way.

Many name brand processed foods are in the database, but for migraine, it's best to avoid confusion and food additives by eating and logging an actual potato rather than Brand X Potato Puffs. Cook from scratch with your own or the 100+ program recipes. Add other items back in later while watching for any change in headache frequency. The calendar included with DietPower can serve as a headache diary. Noting what happened hours or days after eating can reveal important patterns.

Most importantly, the program can tell you exactly where you stand nutritionally. Do you really need to supplement selenium or iron? Are you already getting a dangerous overdose? Do you need supplements? Or just more vegetables? And if so, which ones?

DietPower is not a diet. It is a coach, a checkbook register for whatever diet you choose, or design, to follow. You may not always hear what you want to hear, but in the end, it's all about you and all about you getting better. Entering bad data or ignoring unpleasant truths is like cheating at Solitaire. Eat as much or as little as you want, but eat with your eyes open.

*Do not attempt to log items individually as they wander into your mouth at random.* That way lies madness. Instead, sit down in the morning (or the night before) and log what you will eat that day. DietPower will even suggest food choices to improve your nutritional score. Print the page and you can simply check items off as you eat them, preferably on a schedule. This eliminates the temptation to overdose on coffee, alcohol and snack foods because you have no idea what you are going to eat or when. Food lists can morph into Shopping Lists, which in turn can expand into Menu Plans, which in turn, can change a life.

No time to cook? That usually means that you also have no time to eat healthy meals. That alone can cause devastating migraines. If *time* is the problem, organizing meals will improve that, but it also helps to have the cooking done for you.

## CROCK POTS AND SLOW COOKERS

There is nothing worse than ending a long day too tired to even microwave popcorn for dinner. Whether you spend your days at home or away, a crock pot or slow cooker that has real food ready for you can improve nutrition and reduce stress.

Pre-electric farm wives would bring a pot to boil, then pack it in a box insulated with sawdust and blankets. The food cooked throughout the day at temperatures which turn the toughest cuts of meat tender, with no need to watch it, and reducing hands-on preparation time.

Modern crockpots offer many features. Regardless of price, some are terrible, some terrific. Look for the models with the longest warranties. Check ratings and customer reviews (especially *bad* ones) at www.ConsumerReports.com and www.Amazon.com. Patterns of system failure reported in the one-star reviews reveal that basics are best. The more snazzy electronics, the more can go wrong, but a good slow cooker can be an extremely valuable tool for getting life under control.

Also recommended: the *Saving Dinner* cookbook by Leanne Ely. It is excellent for planning *weekly* meals, and includes at least one slow-cooker meal per weekly plan.

## PEDOMETERS

How much do you move? If it is only a few feet or yards a day, you may have found yet another trigger for your headaches, especially ones diagnosed as "tension." If you are walking and running miles every day but hypothyroid symptoms such as weight gain are dismissed as sedentary life-style or laziness, a pedometer will prove otherwise. You can also plug this information into a food and exercise tracker such as DietPower. Aim for 10,000 steps per day.

## TIMERS

Many chronically stressed and disorganized people have a severely distorted sense of time. Chronic migraineurs are always behind on work and chores (and even fun and recreation). They can never do *anything* because everything will take *too long*.

But *how long is that*? How much time do you actually need to unload the dishwasher or handwash a sink of dirty dishes? Take a shower? Fold a load of laundry? Pay bills?

Set a timer for 15 minutes and do the job to the end to find out. You may be shocked by the answer. A bedroom as unpleasant mess because you don't have time to make the bed is one thing. Finding that it takes just 30 seconds to remove that stress can create a whole new world.

The timer can also focus attention when you are tempted to flit from one thing to another. Is it "impossible" to clean off your desk? Focus on that one thing for 15 minutes and see what happens. If you can't do 15 minutes, then try 10 or 5 — but find out the real value of time. Do this with a real timer, not just a clock on the wall. Something with a real beep or ding keeps us honest and keeps us on track.

## CALENDARS AND DIARIES

This is how you organize and track a life — and all the things that happen in it. If you have a family, get a calendar with spaces big enough for everyone to write their appointments and schedules. Put it on the wall with an attached pencil, not where it is unreachable or can be hidden by clutter. Owning a daytimer and having a calendar on your phone does not replace this. Transfer the information and put it on the central calendar where everyone can see it, where it will not be lost in a purse, left at the office, or inaccessible due to a power outage.

## THERMOMETERS

Get a good digital fever thermometer to check your temperature and provide clues to metabolism. Consumer Reports recommends Vicks and Sponge Bob Square Pants for best accuracy. A good digital cooking thermometer will help turn out better meals, and, the probe, taped to a finger, can double as a home biofeedback monitor.

## BLOOD PRESSURE MONITORS

It is often said that good health does not happen in the doctor's office. Healthy blood pressure is a fine example of that. Best improvement is in patients who monitor their own status at home on a regular basis. Many automatic blood pressure monitors are available. Check them against the one in your doctor's office. They may not be as accurate, but can be close. A reliable brand is Omron.

The Resp-e-Rate, a breath trainer, has been shown to reduce hypertension more effectively than multiple drugs. See website with research papers at: www.resperate.com.

## LIGHT

> The only person who loves sunlight more than someone who loves sunlight is someone who must ration it.
>
> — Andrew Levy

Light is a nutrient. The changing light of day and seasons triggers hormones that control mood, wake and sleep cycles. Of all people, migraineurs tend to suffer depression and disrupted sleep. This can be because, almost by definition, migraineurs tend to avoid the bright light that creates mood-elevating serotonin, the raw material for the sleep hormone melatonin. Even for well-lit migraineurs, if the solution to a migraine attack is to crawl into a dark room and sleep, it can be hard to get back on a regular schedule. An extremely valuable tool is the Philips goLITE, a small portable LED light that emits a specific wavelength of blue, typical of early morning light.

I can attest to its remarkable effect on winter depression here in the Appalachian rain forest where the sun may be hidden behind clouds and mist for weeks or months at a time. I had been in bed for days when I realized I had all the symptoms of a serious depression. I borrowed a goLITE from a friend and used it for most of a day. The next morning I bounced out of bed to find that gangs of unruly children had apparently broken into my house, leaving dishes in the sink, clothes on the floor, scary food in the fridge. The day or week before, I would have rolled over and taken refuge in sleep and despair. But within a couple of hours, all was cleaned and swept and back on track. The goLITE was like flipping a switch on depression. It can also reset sleep cycles thrown off-kilter by odd hours of shift work or migraine attacks.

Also consider a daylight clock. It will wake you up slowly by gradually increasing the light level. It gives you time to finish a dream and to awaken gently and naturally with no screaming alarms or beepy noises. Bio-Brite has been around awhile and worked out most of the bugs. Philips also has several models of daylight clocks, but stick with basics. See reviews at www.Amazon.com.

## FLYLADY.COM

Most organizational materials were written by The Born Organized, a group of people uniquely unqualified to teach the rest of us. www.Flylady.com is a website dedicated to freeing homes and lives from disorganization and clutter. It began with two ladies who once called themselves the Slob Sisters. They were not born organized. They understand the rest of us, and their system works.

Many testimonial letters tell of surviving emergencies — from floods, fires, and hurricanes to the boss dropping in unexpectedly for dinner — because simple but effective routines had been put in place for the first time.

FlyLady does not directly address migraine or brain injury — just the symptoms of drowning in confusion and disorganization. It is applied cognitive therapy, a means of developing the skills to get the chaos under control. It provides a gentle but effective way out of the dark and chaos and confusion, starting with the simplest of baby steps:

- Polish your kitchen sink
- Put on your lace-up shoes.

If you can do that, you're on your way.

Flylady provides tools, techniques, and an international support system. Joining the Flylady community is free; the website is supported by sales at the FlyStore which stocks high quality tools for organization and better life skills. The daily 15-minute assignment (and monthly habit) are on the website.

One of Flylady's favorite mantras is this: *You can't organize clutter.* Flylady gives you tools for getting control of it, but if you need outside help in removing usable household items, the Salvation Army and AmVets provide free pickup.

To remove other items at a moderate cost: www.1-800-GotJunk.com.

If your life and headaches aren't better with these changes, you may need professional help. But what, who, and where to find it?

# Trained Professional Help — What? Who? and Where?

*No one holds the franchise on effective pain treatment. As a pain management practice grows, so does the interdependency of each of the disciplines involved in the diagnostic and therapeutic process.*

First, you *must* see a medical doctor for his or her unique expertise. Eliminate all the things that your migraines are not to be certain that they are not symptoms of an even more serious condition.

Even if you prefer "alternative" health care, nothing will raise red flags for professionals in those fields than announcing that you have come to them because you "don't believe in doctors." No responsible health professional with good reality testing skills will believe for one minute that their niche specialty replaces all that a physician with good diagnostic skills can do. Of course, one thing they can do is write prescriptions. If you need prescription drugs, you must see an MD or DO.

## PHYSICIANS

Physicians today labor under a severe handicap. Not only are appointments often limited to 5 minutes, but an honest physician may also be limited to stating the obvious: eat right, sleep right, exercise. Many patients are affronted by such plain vanilla advice, feeling that if they aren't given drugs, the doctor has failed to do his job.

Nutritionists are in the same boat. Good nutrition is pretty basic stuff. Miracle cures in the form of pills and potions are enticing, and lucrative for the vender, but trying to micromanage nutrition in capsule form is not the best choice.

We are the product of millions of years of evolution. Even if you are in the camp that limits this to a few thousand, that's way bigger than the relatively few short years since WWII when, for many of us, everything has changed, from the jobs we do, to the food we eat, the hours of sleep and even sunlight we get during the day. Your doctor is in the difficult position of trying to unravel how many things have changed for you and how, while attempting to deduce the many possible origins of your head pain.

Your head alone has 22 bones. There are 24 movable vertebrae, some 600 muscles, thousands of blood vessels and nerves, and miles of fascial connections that can be exquisitely painful on their own or trigger pain elsewhere. There are wide variations in personal injuries, lifestyles, genes, anatomy, and crossed wiring. And there is no rule that says only one thing is allowed to go wrong.

There is no possible way that these factors can be sorted out in a brief meeting. There is no one drug that will cover all the possibilities. On the other hand, treating the symptoms can buy you time and enough pain-free space to function while you work through the many factors that may lie behind the headaches.

## BASIC PRESCRIPTION MIGRAINE DRUGS

Drugs for migraine can be enormously useful, they can be life-saving, but they are a balancing act. Sufferers must take enough to stop the attack, soon enough that the medication is effective, but not so often that it triggers serious side effects. Basic options are antidepressants, anti-seizure medications, beta blockers, and triptans.

For migraines with sleep disturbances and depression, tricyclic antidepressants (such as amitriptyline (Elavil) may be prescribed. Sometimes these are poorly received if patients suspect that the doctor is dismissing the migraines as "just depression" or "just in my head." Actually they help sleep by elevating serotonin. This improves mood, but also supplies the raw material to make melatonin, the sleep hormone.

Beta blockers (such as Inderal) block stress hormones and interact with serotonin, possibly decreasing prostaglandin production. They are recommended for migraine associated with panic attacks, high blood pressure, or stress *relief.* That is, you do well under stress but suffer migraines on the weekend *after* the pressure has ended.

Historically, migraine drugs have been heavily based on drugs originally developed for epilepsy. Even if you don't get seizures, they are used in migraine to raise the threshold in sensitive nervous systems. These drugs, such as Topamax, are especially effective in cases which involve Cortical Spreading Depression, a brain behavior common to both migraine aura and seizures (see page 130).

Triptans (such as Imitrex and Maxalt) are used to abort migraines and cluster headaches. They are vasoconstrictors that are effective for many sufferers if taken early, with onset of first headache symptoms. They work by binding to serotonin receptors in the brain and inhibiting release of inflammatory neuropeptides including pain-producing CGRP and Substance P.

All can be helpful, but all come with side effects. All of these drugs have time frames, limits and maximums. Bad things can happen if you don't observe them. Combining migraine drugs with antidepressant drugs can be especially risky. Under the banner of Patient Advocacy, some push more and stronger drugs that in the long run, may be no better than the classic strip of black electrical tape used to "cure" the blinking VCR or engine warning light by covering up the problem. Find the problem.

Using drugs *in place of* finding and eliminating triggers is like wearing bad, ill-fitting shoes then treating the resulting foot pain with pain-killer. You can, but it's inefficient and causes more problems than it solves. Eliminate the triggers, raise the thresholds, and you are on the way to reducing or eliminating the need, expense, and side effects of drugs. For excellent advice on drugs and getting off them, see *Heal Your Headaches*, by David Buchholz (2002).

Migraineurs often complain that their insurance company won't pay for more than a few pills per month. This is not mere churlishness on the part of the insurer. It is that they don't want to also pay to treat dangerous side effects. You shouldn't want them to have to. Even if you try to ignore them, one side effect can be painfully urgent: rebound headaches even worse than the original problem.

## REBOUND HEADACHES

Migraines that worsen while on migraine meds can be a symptom of drug overuse.

**TABLE 13.** DRUGS THAT TRIGGER REBOUND HEADACHES WITH OVERUSE

| Butalbital Compounds | Esgic, Fioricet, Fiorinal, Phrenilin |
|---|---|
| Caffeine Compounds | Anacin, Cafergot, Exedrin, Esgic, Vanquish, Fioricet, Fiorinal |
| Decongestants | Afrin, Dristan, Entex, Sudafed, Tylenol |
| Ergotamines | Cafergot, Ergomar, DHE 45, Migranal, Wigraine |
| Opioids and related | Darvocet, OxyContin, Percocet, Tylenol with codeine |
| Triptans | Amerge, Axert, Imitrex, Zomig and more |

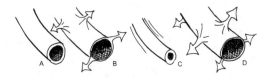

**Figure 106.** DILATION, CONSTRICTION, AND REBOUND

In migraine, normal vessles (A) swell with thinning of the vessel walls (B). Vasoconstrictors constrict vessels (C) relieving the pain but setting up for a rebound headache with all the characteristics of the original migraine (D).

Caffeine is often included in migraine medications because of its relatively gentle vasoconstrictive properties. Unfortunately it is also notorious for causing painful withdrawal headaches when the regular supply stops. Caffeine increases prostaglandin production, worsening PMS symptoms and cramps. It is also believed to dull thyroid function. Is it the caffeine? Prostaglandins? Loss of nutrients in muscle function? The jury is still out, but if you suffer headaches or PMS, try reducing then eliminating caffeine and see if there is any change in symptoms.

So many drinks and drugs contain caffeine that even without coffee and tea you may be getting far more caffeine than you realize and and perhaps far fewer nutrients. A long-time mainstay of dieters, coffee (like alcohol and sodas) is a quick and easy replacement for Real Food.

**TABLE 14.** CAFFEINE IN BEVERAGES AND OTC MEDICATIONS[A]

| Item | Type | Caffeine (mg) | Unit | |
|---|---|---|---|---|
| **Chocolate** | milk | 3-6 | 1 oz | |
| | dark | 2-5 | 1 oz | |
| **Coffee** | instant | 30-120 | 1 cup (8 oz) | 240 ml |
| | brewed | 40-180 | 1 cup (8 oz) | 240 ml |

| Tea | decaf | 3-5 | 1 cup (8 oz) | 240 ml |
|---|---|---|---|---|
| | brewed | 20-110 | 1 cup (8 oz) | 240 ml |
| | instant | 28 | 1 cup (8 oz) | 240 ml |
| | canned, Lipton | 17 | 8 oz | 240 ml |
| **Yerba Mate** | Guayaki | 140 | 16 oz | 480 ml |
| **Soda** | Mountain Dew, reg. | 34 | 7.5 oz | 355 ml |
| | Mountain Dew, diet | 54 mg | 12 oz | 355 ml |
| | Coca Cola | 46 | 12 oz | 355 ml |
| | Dr. Pepper | 41 | 12 oz | 355 ml |
| | Diet Pepsi | 35 | 12 oz | 355 ml |
| | TAB | 45 | 12 oz | 355 ml |
| **Sport/Energy Drinks** | AMP | 71 | 8 oz | 240 ml |
| | Monster Energy | 160[b] | 16 oz | 480 ml |
| | No Fear | 83 | 8 oz | 240 ml |
| | Black Mamba | 160 | 16 oz | 480 ml |
| | Red Bull | 80 | 8 oz | 250 ml |
| | Rock Star | 80 | 8.4 oz | 240 ml |
| **OTC Medications** | Anacin, Exedrin, Extra Strength | 1 tablet | 65 mg | |
| | NoDoz, Vivarin Maximum Strength | 1 tablet | 200 mg | |

a. Data from various sources including product labels and websites.
b. Can does not list caffeine content, but warns to limit consumption to 3 cans per day.

OTHER DRUGS THAT CAN TRIGGER MIGRAINES

Besides migraine drugs and rebound, other common medications have been reported to trigger migraines (Table 15 ).

**TABLE 15.** MEDICATIONS THAT CAN TRIGGER MIGRAINE

| | |
|---|---|
| Hormones | Hormonal contraceptive (birth control pills, injections, and implants) and hormone replacement therapies |
| Stimulants | Bronchodilators for asthma, drugs for ADD, and diet pills. |
| Vasodilators | Nitroglycerin and other nitrates for heart conditions and drugs for erectile dysfunction |
| Other | Some SSRI anti-depressants, acne medications, hair tonics, and statins. |

## DENTISTS

If your headaches are accompanied by clicking and catching in your jaw, relief may be as close as a trip to the dentist. However, be aware that not all dentists are trained to address TMJ disorders and those who are may have radically different approaches. Some emphasize surgery to correct problems in the joint capsule. Others insist that bad bite, muscle imbalances and other problems that create problems in the joint be addressed *first*. And some just fake it.

Regardless of patient testimonials, regardless of reputation or number of articles in the medical journals, be certain that the approach — and the professional you choose — is effective for *you* before investing in massive dental work. Over 20 years, I saw four dentists for treatment of TMJD. Two were terrific, two were disasters.

On discovering my problem with severe TMJD, a temporary splint (made on the opposite side of the country) reduced my headaches by at least 50 per cent. Unfortunately, these excellent results were erased by the dentist who made the permanent splint. He had published several excellent articles on TMJ and head pain in the medical literature and his office was just a few miles from my home. He seemed the perfect choice.

On reporting for my first treatment, the first after office lunch-hour, I was surprised to find a dozen other patients in the one-dentist office with me. We all filed together into an open room with a long line of tables (cheaper than dental chairs) on which the patients lay down. Dr. X jogged, huffing and puffing, from one to another along this assembly-line. He may have been an expert, but nothing he did reflected that.

Most TMJD specialists take great care in establishing correct height of the splint. In contrast, he shoved a mass of soft plastic into the mouth with instructions to bite down. The height was set by the patient (lying supine on the table, which changes bite compared to standing). "How does that feel?" he would ask. A confused "Ok, I guess" from a befuddled patient meant teeth locked into that version of the appliance (no time to shave it down) until the next appointment. The rationale was that this would allow muscles to relax in increments. Each week the base splint would be replaced allowing the jaw to shift forward by a few millimeters, at least in theory. He did none of the tests, measurements, or protocols described in his medical papers to determine whether things were actually moving or changing. He couldn't. He was much too busy.

His approach seems to have worked for some, but not all, and certainly not me. Given the low level of technique involved, those who did improve might have gotten as much relief from a wad of gum. For others, it was sheer disaster. Many therapists in the local bodywork community swore that a large part of their business was in relieving the pain this man had inflicted on his unsuspecting patients.

In my own personal experience, the best approach appears to be the smooth splint combined with myotherapy to relax and balance tight strained muscles. The difference between this and the "toothed" splint seems to be in allowing muscles to relax on their own rather than restricting it to timed, scheduled increments.

Nevertheless, there are problems with the best of splints. Dentists urge you to keep them in at all times, even while eating, as chewing has the most severe impact on TMJD. Unfortunately, chewing anything tougher than scrambled eggs with smooth plastic is near impossible.

The obvious solution is to cap teeth to improve bite and balance but this is not the best first step. In my case, no teeth met except the front ones. Caps meant sawing down and capping nearly *all* my other teeth. (Good teeth, 40 years old before their first cavity.) It also means complete trust that a person knows what he is doing and has your best interest at heart. However, the person who really knows and understands TMJD in terms of will also understand it in the form of a splint for fast results. You shouldn't need to wait for extensive dental work to get relief. In my experience with Dr. X, the headaches returned (including pain in places I'd never had it before) along with substantial bills. I made the mistake of trusting him for $3,000 of damage before I bailed.

If things don't get better within 2-3 sessions, if things get *worse* with treatment, something is wrong and you should get a second opinion with one caveat: *headaches and sinus pain are extremely common after dental work.* Jaw muscles are strained when propped open for long periods during the work. (See Chapter 2.) A good rule of thumb is 5 minutes of work, then relax the jaw for a minute or so. This slows the work but will keep you safe from additional pain and dysfunction.

The American Equilibration Society (AES) deals with diagnosis and treatment of bite problems, TMJ disorders, and associated muscles in hopes of avoiding surgery.

Find a provider at: www.aes-tmj.org.

## HEADACHE CLINICS

After the usual procedures have been exhausted, the next step may be a trip to a headache clinic. I'm sure some are very good, but most reports from my clients have been less than glowing. On the other hand, by definition, I do not see the *success* stories.

In theory, headache clinics specialize in headaches. Some merely specialize in headache patients desperate enough to pay fantastic sums for the treatments and drugs supplied by any family physician with good diagnostic skills and a modest referral network. You may spend a few deliriously pain-free days only to discover, on returning to the Real World, that nothing has changed except your bank balance.

If I were shopping for a pain clinic I would want to see (or have arranged for):

- *Electrolyte Testing*. Not standard blood tests, but via newer tests (such as the Exatest) for free magnesium and Ca:Mg ratios,

- *Endocrine Testing*. Not just TSH, but the full panel including free T3/T4 and reverse T3.

- *Neurotherapy*. Brain mapping / QEEG to evaluate underlying TBI or brain injury.

- *Muscle testing / retraining*. ROM / sEMG to find and treat muscle imbalances.

- *Autonomic training*. Hand-warming, Heart-Rate Variability (HRV), guided relaxation.

- *Hands-on bodywork*. Evaluation for structural distortions (including pelvic and cranial), myofascial distortions, TrPs and the means to treat them. No TrP injections unless there is staff on premises who can actually palpate TrPs and reproduce pain patterns.

- *In-House Research Projects*. The good ones want to be better at what they do, not just run an assembly line. Find out if staff has rpublished any research papers. Read them and compare your treatment and results with what is said in the papers.

Another issue is the Individual Big Name clinic. The bigger the name, the lower the chances of one-on-one appointment time with that person. In-house therapists aren't necessarily there because of outstanding skills. Some Big Names take shameless advantage of this. One charges over $350 per session but travels and lectures so widely that he is rarely at the clinic that bears his name. The actual work is done by interns who charge about the same, but are paid $30 per patient. The rest goes to the Big Name who wasn't there to supervise. All of us have worked for low or no wages in exchange for training, but are interns the best therapists? Too often they therapists in training or lured in by hope of training.

Better to look for instructors (for the technique in question) who have practices of their own. And unless you have extremely good reason to believe that Practitioner X or Clinic Y is your only hope for help, look for help close to home. Expand the geographic circle of possibilities via friends or relatives with a guest room and reasonably functional lives of their own. Always check training and skill levels. A therapist with years of experience (versus a weekend workshopper who hung out a shingle a block away) is worth the longer drive. But too much travel just adds to the stress.

## SURGERY

Headaches may be relieved by surgery, but success depends on the source of the pain.

The discovery that Botox relieved life-long migraines focused attention on trigeminal nerve branches in the forehead and the idea of surgical removal of the entrapping CORRUGATOR muscles. In a study of 60 migraineurs, 17 patients (28 per cent) reported total relief from migraine, 24 (40 per cent) reported an essential improvement, and 19 (32 per cent) reported minimal or no change. Patients with *mild* migraines were most likely (up to almost 90 per cent) to experience improvement or total elimination of migraine (Dirnberger F and Becker K, 2004). Unfortunately, 11 patients with very favorable immediate responses experienced a gradual return of their headaches to pre-op intensity by about a month after the operation. So yes, it can work, but never submit to surgery without an initial trial of Botox.

Chronic headache has also been relieved by cutting the dural bridge, the connection between hypertrophied posterior neck muscles (specifically RECTUS CAPITIS POSTERIOR MINOR) and the dura mater (Hack GD and Hallgren RC, 2004).

When migraines are triggered by the pulsing of an artery next to a nerve in head or neck, surgical decompression has offered great relief to some patients (but not all). One potential trigger is the interaction between the superficial temporal artery and the auriculo-temporal nerve. In 34 per cent of heads studied, anatomical variations were found suggesting a definite source of migraines. Another may be the greater greater occipital nerve and artery, found in a study of 50 heads to cross each other 54 per cent of the time. The relationship varied from a single crossing to a twining. In either case, pulsing of the artery could irritate the nerve and provide a possible explanation for migraines triggered in the occipital region (Janis and others, 2010).

Surgery should always be the last resort. If muscles are involved, as in SUBOCCIPITAL / dural strain or Thoracic Outlet Syndrome, conservative options should always be tried first. (See page 97.) On the other hand, no muscular technique will untangle entwined nerves and blood vessels or correct aberrant anatomical relationships. Choose a surgeon carefully, and check all options.

## WESTERN OR ALTERNATIVE MEDICINE

> It is generally agreed that the ability to perform a skilled physical examination has become a lost art in modern medicine.
>
> —Allen B. Weisse, MD (2010)

"Western" or "Alternative / Complementary" medicine? Which to choose? The supposed choice between one or the other is a gross over-simplification. But as long as we are simplifying grossly, let's reduce it to: "Hands-Off" versus "Hands-On Medicine."

Hands-Off Medicine can be thought of as Automated Insurance Company Medicine. It hardly does "Western" Medicine justice. It just hasn't got the time. Consider the woman who wanted to try biofeedback for her "anxiety and shaking." Her doctor had prescribed Valium, but she wanted an alternative to drugs. Would biofeedback help? Perhaps, but that depends on the source of the problem.

"What brings on this shaking and anxiety?" I asked.

"It happens when I turn my head to the right," she said.

What happened when she turned her head to the *left*? Nothing.

Straight ahead? Occasional minor symptoms.

On turning her head to the *right* she lost all motor control. This was not anxiety, it was a blatantly obvious neurological problem. It was nerve compression by vertebrae so severely misaligned that the problem could be seen from across the room. Biofeedback was *not* the answer but neither was Valium. I walked her down the hall to a chiropractor who resolved the problem, not because he was a master of exotic Eastern arts, but because he had the training to deal with neurological problems of cervical origin, and the time and concern to evaluate and treat the situation properly.

Five-minute appointments with an overworked MD are not unusual. Many of our former gods of medicine have been demoted to altar boys serving stockholders and the bottom line. Result: critical medical decisions are being made by insurance company clerks with no medical training who are afraid the bad patients will take away their Christmas bonuses. This is not what Western Medicine should be.

Chiropractic and Osteopathy come under particular fire as part of the turf wars. But these are also Western Medicine, as is biofeedback. Pushed to the wall, many will say that it isn't the modality that constitutes "Western Medicine," it is the rigorous testing and evaluation by the Western Scientific Method. Unfortunately much of the Western Scientific Method has been shanghaied by Western Big Business[1].

The enormous possibilities of hands-on medicine and biofeedback are dismissed by persons who freely admit they have never looked into it while prescribing drugs with

---

1. For a painfully detailed review of modern "scientific rigor" and how studies are actually run, see Carl Elliot's *White Coat, Black Hat (2010)*.

an efficacy rate of 10 per cent above placebo accompanied by debilitating side effects, and untested techniques with little but tradition or profits to recommend them.

This is not scientific rigor. It isn't even scientific. Sadly, if you want scientific rigor, the best source may be East of here — in Great Britain. American journals and TV trumpet what's profitable (or has not yet killed an overly embarrassing number of patients). British journals tend to report what has actually been proven to work. The differences are heavily based on international differences in insurance coverage ("what pays, stays") and different medical traditions.

Acupuncture might be considered the most un-Western art, yet there is the surprising evidence of "Otzi the Iceman." In 1991, his freeze-dried 5,000-year-old remains were found melting from a glacier in the Otz Valley between Austria and Italy. On his body were 15 tattoos, 11 located on traditional acupuncture points or along a meridian. One point was a local point and 3 had apparently deviated with distortion of the skin in the course of freezing and drying. Nevertheless, the points correspond remarkably well to conditions from which Otzi suffered as revealed by forensic analysis. Otzi, the oldest mummy ever found, altered many of our ideas of life at that time including proof that acupuncture originated at least 2,000 years earlier than previously believed, and that it was practiced in *Western* Europe.

Perhaps these different paradigms are different views of the same elephant. For example, Chinese medicine attributes headaches to the gallbladder meridian. If we "don't believe in meridians," we will ignore that observation. But what does this actually mean? The gallbladder meridian runs along the fascia lining the borders of muscles involved in headaches, shortness of breath, and yes, even areas of pain referred by problems in the gallbladder (see page 256).

Different medical systems, varying from country to country, have different strengths and weaknesses. Ideally, they work together, each complementing the other[1]. Unfortunately, many critics stick to rigid categories, assuming that anything missing from the syllabus when they graduated back in 1957 must be superstition and quackery. The Alternative Medicine version of that is the extremely sweeping and incorrect statement: "Doctors don't know anything."

Nonsense. See a doctor. Go from there.

---

1. Many traditional Eastern remedies have lost out to Western drugs for good reason. Despite ongoing popularity of rhinoceros and tiger parts, Western Viagra (a powerful vasodilator) definitely works better. On the other hand, it is also more likely to give the men who take it heart attack or stroke, because it actually does work and because the one-size-dose-fits-all favored by Western Automated Medicine may work all too well.

## HANDS-ON BODYWORK

> If you go around for years with something tight, you can't just say "Ok, now get loose."
> —Dr. Mary Lee Esty

While writing this book, I worked with many manual therapists and observed their techniques, some similar and some different from the ones in which I was trained. On watching bones realigned, restrictions eased, neurovascular function restored, there has been a persistent refrain in the back of my mind: "Drugs can't do that."

Why the many muscular and postural inputs to migraine are not more widely considered and treated with manual therapy is often simple economics. It takes *time* to evaluate. It takes *time* to work out tangles and restrictions in fascia and muscles. It takes *time* for the tissues to relax. But *time* is *money*.

Drugs to block symptoms may be faster, cheaper, and easier for both physician and patient. They fit the Automated Medicine Model. Manual therapy does not. To survive with insurance, a therapist must pack in patients, good for the bottom line, not for you. A skilled therapist may be able to treat 1-2 patients per hour, but more is iffy and 40 patients before lunch is not good therapy.

How do you know the length of appointments? Ask. If given a choice of 5:30, 5:35, or 5:40, go elsewhere. If you want real attention, an hour or more of time, you're looking at private pay[1]. Every bodyworker has heard some version of: "Your treatments work better than what my doctor does, but you don't take insurance and he does." If it doesn't work, why do it at all? Don't opt for bad therapy just because "insurance covers it." Don't waste your time or money — or anyone else's.

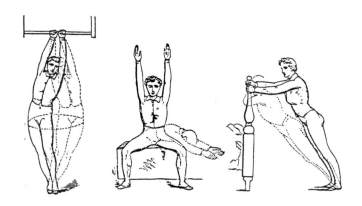

**Figure 107.** THE SWEDISH MOVEMENT EXERCISES OF 1860

---

1. Health Savings Accounts (HSA) and Flexible Spending Accounts (FSA) may cover what standard health insurance will not.

We might think of hands-on bodywork as Paleolithic Medicine, arising in some form in almost all cultures worldwide. Its ancient roots now reach into disciplines now pigeonholed as massage, osteopathy, physical therapy, and more, but now with a tremendous amount of cross talk and interdisciplinary cross-pollination.

For example, what we today call "Swedish Massage" was once known as the "Swedish Movement Cure" and included stretching and strengthening exercises. In 1860, Dr. George Taylor laid these out in *An Exposition of the Swedish Movement-Cure* with: "Examples of Single Movements, and Directions for Their Use in Various Forms of Chronic Disease, Forming a Complete Manual of Exercises" (Figure 107). Modern "Swedish Massage" retains massage techniques, but has abandoned its therapeutic exercises. Both tools are used by myofascial therapists who tend to focus on muscles rather than their connective tissue, ligaments and tendons. That's done by the physical therapists who have expanded from hot packs and strengthening exercises to spinal manipulations but whose basic training does not include osteopathic skills that relieve pressure and restrictions within the skull.

Many headaches come from the neck. The curve of a normal acts as a spring. In motion, discs and vertebrae compress and rebound vertically and obliquely forward. In the straight ("Military") neck (Figure 108-B), discs are vertically compressed with every step, leading to disc narrowing , bone spurs, and nerve compression. Individual vertebrae may also be rotated out of alignment. Painkillers, muscle relaxants and other drugs do not rotate misaligned bones back into place.

All of these skills tend to be dismissed as "alternative," but alternative to what? To not having them available to use when appropriate? Part of the problem is turf wars. Turf is money. Notice how many articles on "alternative" treatments start with an estimate of how many millions of dollars are wasted on these treatments. (Read: in "their " offices rather than "ours").

What matters is what works and what works best for you.

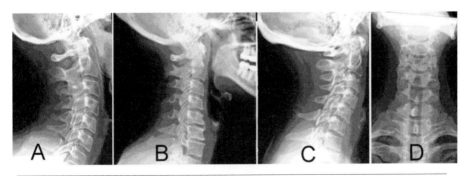

**Figure 108.** CERVICAL CURVES

A Normal, B Straight or ("Military") with reverse curve, C Partially reversed, D Rotated 7th vertebra

## MASSAGE

Massage can be enormously beneficial for both tension and migraine headaches. But for best results find someone who is actually trained and certified. There's more to massage than pushing lotion around, more to "therapeutic" than wind-chime music. Ask about training and certification. Some states do not require it. Some states, such as New York, are extremely strict as the actual intent was to block prostitution. Ask about the actual school attended and its pass/fail rate for students undergoing the National Certification exam.

For example, the Pittsburgh School of Massage offers excellent high-quality training. Its graduates have an almost 100 per cent pass rate on the National Certification Exam, far above State and National averages. In vivid contrast, at a local trade school, applicants who failed the entrance exam were not rejected but automatically sent to the massage program. Some students took advantage of every opportunity to learn, but overall I would not seek out graduates of that school.

Massage schooling and licensure are controlled by the states but there is also a national certification exam for massage (www.NCBTMB.org). Your best approach is to get a recommendation from a trusted friend but work with the therapist with whom you feel most comfortable and who can give the most lasting results. When you are looking for therapeutic massage (versus "spa massage") look for a history of interest and training in therapeutic disciplines.

That said, good massage can reduce stress, lower blood pressure, relax knotted muscles, and feedback loops of pain and dysfunction. Migraine can be heavily neurological, but most often it involves muscles as well. If the problem is primarily muscles, then someone who can deal with muscles is the best person for the problem.

## CHIROPRACTIC

Many migraines come from the neck. Does your neck hurt or feel stiff? It may not be a symptom, it may be a cause. Slide your fingers firmly down the back of your neck, from the base of the skull to nape of the neck. If you feel a prominent bump on one side (but not the other) it may indicate a vertebra rotated out of position and you may have found a major trigger for your migraines.

Chiropractic addresses these and neurovascular relationships particularly in cervical areas which are so heavily involved in head pain. Yet today many people still consider chiropractic to be a quack profession, somewhere in the realm of magical thinking and outright fraud. This notion dates to the time when standard medicine treated nearly every condition with arsenic or opiates but controlled the turf. In fact it is chiropractic that has been relentlessly tested and found effective for back and cervical pain. It is actually many of the "mainstream" treatments that have never been formally evaluated because of long unquestioned tradition. RA Deyo, MD (1983) concluded that there was no good evidence to support the efficacy of corsets, bed rest, TENS, conventional traction, or muscle relaxants on back pain. Gilbert and others (1985) agreed that bed rest and some standard physical therapy exercises actually do more harm than good. In 1994, the Agency for Health Care Research and Policy[1] reported that despite chiropractic's derogatory label as "alternative care," manipulation gave clearly superior results in low back pain compared to standard modalities.

Turn-of-the-century medicine has become Modern Medicine.

Turn-of-the-century chiropractic has become Hands-On Neurology[2].

Many people resist the suggestion that their headaches may come from misaligned vertebrae, and that chiropractic might help. "I would *never* go to a chiropractor!" said a chronic migraineur. "I hear they *kill* people." Palpation revealed a prominent lump on the right side where the C3 vertebra was severely and obviously rotated. Her MD never noticed the problem and it was never treated beyond painkillers and migraine meds which didn't work very well.

Some years ago, intrigued by the notion of Killer Chiropractors, I researched reports of vertebral artery dissection in the on-line archives of the respected journal *Stroke*. There were indeed reports of chiropractor induced injures but as always, there was more to the story than we usually hear.

- There were injuries from MDs who *did* recognize cervical problems and attempted to correct them, but without appropriate training. Oddly, these failed attempts are labeled as "chiropractic manipulations" despite not having been done by a chiropractor.

---

1. Under the US Department of Health and Human Services.
2. Observe the medical textbooks at www.Lww.com. Take a close look at the anatomy, physiology and neurology textbooks listed under "Chiropractic." It is hardly "aromatherapy."

- There was a report of a man who died at a health club. Apparently the owner would "crack" his customer necks if requested. One day when he was out of town, the owner's wife tried it. She had seen it done many times. Unfortunately, *seeing* it done is not the same as years of chiropractic training.

- The bulk of the articles were on searches for a *genetic marker* thought to underlie "spontaneous vertebral artery dissection."

Yes, there are accidents, but chiropractic is not high risk *provided* the practitioner stays within training boundaries *and* the patient is honest about his condition. For example, chiropractic adjustments are dangerously inappropriate following recent skull fracture, brain hemorrhage, stroke, aneurysm, or brain stem injury, systemic infections or extremely high blood pressure. Some problems are due to anatomical oddities. A local chiropractor, noticing an odd neck instability in one of her patients, ordered an MRI which revealed that the patient had no odontoid process (the pivot point in the C2 vertebra around which C1 (the atlas) rotates.

Risk is always best addressed by the insurance industry. Malpractice insurance for chiropractors is about the same as for veterinarians, around $2,000 per year (less than some of us pay for auto insurance) compared to around $200,000 for physicians. The comparison is not exactly fair as chiropractors do not deliver babies or deal with burst appendixes. They cannot do injections or surgery so there is no risk of infection. They cannot prescribe pharmaceutical drugs which kill thousands of people per year[1] even when used correctly. Chiropractic is a relatively low-risk profession.

"Quackbuster" websites are strangely concerned about *subluxations*, a fighting word among turf warriors, but largely a matter of definition. This venerable old medical term simply means shifts in position of a bone or joint that are "less" (*sub*) than a true, blatant dislocation (L. *luxatio*). These may involve slips along a plane, rotations and tilts around any available axis, and resulting strain on connecting fascia, vessels and nerves. These are easily seen in the pelvis, easily felt in the neck.

You can see these for yourself at the beach or the bathroom mirror while standing up straight. The two dimples in the lower back are actually bony *high* points of the pelvis. Normally, they should be level. One higher than the other is a shift in the relationships between the pelvic bones. Returning bones to proper alignment can provide enormous relief. In the Sacro-Iliac (SI) joint or pubic symphysis, it may be the difference between being able or unable to walk. In the neck (see Figure 108), it may be the difference between migraine pain and being pain free.

If you are concerned about "neck cracking" be aware that chiropractic has developed some exquisitely gentle techniques (such as the Cox method), in contrast to old-style

---

1. In 1871, on an expedition to the North Pole, explorer Charles Hall became violently ill after drinking a cup of coffee given to him by a rival. In 1968, tissue samples from the still-frozen corpse revealed "an intake of considerable amounts of arsenic by Hall in the last two weeks of his life." Murder? Maybe. Or maybe just medicine, for in those days, arsenious acid was standard treatment for everything from headache to ulcers to gout (Loomis CC, 2000).

high velocity thrusts. You may feel a "ping" rather than a crunch. And no, this does not "kill people."

The strong chiropractic presence at the Olympics and PGA golf tournaments is because their chiropractors ("Certified Chiropractic Sports Physicians," CCSPs), treat without the drugs or bed rest that would remove athletes from competition. Top-level athletes need top-functioning bodies and they need them right *now*. They do not fight their way to the Olympics only to be murdered by their health care providers.

Personally, I have always considered a good chiropractor a critical part of my sports bag. In falls I have knocked pelvic bones so badly out of place that I couldn't walk for the sciatic pain. But the chirodoc had me back on the mat the next day, something that my MD would have been unable to treat in any other way. Bones and joints displaced by a blow are best treated by simply putting them back where they belong rather than spending weeks in bed on muscle relaxants.

That said, if bones continuously go "out," something else is needed. Bones do not move alone. They are *moved*, pulled by dysfunctional muscles and fascia, poor posture, and other stresses. Every muscle that attaches to a vertebra can potentially pull it out of alignment. Consider LEVATOR SCAPULA (Figure 30 on page 61). This muscle, with the help of hunched shoulders or a tote bag, can pull on and distort all of the upper cervical vertebrae including the atlas (C1). Shoving them back several times a week won't fix the source of the problem. Address the source.

Be skeptical of those who require treatments several times a week, push special supplements, and who require payment in advance for a long series of treatments.

A big red flag is full-spine X-rays. This is 1950s technology with all that implies about consumer safeguards. I fell for that once, when told they were needed for diagnostic purposes. For good information you need good X rays. These aren't Fortunately, the risk of irradiating brain, thyroid, liver and more for a low back problem was offset by a beam of such a low energy and high scattering that it was blocked by muscles and even clothing. The amazingly poor quality film that resulted was useless for diagnosis. Even if it had been clear, X-rays should never be done at random. If they are needed, limit them to the area of concern and have them done at a hospital or radiology center.

## OSTEOPATHY

> Joints are usually "slaves" to soft tissue rather than the other way around.
> —Upledger, John, D. O. (1987)

The health care professional who stands between the AMA physician and chiropractic is the Osteopathic Physician.

Ask an osteopath the difference between a medical doctor and doctor of osteopathy and you will probably be told that they are the same "except that the DO has more training": medical skills plus hands-on manipulative skills. Doctors of Osteopathy are trained in all the particulars of standard medical school; they have also been trained in the techniques of manipulation and palpation skills used in chiropractic. Their work laid the foundation for much manual technique seen today.

Unfortunately, in attempting to make themselves acceptable to the AMA, osteopathy in the US has largely lost the manipulative skills for which it was once renowned. Your best chance of finding practitioners with these skills is in areas of old osteopathic colleges especially those close to Canada, such as Michigan State University or Erie, Pennsylvania.

Today, older osteopaths complain that many students entering osteopathy school are after the medical degree only, with no interest in doing manipulative techniques. And graduates who do train in manipulation find it difficult to apply their skills within the time frames mandated by insurance companies. Some have actually had limits on numbers of patients written into their contracts. They cannot do what they do in 5 or 15-minute blocks.

To find a DO with manipulative skills, see: www.academyofosteopathy.org

## CRANIO-SACRAL THERAPY

Craniosacral Therapy was developed by osteopath John Upledger who (like many osteopaths) feared that the skills of osteopathy were dying. Craniosacral techniques are the basic osteopathic cranial manipulation techniques. By analogy with Chinese bare-foot doctors, he loosed on the world an army of bare-foot osteopaths. Skills vary however. Some have merely taken a weekend workshop and hung out a shingle. Others have trained for decades. One can hurt, the other can help.

Many years ago, when a friend suggested I try cranial work, I picked a therapist out of the phone book. I still remember the horrific headache that resulted from her treatment. I spent several days vomiting and seriously considered leaving the planet. Later I learned that the Upledger Institute tracks training for their students and these records are available on the Internet. I searched out a list of names with the most training and checked them out one by one. This time I struck gold.

Although my random migraines (and their triggers) had resolved with neurofeedback, barometer headaches remained. I could still predict every incoming storm front and could even trigger a migraine by driving too fast up and down hilly highways. An excellent cranio-sacral therapist changed all that. It was the most amazing thing in the world to me to wake up to pouring rain or to find 2 feet of snow on the ground — and not to have known about it days before. No headache, no pain, no feeling of overwhelming exhaustion and fatigue.

The best therapist I found was also trained in Visceral Manipulation which treats deep fascia that surrounds, suspends, and restrict organs. Fascial fibers run continuously from the top to the bottom of the body, literally connecting your forehead to the bottoms of your feet. It also links cranial bones to the rest of you. Pushing cranial bones to relieve fascial strain in head and neck impacts other areas in surprising ways. There is nothing more startling than having a therapist work on your head but feeling it in your low back.

Find a practitioner through www.Upledger.com or the International Association of Healthcare Practitioners (www.IAHP.com) under "Search Practitioners." For best results, enter the first three digits of your ZIP code in the search box.

Notice the many people who have taken one class and hung out a shingle. You deserve better. Look for the person with the most training, preferably someone with *several* classes in craniosacral and several classes in visceral manipulation.

Regardless of licensure, never rely on a therapist with just one class. Figure 109 shows training records for two practitioners. Which one is the better bet?

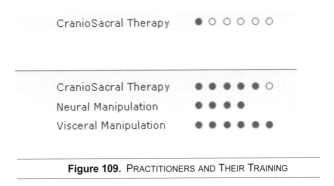

**Figure 109.** PRACTITIONERS AND THEIR TRAINING

Practitioners are not listed in order of coursework or years of experience. Higher rankings on the list are available for a fee, so excellent therapists with extensive training may show up at the bottom, alphabetically below dozens of one-class students.

Find someone you trust and feel comfortable with and who gets good results.

## PHYSICAL THERAPY

> Traditional PT is best for acute injuries: a torn hamstring, a car accident, occupational injuries, and getting stroke victims up and moving. It is severely limited when it comes to long-term chronic conditions.
>
> —Brian Tuckey, PT, OCS, JSCCI

> I started my own practice because I was dissatisfied with being unable to spend the appropriate amount of time required to evaluate, diagnose and treat my patients.
>
> —Todd Kotyk, M.P.T.

Physical therapists (PTs) are the experts on movement. Traditionally, they have been wonderful for dealing with disuse syndrome, and rehabilitating stroke victims to get them up and out of the hospital and back into active life. But muscular issues in reasonably normal patients are a bit different.

In the US, PTs were long under the control of the MD who might be an expert on heart disease or infection but knew little about muscles. Although seen as the muscle experts, they were often forbidden to treat effectively, restricted to the MDs specific prescription, even if they knew the problem was coming from somewhere else.

Emphasis has long been on *strengthening* even where the muscle was already shortened. "Weakness" can be due to poor muscle development (Life as a Couch Potato), it may also be due to the nerve damage and wasting which occurs in polio (the traditional PT paradigm). In otherwise healthy, active persons, weakness is more likely due to overshortening or overstretching. Exercises that require an already shortened muscle to contract further only make the problem worse. What is needed is stretching and lengthening to restore the ability of the muscle to contract at all.

Dr. Travell insisted that patients should be able to do 10 pain-free repetitions through full range of motion for 2 weeks *before* starting strengthening exercises. Her constant refrain was: *First* lengthen *then* strengthen. Strengthening exercises should never be done on a muscle inhibited by pain. Overriding these protective inhibitions sets up inappropriate movement patterns. Other muscles must then subsitute in jobs they aren't intended to do resulting in more strain and pain. And that was my long-held image of PT. More strain, more pain.

Until a couple months ago, I frankly had nothing good to say about PT and would never have seen or recommended it for headaches, certain that it would only make them worse. Nevertheless, in hopes of finding *something* good to say, I interviewed several PTs for this section, Brian Tuckey, Peter Coppola, and Todd Kotyk[1]. These excellent therapists gave me a whole new appreciation for what PTs can do — or what they can

---

1. Brian Tuckey is with Tuckey & Associates in Frederick, Maryland, an instructor for the Jones Institute on strain-counterstrain techniques developed by osteopath Dr. Lawrence Jones. Peter Coppola, with Backways Physical Therapy in Prescott, Arizona, and Todd Kotyk with Appropriate Physical Therapy in Canonsburg, Pennsylvania, teach fascial and visceral techniques developed by French osteopath Jean-Pierre Barral.

do having added osteopathic techniques to their tool sets, well beyond (as all of them agreed), basic PT training.

In the US, until recently, PTs weren't allowed to manipulate vertebrae directly, turf reserved for doctors of osteopathy and chiropractic. PTs could work with muscles, tendons and ligaments. As a result, misaligned vertebrae might "accidentally" pop back into place. Oops! "Well, that just happens sometimes," was the cover story. Now that PT is a doctoral program, direct manipulation fits more openly under the PT umbrella. Kotyk demonstrated correction of rotated cervical vertebrae on my computer-strained neck. He did it by treating muscles and tendons. These are the tissues that actually move bones in or out of place often with painful results. "In all headache patients," says Tuckey, "the C1/C2 vertebrae are the first thing I check."

Is this now standard PT? *It is not.*

PT has three basic tools: Manual (hands-on) techniques, exercise, and *modalities* (anything mechanical). To move away from the unprofitable hands-on end of the scale, many PTs have become increasingly reliant on machines such as TENS units or ultrasound. Sometimes these help, sometimes they don't.

"But here's the decision point," says Tuckey. "If you don't see improvements within 6 sessions, and if the therapist is doing the same thing each visit, you're wasting your time and money. Before you start, ask the therapist how much of the practice is machine-based modalities. If more than half, go elsewhere. And yes, you can do this. It is your choice. Because PT is now a doctoral-level program, in most states, patients have direct access and a legal right to see any PT they choose." [1]

If your physician insists that you see a specific PT ask why. "Does he work for you? Do you have a financial interest in this group? You may hear "yes," you may hear "no," but evaluate for yourself. Sometimes, in the same suite, the relationship is obvious. Sometimes they are on the other side of town, disguised by a different name.

Whoever you choose, be sure that hands-on manual therapy is available as the bulk of the treatment. Many claim that every problem can be corrected by exercise alone. That is simply not true, although it is certainly more profitable.

This does not diminish the importance of exercise, but it does not stand alone.

Exercise *combined* with hands-on therapy can work wonders.

---

1. Exceptions: Medicare will not cover physical therapy without a referral from an MD or DO. Insurance in general will not cover PT without authorization by a doctor, but with self-pay you should be able to see anyone you choose.

## MYOFASCIAL TRIGGER POINT THERAPY

> When I asked the staff at the tuberculosis hospital what caused the pain, they would say, "It comes from the infected lung, of course." On the cardiac service. . . "It comes from the heart, of course." On the medical service. . . "It's an emotional, psychogenic pain." All the patients had identical patterns and we mapped these patterns. We began injecting the trigger points with procaine and got good results.
>
> —Janet Travell, M. D.

Trigger Point Therapy is recognized as a highly effective treatment for pain and dysfunction by the highly regarded American Academy of Pain Management.

The term *myotherapy* was coined by Massachusetts physician Dr. Desmond Tivy to describe the pressure technique popularized by Bonnie Prudden (1980) based on work by Dr. Janet Travell, Dr. David Simons, Hans Kraus, and many others throughout the years. Prudden had assisted Dr. Tivy when he treated TrPs with procaine injection. Her job was to probe for sore spots in muscles then mark them for treatment. Prudden quickly rediscovered what *shiatsu* practitioners and other bodyworkers learned centuries ago; pain may disappear in response to direct pressure. Very often the pain had vanished by the time the patient made it down the hall to the treatment room.

Myofascial Trigger Point Therapists are trained in musculoskeletal dysfunction, basic kinesiology, ROM testing, and corrective and therapeutic exercises. They do not diagnose medical conditions. Before beginning treatment, most will require referral from a medical doctor, to check for any underlying medical condition.

This technique is a specialty in the bodywork community. Many massage therapists claim to "know trigger point" but in general I have not found this to be true without specific training. The term has gone from unknown to marketing buzzword in the last few years, but effective ttherapy requires familiarity with referred pain patterns and a thorough knowledge of the muscle anatomy and neurology behind them.

Trigger point therapy was the first thing I found that actually helped or halted a migraine. I was so impressed that I took two years off to study the technique. I had definite neck and jaw problems, but was learning to treat those and so was surprised and disappointed when headaches got *worse*. Instead of waking up every Tuesday with a migraine, I was waking up every Wednesday with a migraine[1]. Why?

Tuesday was a 12-hour day. From 9 in the morning until 9 at night, 2 hours of cadaver anatomy then one exercise class after another, done barefoot ("We must exercise the feet!") over concrete covered with wood topped with a formaldehyde-based finish. A fellow student broke out in hives if her skin touched that floor. I got stuffy just walking into the room. Years later I learned that I have a severe case of Morton Foot. At home, I could adapt in my running shoes. Barefoot over concrete and formaldehyde fumes I could not. But it was there that I first realized the link between tight, strained leg

---

1. See Tuesdays and bad chemical hood design on page 212.

muscles and migraines, and that treating thighs and calves could halt the attack even after treating the apparently "correct" muscles of neck and head did not help.

Treating the actual source of pain is a challenge for both therapist and patient. It's always tempting to try to help what hurts by working where it hurts. Treatment, however, is best done by treating the source rather than the symptom. Have your therapist explain the referral patterns behind your headaches and be sure to do your stretching as assigned. These are as important as the TrP treatments themselves.

The National Association of Myofascial Trigger Point Therapists (NAMTPT) requires an examination. Find certified practitioners at: www.myofascialtherapy.org.

### Strain-Counterstrain

Strain-Counterstrain is a related hands-on manual therapy developed by osteopath Lawrence Jones. It alleviates tightness and spasm in muscle and connective tissue through "positional release," finding the position where the muscle is slackened and pain decreases (usually the opposite of the ROM stretch). These positions are held for up to 90 seconds relaxing the spasm and apparently reseting the sensors and reflexes. This allows local areas of inflammation within the painful tissue to dissipate, restoring joint mobility and circulation. Find a practitioner at www.JISCS.com.

### Trigger Point Injection

Intermuscular trigger point injection is intended to halt the pain signals between the area of shortened muscle and pain receptors in the brain. It is useful for stubborn or very deep trigger points that do not respond to or are out of reach of pressure techniques. Injection should never be seen as *treatment*. It is equivalent to novocaine at the dentist's office, providing a window of opportunity for the real work to follow. Injection provides temporary pain *relief* and a window of opportunity for the actual treatment: the range-of-motion and muscle lengthening to follow.

On pain charts, the Xs indicating TrPs are only general guides. Steroid injection of a sore elbow, knee or shoulder has long been a standard treatment. Besides the dangers of steroids themselves, another issue is the injection site. Some 85 per cent of pain of myofascial origin is referred from elsewhere, several inches or several feet away. Hence attempts to relieve pain by injecting the area where it is actually felt will fail some 85 per cent of the time.

This is an important issue should you opt for trigger point injection for headaches. A trigger point is the point that actually "triggers" and refers pain elsewhere. I've heard reports of patients receiving 100 and more supposed trigger point injections with all their associated risk of bruising, infection, and post-treatment pain. These were not all trigger points. A trigger point is not just a point that hurts. It is not the same as a taut band. No one should be doing "trigger point injection" unless they can actually palpate the point and trigger (reproduce) the pain.

A dry needle (as in acupuncture, or even a dry insulin needle) inserted into a trigger point is as effective as a hypodermic needle with injection. The needle seems to short out aberrant electrical impulses and can also break up scar tissue. Injection helps to relieve the pain, but what is injected is also important. Different drugs vary widely in effectiveness and toxic side effects on muscles (Travell & Simons, 1999).

- *Procaine (novacaine).* Travell's original protocol was developed using procaine hydrochloride at concentrations of no more than one percent, never more than 1 gram of solution, and never with epinephrine. Procaine is the least myotoxic of compounds used for muscle injection. A vasodilator, it improves blood flow in trigger points and induces muscle relaxation but not paralysis. Procaine breaks down in the bloodstream so its effects fade quickly with no strain on the liver.

- *Lidocaine, marcaine.* Cheaper than procaine, lasting twice as long, but more myotoxic. "Longer-lasting" sounds good, but if the needle hits a nerve, expect to do without the body part that nerve supplies for the next 12 hours or so. Because these substances are broken down in the liver, they can be toxic to anyone with impaired liver function.

- *Saline Solution.* Injection of TrPs with *isotonic* saline solution (with the "same" saltiness as blood) has been found helpful. *Hypertonic* saline solution ("more" salty than blood) has been used specifically to *irritate* muscles. Why? TrP pain referral charts were made by injecting specific muscles with hypertonic saline. The painful results were mapped and documented.

- *Steroids.* Injection with steroids may be more effective than lidocaine alone but also more dangerous (Simons, DG and others, 1999, p. 610). Steroids break down connective tissue, one of several reasons why patients are limited to a few shots per year.

Done correctly, TrP injection can be extremely useful but it does not replace the rest of the protocol: intermittent cold and passive stretch followed by moist heat, followed by active ROM stretching to return shortened muscle fibers to their proper resting length. (See Chapter 2.)

The "pain clinic" that does trigger point injections but ignores perpetuating structural and life-style factors, muscle health, and muscle lengthening, is providing only short-term relief of symptoms. If TrPs return, requiring continuing injection, something else is wrong. The persistent TrP in the left TRAPEZIUS may be coming from a disturbed gait pattern in the right hip, from work injuries, dehydration, hypothyroid, and many possible nutritional deficits. Look for TrPs, but also look for their causes.

## ROLFING AND KINESIS

Rolfing® is named for its American creator, Dr. Ida P. Rolf (who called it "Structural Integration"). Dr Ida P. Rolf earned her PhD in biochemistry though Columbia University in 1920, studied particle physics and math in Switzerland. Back in New York, she met a Dr. Morrison, a blind osteopathic physician, and began to develop concepts of structural integration rooted in gentle, soft-tissue osteopathic technique.

Today Structural Integration (SI) is a hands-on practice involving manipulation of fascia combined with movement education to restore balance and functionality. It has a painful reputation, due to impatient early efforts, and improperly trained individuals who assume that any forceful technique must be Rolfing. I heard a first-hand report of broken ribs and a fractured sternum suffered by a man who was himself a Rolf practitioner, yet when I went to experience it for myself, what I found was gentle pressure. Individual practitioners fall between the two extremes, but in general, over the last 15-20 years, the Rolf Institute, particularly in Europe, has taught a lighter more patient approach. "Now," says practitioner Emily Dolan Gordon, "we have learned to listen to tissue, rather than trying to boss it around."

Force varies by client and practitioner. On revisiting the technique for this book, I worked with Brian Joly of Pittsburgh who has what I must describe as a firm approach. But any temporary discomfort is well worth it when just minutes of work produces major changes in posture and comfort in standing and walking.

Rolf's original work has evolved in various directions through her students, from the work of Joseph Heller, "Hellerwork" to Tom Myers' Kinesis Myofascial Integration (KMI), Bill Williams' SOMA, Ed Maupin's International Professional School of Bodywork in California, the Guild for Structural Integration. The trademark holder, the Rolf Institute for Structural Integration, strives to retain Rolf's original techniques.

Find US practitioners at: www.rolf.org, European at: www.rolfing.org.

For the international association see: www.theiasi.org.

KMI practitioners can be found at: www.anatomytrains.com/kmi.

To learn more about fascia and fascia research in general, see www.fasciacongress.org.

## ACUPUNCTURE

Regardless of origin, acupuncture was formalized and preserved into modern times by the Chinese, a situation which led to a truly astonishing example of Western Medical prejudice. Many observable effects were routinely dismissed as Communist brain-washing at least until after President Richard Nixon's trip to China in 1972 and opening of trade negotiations.

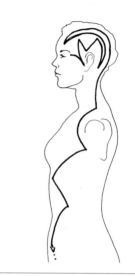

Traditional Chinese medicine attributes headaches to the gallbladder meridian which runs along fascia lining borders or bellies of TRAPEZIUS, STERNOCLEIDOMASTOID, TEMPORALIS, OCCIPITOFRONTALIS and other muscles that can cause severe headaches regardless of your politics.

**Figure 110.** GALLBLADDER MERIDIAN

Acupuncture has been tested on headaches using traditional points along traditional meridians with "sham" points as controls. Headaches got better with needling of traditional points. But, to the consternation of the researchers, they also got better with needling of the "sham" points. Results of this sort tend to be attributed to "placebo effect" but also fit well with the idea that meridians are lines of fascia. Whether a needle is on a formally described meridian or not, fascia, our first nervous system, is *everywhere*.

Modern research supports the idea that meridians are lines of fascia, and that traditional points communicate with deeper fascial planes. Langevin HM and Yandow JA (2002) found that major points correlated with fascial planes between muscle as verified by ultrasound imaging. These points were found at fascial boundaries and showed all the traditional attributes to a far greater degree than control points a short distance away.

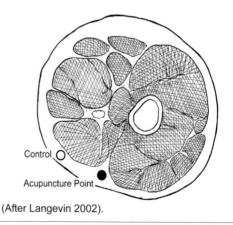

Control

Acupuncture Point

(After Langevin 2002).

**Figure 111.** ACUPUNTURE POINTS AND FASCIA

Acupuncture may be another means of manipulating and realigning fascia, a means of improving communication signals through the fascial network. Changes may occur no matter where the needle is placed but results may be enhanced at acupuncture points of intersecting fascial planes. Table 16 summarizes Langevin and

Yandow's many correlations between traditional Eastern terms / concepts and traditional Western anatomy / physiology.

**TABLE 16.** ACUPUNCTURE CONCEPTS IN WESTERN TERMS

| | |
|---|---|
| Acupuncture meridians | Fascial planes. See "The Fascial Connection" on page 39 and Myers' lines. |
| Acupuncture points | Convergence / intersections of fascial planes |
| Qi / ki | "Sum of all body energetic phenomena (metabolism, movement, signaling and information exchange)" |
| Meridian qi / ki | Biochemical/bioelectrical signaling and information exchange travelling along fascial planes. |
| Blocked / Restored qi flow | Impaired / improved signaling along fascial lines due to alterations in fascia or its collagen fibers. |

Medical acupuncture specifically represents the use of acupuncture by fully trained and licensed physicians. The American Academy of Medical Acupuncture includes more than 1,500 physicians who also do acupuncture. The AAMA has developed standards (200 hours of formal acupuncture training plus Continuing Education requirements), proficiency examinations and certification requirements for its members. Find a provider in your area at: www.medicalacupuncture.org.

## BIOFEEDBACK

> The stronger the imagination, the less imaginary the results.
> —Rabindranath Tagore

Biofeedback in its many forms is a major tool in the headache tool kit.

The formal laboratory studies of biofeedback began in the 1960s at the acclaimed Menninger Clinic observing yogis from India. It continued with such flaky New Age folk as the US Air Force and NASA scientists, physicists and psychophysiologists from UCLA. Despite a long history (far longer and older than antidepressants and most migraine drugs), biofeedback is still considered an "alternative" treatment or training, sometimes described as "controversial."

I know firsthand that it can work amazingly well. No controversy there. The debate seems to be whether brains and behavior can be altered without drugs. We know they can, simply with food and changes in blood sugar, sound and music, light, and even the thoughts and activities you choose to engage in.

The real concern seems to be the usual: It Will Destroy Civilization As We Know It. Drug companies fear loss of profits, psychologists and psychiatrists fear loss of patients. But biofeedback doesn't replace proper medical or psychiatric care. It is not a commodity, it is hands-on brain training. It takes time and effort. No one gets rich doing biofeedback.

People who haven't read the research literature typically claim that there is no research literature. Studies tend to be small and clinical and probably always will be. There is no multi-billion-dollar international biofeedback cartel. Doctors don't get trips to Hawaii as reward for prescribing handwarming. No one hires mega-buck advertising firms to ghostwrite phony research articles to place in medical journals, nor do they have the money to bribe MDs to sign off on them as pharmaceutical companies have done in several recent notorious examples.

One "quackbuster" website (widely believed to be funded by drug companies) includes biofeedback on their list of questionable treatments. Grudging admission that it does work is quickly followed by speculation that patients could probably have obtained equally good results without the electronic equipment. Perhaps. The same can be said of flight simulators.

For those who want fast and effective results without crashing and burning, a course of biofeedback with a knowledgeable flight instructor can be enormously helpful in headaches of all kinds. And, while there's much more to it than handwarming, that is a great start.

### Handwarming

Hand-warming as therapy was once spoken of by practitioners in hushed under-the-table tones. Today it's a standard. Most headache clinics and many psychotherapists teach handwarming.

Handwarming may seem a small thing, but it is far from trivial. Simply holding hands under warm water or warming with microwaveable hand mitts can improve circulation and decrease number and intensity of migraines[1]. Handwarming done with the mind alone becomes an exercise in calming the entire autonomic nervous system.

One of its many advantages is that it can be practiced at home with nothing more than a comfortable chair, some pleasant music, and a digital thermometer such as the Stress Thermometer ($19.95 from www.Amazon.com).

Also consider the computer "game" Wild Divine. Finger sensors track heart rate, temperature, and galvanic skin response similar to old professional systems once costing thousands of dollars. To play you must breathe, you must relax. See www.wilddivine.com.

### sEMG and Muscle Retraining

Muscles lurk behind many kinds of headaches. One can often deduce the source and location of a classic one-sided migraine just by observing a patient's posture. Head-Forward posture is very common in migraineurs. One shoulder may be higher than the other, one side of the muscle may be remarkably weaker or stronger than the other, may recover more slowly or incompletely after work. A patient, from simple habit or a misguided attempt to guard against pain, may never allow muscles to relax completely, yet be entirely unaware of this behavior.

Surface Electromyography (sEMG) is a painless, non-invasive method of observing and documenting muscle behavior, strength, and balance. It is used to guide rehabilitation, exercise programs/prescriptions, and decisions on returning to game or work. sEMG picks up and amplifies the signals on the skin surface which are generated by the nerves in area of the sensor. The resulting EMG signals are displayed and graphed (on computer screen or paper). This quantifies the exact degree of the problem while making it clearly visible to the patient, and allowing correction of dysfunctional patterns and therapies.

For headaches (where myofascial issues have long been ignored or denied) sEMG can be extremely useful in showing that there is a problem *at all,* what that problem might be, and ways of best resolving it through manual treatment and muscle retraining, guided biofeedback, and awareness.

How do these differ? Some contractions are under the direct control of the client and once they are aware of the problem, they can correct it. Some are not, but sEMG reveals

---

1. It is less reliable for aborting attacks after they have started, especially for beginners new to the technique but warming can be done mechanically and some migraines aborted by working legs and calves. See page 94.

the difference[1]. For example, the simultaneous but inappropriate contraction of two adjacent muscles (*co-contractions*) suggests the presence of adhesions between the two. All the biofeedback and positive mindset in the world will not break those adhesions or realign scar tissue. Direct hands-on treatment will.

*Neurofeedback*

In my opinion, if any medication had demonstrated such a wide spectrum of efficacy it would be universally accepted and widely used . . . [Neurofeedback] is a field to be taken seriously by all.

—Frank H. Duffy, MD
Harvard Medical School

*Neurofeedback* is biofeedback applied to the brain, or more specifically, to the brainwave signals which appear at the scalp as a result of firing of cortical neurons.

There is no question that altering brainwaves can alter behaviors. This is, after all, one of the foundations of drug therapies. Speeding up a slow brain with antidepressants will kick it out of its depressed state. Slowing down a brain in hyperdrive with anti-anxiety meds will relieve panic attacks and night terrors. The problem is that drugs are not hemispherically or location specific. They can't treat just one side or one area of the brain.

In contrast, neurofeedback can be very targeted, very specific, and very effective. It can reawaken the brain, and get brain and body back on the road to recovery. Clients routinely report greatly reduced pain and anxiety, with greatly improved clarity, organizational skills, and self-control. You can expect improvement in a range of conditions as diverse as traumatic brain injury (TBI), PTSD, fibromyalgia, PMS, epilepsy, autism spectrum, and migraines. If present, depression and ADD often improve as side-effects of treating the more apparently physical disorders.

One of the problems with the current paradigm of Automated Medicine is the attempt to fix everything that's wrong with your earth vehicle by pouring yet another additive into the gas tank. Sometimes this works. Sometimes the problem is not the gas or the tires or the fenders. Sometimes it is the electrical system.

Neurofeedback is a painless and drug-free way of helping the brain return to a healthy state, to do a better job of regulating itself and the body. The goal of neurofeedback is not so much *relaxation* as resetting less-than-optimal patterns in the Central Nervous System (CNS). Relaxation is a side effect — as is relief of migraine and other seemingly physical symptoms such as fatigue and pain.

Although there are many forms of neurofeedback, they fall into two basic categories.

---

1.   sEMG is now reimbursed by several insurance companies including Aetna and Cigna, for several pain problems including headache and TMJD.

Traditional ("classical") NF is a learning process, like standard operant conditioning. The brain learns to recognize a desired brainwave or state and produce it on demand. The reward is a food pellet in the form of a light or tone. Examples include:

- Brainmaster (from www.Brainmaster.com)
- Cygnet (from www.EEGInfo.com)

The newer stim systems feed back an extremely tiny, consciously imperceptible, electrical signal. But the brain hears it, and these systems typically produce results far more quickly than Classical NF techniques. Examples include:

- Flexyx (the system on which much early research was done, still in use, but no longer commercially available),
- LENS (available from www.Ochslabs.com),
- Neuro-Gen (available from www.Neuro-Gen.com).

There can be advantages to each of these approaches.

Traditional neurofeedback is a training process. It teaches your brain (typically below the level of consciousness) to recognize, control and work with your own brainwaves, in meditation and in daily life. Training is expected to take 20-40 sessions.

Stim neurofeedback requires no special effort or attention from the client (an advantage in young or Autistic Spectrum children). Like AAA, it is a rescue service, intended to pull you out of the ditch and speed you on your way. It doesn't teach you how to drive, it simply rescues and repairs, but it can do this very quickly. Positive results should begin to appear within the first 3-6 sessions, others within 12-20 sessions.

Either approach is a feather compared to the baseball bat of drugs or surgery. You can move a person very effectively by tickling him with a feather, but not through a locked and barred steel door. The feather won't work if bones are misaligned or jammed too tightly to allow proper neurovascular function. Clients who fail to improve with neurofeedback (especially those who have been hit in the head with a windshield or a planet) are referred for bodywork.

Either approach can work miracles for *some*, but not for *all* simply because neurofeedback can't do everything. It doesn't replace proper medical care, appropriate psychotherapy, or supply missing nutrients. It doesn't work well if there is chronic systemic infection. It can reduce spasticity and relax muscles caught in flight-or-fight loops of stress and tension, but it does not remove scar tissue or adhesions. It does not fix the bad posture that inhibits breathing and blocks blood supply to muscles and brain.

Case in point: At a seminar, we were shown a video of a young man being wired for biofeedback in hopes of training him to control his headaches. What kind of headaches and where? They didn't say, but one could guess based on his severe Head-Forward posture, round shoulders, collapsed chest, extreme swayback, the Doonesbury slouch of a serious computer geek. He did not need biofeedback, at least not as the starting point. He needed to quit slouching and stand up straight. But at some point muscles and fascia become so shortened, overstretched, adhesed, and unbalanced that standing up straight becomes physically impossible.

As mentioned under sEMG, some muscle contractions and their release are not under the client's control. Simultaneous but inappropriate contractions in adjacent muscles (*co-contractions*) suggest the presence of adhesions, that is, different layers of tissue glommed together, no longer able to slide past each other as they must do for proper function. In such a case, the only way to correct the problem is direct hands-on bodywork to relieve restrictions. Drugs won't do it. sEMG reveals the problem, bodywork will relieve myofascial and structural problems, and biofeedback will keep things functioning as they should if combined with proper food, sleep, and exercise.

Nevertheless, neurofeedback alone has restored function, relieved headache, body pain, and depression after traumatic brain injury. Popular wisdom is that how you are a year after the injury is as good as you're going to get. As I know all too well, with neurotherapy this just isn't so.

In 1996 I stepped off an icy curb in a storm and smashed the back of my head on the curb. It was a skull fracture, it was a severe concussion, and it was the end of my life as I knew it. The migraines changed sides but were even worse and more constant than before. In addition, I couldn't remember how to cook, how to program, or how to stay awake for more than 3 hours at a time.

After years of living in head injury hell, I happened to stumble across references to neurofeedback and resolved to give it a try. Dr. Mary Lee Esty had applied the Flexyx Neurotherapy System to Iraq/Afghanistan veterans suffering from serious Traumatic Brain Injury (TBI) and Post Traumatic Stress Syndrome (PTSD). These vets had already received the best the military had to offer with little result, but neurotherapy worked for them (Esty ML and Nelson DV, 2009).

And it worked for me. Dr. Esty saved my life and sanity 7 years after severe TBI, long after improvement was thought to be no longer possible, and long after I had done everything I was supposed to have done — to little or no avail. Suddenly I could stay awake for 5 or 6 hours, then 8, then 16. I could shop for groceries and remember to put them away. Rather than turning in circles trying to remember how to microwave a potato, I could remember how to cook again.

Losing the devastating fog and confusion of head injury was miracle enough, but the real surprise was that my life-long problem with random migraines began to disappear, as did some of the once-ferocious food sensitivities and other triggers. I was still sensitive to weather and and pressure changes. But even migraines from those sources were nothing compared to what they had been.

Sites below list practitioners using various systems. You can also find many videos on migraine, biofeedback and neurofeedback at: www.YouTube.com.

- For practitioners in traditional biofeedback, Biofeedback Certification International Alliance (BCIA) see wwwBCIA.org.

- For information on mlitary / combat injuries including TBI and PTSD treated with biofeedback, see www. brainwellnessandbiofeedback.com. Dr. Esty's practice in Bethesda, Maryland, is the only one I currently know of that offers biofeedback, neurofeedback, and muscle retraining via sEMG.

- For extensive information on neurofeedback in epilepsy and other conditions, see www.EEGInfo.com and wwwMind-BrainTraining.com/NeurofeedbackStudiesandLinks.html

- For a bibliography of research papers on biofeedback and neurofeedback see www.ISNR.org and www.AAPB.org.

In retrospect, it is astonishing that neurofeedback worked as well for me as it did. Neck and head had suffered a wide variety of sports injuries. The fall in the ice-storm was just the final devastating blow to the system. While working with two excellent craniosacral therapists, both commented on severe cranial distortion. Relieving that eliminated the extreme sensitivity to weather and pressure changes and seems to have been the final missing piece to the mystery.

It's not the last step however. Stress and strain on muscle and bone is constant and changing, often inappropriate and damaging. Do you tense your neck when walking, writing, talking, sleeping? Learn to recognize it, adapt, and flow to help the body work in the way it was intended.

## ALEXANDER AND FELDENKRAIS

Frederick Matthias Alexander (1869-1955) was an Australian stage performer and Shakespearean actor. The sudden and catastrophic loss of his voice inspired him to discover what he was doing to cause his affliction. His methods expanded to become known as Alexander Technique (AT).

AT teaches tools for discovering, stopping or transforming behaviors that get in the way of optimal function of the body "in ordinary actions of living — rising, sitting, walking, standing, using arms, hands, voice, tools, instruments of all kinds." How you perform these everyday activities may offer you and an AT teacher many clues to the physical origins of your migraines.

Moshe Feldenkrais (1904-1984) was an engineer, physicist and a "player" of Judo, a martial art that teaches balance, coordination and efficiency of motion. A knee injury inspired him to investigate human movement and neurophysiology. He studied with Alexander, adding work in biology, cybernetics, and learning theory, developing a method of muscle education that explores and develops mind/body coordination.

Both approaches improve flexibility, strength, coordination, and balance. Many consider them critical to avoiding pain and injury.

Improved awareness of body mechanics has led to major changes in arts education. Alexander Technique is now standard training in many schools of music, drama, and dance.

Alexander practitioners can be found at: www.ati-net.com.

Feldenkrais practitioners can be found at: www.feldenkrais.com.

# YOGA

It pays to know methods of prevention and treatment for orthopedic problems that are low-cost and rely almost entirely on self-care.

—Jane E. Brody (2011)

Yoga is stone-age physical therapy. Illustrations of poses have been found dating to 3,000 B.C., but the practice is certainly older while our bodies are very much the same. It is excellent exercise for mind and body.

Yoga came to the U.S. in the 1890s, but as it became most familiar during the 1960s, it has never quite escaped its "counter-culture" image. This may be changing as its value has been documented in clinical tests by physicians who are both "mainstream" and yoga practitioners. One of these is Dr. Loren Fishman, physiatrist and yoga practitioner, of the very mainstream New York-Presbyterian/Columbia Hospital.

Dr. Fishman has treated a range of common and painful conditions ranging from Rotator Cuff Syndrome (a shoulder injury) to Piriformis Syndrome (entrapment of the sciatic nerve by the piriformis muscle of the hip) with classic or modified yoga exercises in place of standard treatments often involving tens of thousands of dollars of surgery (Brody JE, 2011). He has also written several books on yoga applied to skeletomuscular problems.

Researchers at Boston University School of Medicine studied the effects of yoga on mood, anxiety, and GABA levels in the brain (Streeter and others, 2010). Simply getting out and walking is known to decrease depression and improve muscle fitness, but yoga was found to do it even better.

# The End of Migraines

Are my headaches gone forever? Well, not exactly. Once or twice a year, usually during mold or pollen season, I still get the old familiar 2-3 days of nauseating migraine pain.

But this stands in stark contrast to severe incapacitating migraines 2-3 times a week, lasting 2-3 days or even 2-3 weeks at a time. There were entire years when I was shocked and surprised if I woke up without a headache. Today I am shocked and surprised if I wake up *with* a headache, but they might last a few hours at most.

It isn't simply a matter of avoiding triggers. Many serious triggers lost their power, not over years, but over weeks and months. Some vanished overnight.

- Bright sunlight was once a sure trigger. When I had to go out in bright sun I wore glacier glasses, the darkest lenses possible with wrap-around sides to block any leaks. Light sensitivity is often attributed to eye color, but also a common symptom of migraine and head injury. I had all of these.

  Now I enjoy sunny days and am unaffected by the brightest light even though I have the same genetically blue eyes today that I've always had. I wear a brimmed hat in bright, hot sunlight. But sunglasses? Not needed. I don't even own a pair.

- Onions were once one of my deadliest triggers. A single accidental bite of onion lurking in a salad or the wrong hamburger, could trigger a ferocious 2-3 day migraine.

  Today I enjoy the occasional order of onion rings. Too many will trigger upset stomach and restless sleep, but not migraines.

- Cheese and chocolate used to be deadly.

  Today Jarlsberg (a Norwegian "baby Swiss") is a diet staple, while a deliciously moldy brie, blue cheese, and chocolate are delightful treats.

- Red wine is a standard on all the migraine food lists. Once I would check the calendar, pollen levels, and incoming weather fronts before risking a sip or two.

  Today I can merrily guzzle way too much with no visible ill effects. Stupid behavior will reward me with a hangover like anyone else, but a glass or two of wine never brings the horrific consequences it would have a few years ago.

- Barometric changes were a constant threat. I would land in bed with a migraine 2 days before the weather front arrived. Riding a high-rise elevator or the subway, flying, or even driving too fast up and down hills was risky.

  Today I am surprised to wake up to 2 feet of snow or pouring rain. If I am *not* surprised, if storms are again heralded by head pain, I know it is time to go back for a tune-up of neck and cranial bones.

- For decades I never went anywhere without my medications. There was the office stash, the purse and backpack stash, the home stash. And I never left home without a plan for how to get back or sleep it off safely if an uncontrollable migraine should strike at work or during travel. This seriously restricted life, work, and travel.

  Today I have no prescription drugs. I do have several small dusty bottles of Excedrin and Aleve somewhere in the house. These were purchased on the fly for the rare occasions when a headache did strike while I was out and I was caught by surprise because I don't even think to keep the pills with me anymore.

So now, with the same set of genes, I can play in the sunshine, eat cheese, chocolate, and the occasional onion ring washed down with red wine regardless of the weather. I still have jaw issues, but when my TMJ splint broke (under a tire in the parking lot) I never bothered to replace it. I probably should and will one day, but meanwhile, the ability to recognize muscle problems and correct them is enough.

What do I still avoid? Fast-foods, processed foods, and tough foods. I cook from scratch, avoid MSG, artificial sweeteners, sulfites, and other preservatives. Shampoo is no longer laced with formaldehyde like it was 20 years ago, but new carpet is and I avoid it. If a building or a room makes me sick, I no longer assume that the problem is entirely with me. I no longer spend hours every day playing the piano, but when I do (or during computer time) I watch posture, and am much more attentive to how I am using my body. Learning to play the violin has made the relationship between shoulders, neck and migraines painfully clear.

Some improvement can be attributed to getting older when some migraines tend to resolve, but that explanation does not cover all the bases. Age can't explain *overnight* loss of symptoms and sensitivities after biofeedback and bodywork. It doesn't explain improvement of TMJ symptoms within *minutes* of sEMG retraining of unbalanced jaw muscles.

Yes, I *can* still get migraines. The combination of wild weather, mountains, highway food, computer work and too much coffee, still puts me at risk. Simple dehydration and too much violin time will do the job but many of these triggers are optional.

For me, drugs worked poorly but given the many factors that combined to produce the migraine symptoms, I now know why. I also know that there are many choices beyond life in horrific pain or zonked out on drugs.

For those of you who still face those choices, I sincerely hope that my journey will be of help in yours.

# Research and References

Here's a short list of recommended books.

- On identifying the problem:
  - *10 Simple Solutions to Migraines: Recognize Triggers, Control Symptoms, And Reclaim Your Life*, by Dawn Marcus, MD, Includes many charts and checklists for evaluating headaches and finding patterns.

- The relationship between triggers and pain, migraine drugs and how to get off them:
  - *Heal Your Headache*: by David Buchholz, MD.

- On toxic chemicals in personal care and other products. Why your headaches may be coming from your shampoo, hair straightener, creams and lotions.
  - *Not Just a Pretty Face: the Ugly Side of the Beauty Industry*, by Stacy Malkin

- On hypothyroid, history and treatment:
  - *Hypothyroidism:The Unsuspected Illness,* by *Broda* Barnes, MD, and Lawrence Galton
  - *What Your Doctor May Not Tell You About Hypothyroidism*, by Ken Blanchard, MD, and Marietta Abrams Brill

- What it's like, if you have not suffered migraines yourself:
  - *A Brain Wider Than the Sky,* by Andrew Levy, Ph.D.
  - *Migraine Art*, by Klaus Podoll, MD, and Derek Robinson

- What actually goes on in there, under the hood (for medical professionals):
  - *Travell & Simons Myofascial Pain and Dysfunction: The Trigger Point Manual*, by Janet G. Travell, MD, and David G. Simons, MD. A hefty two-volume set for medical professionals, with superb illustrations understandable by anyone.
  - *Tension-Type and Cervicogenic Headache: Pathophysiology, Diagnosis, and Management*, by Cèsár Fernández-de-las-Peñas, P.T., D.O., Ph.D, Lars Arendt-Nielsen, Ph.D., and Robert D. Gerwin, MD.

For more up-to-date information, see www.PubMed.com.

# References Cited

Adison, AW (1951), Cervical ribs: symptoms, differential diagnosis and indications for section of the insertion of the scalenus anticus muscle. *Journal of the International College of Surgeons*, Vol. 16, pp. 546-559.

Adler I (1900), Muscular Rheumatism: *Medical Record*, Vol. 57, pp. 529-535.

The classic paper on what we now call "Trigger Points." Adler noticed these in the late 1800s and reviewed the same symptoms reported in German medical literature dating back to 1840.

Ahluwalia N, Sun J , Krause D, Mastro A, Handte G (2004), Immune function is impaired in iron-deficient, homebound, older women: *American Journal of Clinical Nutrition*, Vol. 79, pp. 516-521.

Alix ME, Bates DK (1999), A proposed etiology of cervicogenic headache — the neurophysiologic basis and anatomic relationship between the dura mater and the rectus posterior capitis muscle. *Journal of Manipulative Physiological Therapeutics*, Vol. 22, pp. 534-539.

Amen DG (2004), *Images of Human Behavior: A Brain SPECT Atlas*. Mindworks Press, 121 pp.

See what goes on in a brain with ADD / ADHD (and many other conditions long thought to be more or less imaginary, such as lingering head injury or PMS). See also what happens when a brain is dosed with heroin, marijuana, alcohol and nicotine perhaps in an attempt to relieve pain or anxiety. Many images available on-line at www. brainplace.com/bp/atlas/.

Artenian DJ, Lipman JK, Scidmore GK, and Brant-Zawadzki M (1989) Acute neck pain due to tendonitis of the longus colli. *Journal of Neuroradiology:* Vol. 31, n. 2, pp. 166-169.

Baker AJ and others (1993), Excitatory amino acids in cerebrospinal fluid following traumatic brain injury in humans. *Journal of Neurosurgery,* Vol. 79, pp. 369-372.

Baker BA (1986) The muscle trigger: evidence of overload injury. *Journal of Neurology and Orthopedic Medical Surgery*, Vol. 7, pp. 35-44.

Data on muscles that are almost *always* injured in traffic accidents.

Bakris G, Dickholtz M Sr, Meyer PM, Kravitz G, Avery E, Miller M, Brown J, Woodfield C, Bell B (2007), Atlas vertebra realignment and achievement of arterial pressure goal in hypertensive patients: a pilot study. *Journal of Human Hypertension*, Vol. 21, n. 5, pp. 347-352.

Barnes, Broda O and Galton, Lawrence (1976) *Hypothyroidism: The Unsuspected Illness*. Harper & Row, Publishers, 308 pp.

A history of thyroid treatment from one of the pioneers. A tireless researcher, Barnes originated the idea that waking (basal) body temperature is the most accurate measure of thyroid function, backing it up with thousands of case histories. See also Blanchard, Ken (2004).

Beasley R, Heuser P, Raymond N (2005) SIT (seated immobility thromboembolism) syndrome: a 21st century lifestyle hazard. *New Zealand Medical Journal*, Vol. 118, n. 1212, U1376.

Becser N, Bovim G, and Sjaastad O (1998), Extracranial nerves in the posterior part of the head: anatomic variations and their possible clinical significance. *Spine*, Vol. 23, p. 1435.

Bergman RA, Afifi AK, Miyauchi R (1995), "'Circle of Willis" in *Illustrated Encyclopedia of Human Anatomic Variation*, an on-line digital atlas. Accessed Jan 9, 2011.

www.anatomyatlases.org/AnatomicVariants/Cardiovascular/Text/Arteries/CircleofWillis.shtml.

On variations in the Circle of Willis. Based on a study of 1,413 brains, the classic textbook image of the circle was seen in less than 35% of cases. In one variation, both anterior cerebral arteries are supplied by a single internal carotid artery. If that is blocked, you're in trouble.

Berguer R, Higgins R, Nelson R (1980), Noninvasive diagnosis of reversal of vertebral-artery blood flow. *New England Journal of Medicine*, Vol. 302, n. 24, pp. 1349-1351.

Bernstein, Carolyn (2008), *The Migraine Brain*, Free Press, 353 pp.

Beil, Laura (2011), In Eyes, a Clock Calibrated by Wavelengths of Light. *The New York Times*, Health Section, July 4, 2011.

Current research on different types of light and its effects on melatonin and sleep. LED computer screens which tend towards the blue end of the spectrum may wake you up in the morning. Before bedtime, they may keep you awake and sleepless for hours compared to old-style CRT monitors. Available on-line at: www.nytimes.com/2011/07/05/health/05light.html.

Blanchard, Ken and Brill, Marietta Abrams (2004), *What Your Doctor May Not Tell You About Hypothyroidism: A Simple Plan for Extraordinary Results*. Grand Central Publishing, 252 pp.

Blaylock, Russell L (1996), *Excitotoxins: The Taste that Kills*. Health Press, 320 pp.

Blumenthal HJ, Vance DA (1997), Chewing gum headaches. *Headache*, Vol. 37 n. 10, pp. 665.

Case reports on migraines provoked by chewing sugarless gum with aspartame.

Bogduk N (1992), The anatomical basis for cervicogenic headache. *Journal of Manipulative and Physiological Therapeutics*, Vol. 15, n. 1, pp. 67-70.

On headaches caused by structures innervated by spinal nerves C1-C3 including muscles, joints and ligaments of the upper three cervical vertebrae, the dura mater, and the vertebral artery.

__ (1982), The clinical anatomy of the cervical dorsal rami. *Spine,* Vol. 7, p. 319.

Bovim G, Bonamico L, Fredriksen TA (1991), Topographic variations in the peripheral course of the greater occipital nerve: autopsy study with clinical correlations. *Spine*, Vol. 16, p. 475.

Brody JE (2011), Ancient Moves for Orthopedic Problems: *The New York Times*, August 1, 2011, page D7. Available on-line at:www.nytimes.com/2011/08/02/health/02brody.html

Brown WA, Meszaros Z (2007), Hoarding. *Psychiatric Times*, Vol. 24, n. 13.

Buchholz, David (2002), *Heal Your Headache.* Workman Publishing, 246 pp.

We disagree on muscular inputs, but here is excellent information on the physiology of headache, personal triggers, and how to get off the drugs that may actually be making your migraines worse.

Brenton BP (2000), Pellagra, Sex and Gender: Biocultural Perspectives on Differential Diets and Health: DOI:10.1525/nua.2000.23.1.20

A proposal that niacin deficiency may be modulated by estrogen. Available on-line.

Buse D, Manack A, Serrano D, Turkel C, Lipton RB (2010), Sociodemographic and comorbidity profiles of chronic migraine and episodic migraine sufferers: *Journal of Neurology, Neurosurgery & Psychiatry*, Vol. 81, pp. 428-432.

Carod-Artal FJ, da Silveira Ribeiro L, Braga H, Kummer W, Mesquita HM, Vargas AP (2006), Prevalence of patent foramen ovale in migraine patients with and without aura compared with stroke patients: a trans-cranial Doppler study. *Cephalgia*, Vol. 26, n. 8, pp. 934-939.

Csapo R, Maganaris CN, Seynnes OR, Narici MV (2010), On muscle, tendon and high heels. *Journal of Experimental Biology*, Vol. 213: pp. 2582-2588

Cavallotti D, Artico M, De Santis S, Lannetti G, Cavallotti C (1998), Catecholaminergic innervation of the human dura mater involved in headache. *Headache*, Vol. 38, pp. 352-355.

Chaitow, Leon (2007), *Positional Release Techniques: Churchill Livingstone, 288 pp.*

On the remarkably effective osteopathic technique for releasing tense or spasming muscles and resetting (rather than exacerbating) tendon reflexes.

__(2002), *Multidisciplinary Approaches to Breathing Pattern Disorders:* Churchill-Livingstone, 288 pp.

Christiansen I, Thomsen LL, Daugaard D, Ulrich V, Olesen J (1999), Glyceryl trinitrate induces attacks of migraine without aura in sufferers of migraine with aura. *Cephalalgia*, Vol. 19, pp. 660-667.

Cohen, JS (2004), *The Magnesium Solution for Migraine Headaches: How to Use Magnesium to Prevent and Relieve Migraine and Cluster Headaches Naturally.* Square One Publishers, 64 pp.

This tiny book is an extensive review of research on magnesium, migraine and cluster headaches.

Davies, Clair (2006) *The Frozen Shoulder Workbook: Trigger Point Therapy for Overcoming Pain & Regaining Range of Motion*. New Harbinger Publications, Inc., 285 pp.

__and Davies, Amber (2004), *The Trigger Point Therapy Workbook: Your Self-Treatment Guide for Pain Relief. New Harbiner Publications, Inc.*, 323 pp.

Davis DR, Epp MD, and Riordan HD (2004), Changes in USDA Food Composition Data for 43 Garden Crops, 1950 to 1999. *Journal of the American College of Nutrition*, Vol. 23, pp. 669-682.

Available on-line at: www.jacn.org/cgi/content/full/23/6/669#F1. Our food is changing.

Dean NA and Mitchell BS (2002), Anatomic relation between the nuchal ligament (ligamentum nuchae) and the spinal dura mater in the craniocervical region. *Clinical Anatomy*, Vol. 15, n. 3, pp. 182-185.

DeJung, Beat (2002), *Triggerpunkt-Therapie.* Huber, Bern.

A German text on trigger point therapy emphasizing dry needling.

Delgado-Sanchez L, Godkar D, Niranjan S (2008), Pellagra: rekindling of an old flame. *American Journal of Therapeutics,* Vol. 15, n. 2, pp. 173-175.

DeRubeis RJ, Hollon SD, Amsterdam JD, Shelton RC, Young PR, Salomon RM, O'Reardon JP, Lovett ML, Gladis MM, Brown LL, Gallop R (2005), Cognitive therapy vs medications in the treatment of moderate to severe depression. *Archives of General Psychiatry*, Vol. 62, pp. 409-16.

Dirnberger F and Becker K (2004), Surgical treatment of migraine headaches by corrugator muscle resection. *Plastic and Reconstructive Surgery*, Vol. 114, pp. 652-657.

Duffy FR (2000), Editorial. *Clinical Electroencephalography, Vol. 1, n. 1, pp. v, vii.*

Source of the famous statement by Harvard Medical School professor and pediatric neurologist on the value of neurofeedback in many difficult areas.

Durham PL, Vause CV, Derosier F, McDonald S, Cady R, Martin V (2010), Changes in salivary prostaglandin levels during menstrual migraine with associated dysmenorrhea. *Headache*, Vol. 50, n. 5, pp. 844-851.

Doepp F, Schreiber SJ, Dreier JP, Einhäupl KM, Valdueza JM (2003), Migraine aggravation caused by cephalic venous congestion. *Headache*, Vol. 43, n. 2, pp. 96-98.

Edeling H and Hack, GD (1998), Cervicogenic headache: a new surgical procedure [abstract] *in: Proceedings of the American Association of Neurological Surgeons*, Philadelphia, PA.

Egger J, Carter, CM, Soothill, JF, and Wilson, J (1989), Oligoantigenic diet treatment of children with epilepsy and migraine. *Journal of Pediatrics*, Vol. 114, n. 1, pp. 51-58.

Further study on the role of food allergies in migraine. See Egger J (1983) and Monro J (1984).

___, Carter CM, Wilson J, Turner MW, Soothill JF (1983), Is migraine food allergy? A double-blind controlled trial of oligoantigenic diet treatment. *Lancet*, Vol. 2, n. 835, pp. 865-869.

Elliot, Carl (2010), *White Coat, Black Hat: Adventures on the Dark Side of Medicine*. Beacon Press, 224 pp.

Esty ML and Nelson DV (2009), Neurotherapy of TBI/PTSD in OEF/OIF veterans. *Journal of Neuropsychiatry and Clinical Neurosciences*, Vol. 21, pp. 221-223.

Featherstone, HJ (1985), Migraine and muscle contraction headaches: a continuum. *Headache*, Vol. 24, p. 194.

Tension, migraines, and cluster headaches have long been considered separate entities. This paper suggests they are not so different after all. Cohen (2004) and Seelig M (2003) suggest a deficiency of magnesium as a common cause. Blaylock (1997) notes that destruction of brain cells by MSG, aspartame and other excitotoxins is more severe when magnesium levels are low.

Ferguson, Lucy Whyte, and Gerwin, Robert (2004), *Clinical Mastery in the Treatment of Myofascial Pain*. Lippincott, Williams & Wilkins, 608 pp.

Case histories of myofascial pain and effective treatment by a chiropractor and a neurologist.

Fernández-de-las-Peñas, Cèsar, Arendt-Nielsen, Lars, Gerwin, Robert D (2010), *Tension-Type and Cervicogenic Headache: Pathophysiology, Diagnosis, and Management*, Jones and Bartlett Publishers, 509 pp.

From the physiology of muscle pain, trigger point pain patterns, patient interviews and evaluation of cervical vertebrae dysfunction to various treatments and therapies.

Fields WS, Lemak NA (1972), Joint Study of extracranial arterial occlusion, VII. Subclavian steal: a review of 168 cases. *Journal of the American Medical Association*, Vol. 222, pp. 1139-1143.

Findley, Thomas W. and Schleip, Robert (Eds) (2007), *Fascia Research: Basic Science and Implications for Conventional and Complementary Health Care*. Elsevier, 282 pp.

Finn R and Shifflett CM (2003), *Range-of-Motion Testing*. Round Earth Publishing [charts].

A set of two charts (Upper Body and Lower Body) illustrating ROM tests, including those shown in this manual. Website: www.round-earth.com

Franklin, Eric (2003), *Pelvic Power: Mind/Body Exercises for Strength, Flexibility, Posture, and Balance for Men and Women*. Princeton Book Co, 127 pp.

Fried, Robert (1993), *The Psychology and Physiology of Breathing in Behavioral Medicine, Clinical Psychology, and Psychiatry:* Plenum Press, 374 pp.

The mechanics of breathing and its effect on *all* body systems. See also Chaitow (2002).

Gaby AR (2002), Intravenous nutrient therapy: the "Myers' cocktail". *Alternative Medicine Review* Vol. 7, n. 5, pp. 389-403.

A review of the efficacy of a modified "Myers' cocktail" in migraine, fibromyalgia, asthma, cardiovascular and other conditions with clinical experience, precautions and potential side effects.

Garber, Greeg (2005), *A Tormented Soul*. ESPN.com.

Online at: www.sports.espn.go.com/nfl/news/story?id=1972285

Gard G (2009), An investigation into the regulation of intra-cranial pressure and its influence upon the surrounding cranial bones. *Journal of Bodywork and Movement Therapies*, Vol. 13, n. 3, pp. 246-254.

On the arterial and venous anatomy inside and around the skull and spinal column.

Gasbarrini A, De Luca A, Fiore G, Franceschi F, Ojetti VV, Torre ES, Di Campli C, Candelli M, Pola R, Serricchio M, Tondi P, Gasbarrini G, Pola P, Giacovazzo M (1998), Primary Headache and *Helicobacter Pylori*. *International Journal of Angiology*: Vol. 7, n. 4, pp. 310-312.

Gonçalves DA, Camparis CM, Speciali JG, Franco AL, Castanharo SM, Bigal ME (2011) Temporomandibular disorders are differentially associated with headache diagnoses: a controlled study. *The Clinical Journal of Pain*, Vol. 27, n. 7, pp. 611-615.

Graff-Radford S, Jaeger B, Reeves JL (1986), Myofascial pain may present clinically as occipital neuralgia. *Neurosurgery,* Vol. 19, n. 4, pp. 610-613.

Three case reports to consider before irreversible surgical interventions.

Grosser K, Oelkers R, Hummel T, Geisslinger G, Brune K, Kobal G, and Lötsch J (2000), Olfactory and trigeminal event-related potentials in migraine. *Cephalalgia.* Vol. 20, n. 7, pp. 621-631.

This study investigated trigeminal nerves and — for the first time — *odor* as a trigger for migraine.

Grossinger R (2006), *Migraine Auras: When the Visual World Fails.* North Atlantic Books, 264 pp.

One of the few books on a common symptom of migraine; reviews historical literature and the many proposed causes for the phenomenon. See also Podoll K and Robinson D (2009).

Grotheer P, Marshall M, and Simonne A (2005), Sulfites: Separating Fact from Fiction: Document FCS8787, Florida Cooperative Extension Service, Institute of Food and Agricultural Sciences, University of Florida. Available on-line at www.edis.ifas.ufl.edu/fy731.

Gudmundsson G (2010), Infantile colic: Is a pain syndrome. *Medical Hypotheses,* Vol. 75, pp. 528-529.

A suggestion that infantile colic begins with pain in the masticatory muscles in the course of sucking. Crying leads to swallowing of air and abdominal pain.

Gursoy-Ozdemir, Yasemin and others (2004), Cortical spreading depression activates and upregulates MMP-9. *Journal of Clinical Investigations,* Vol. 113, pp. 1447-1455.

On finding that cortical spreading depression damages the blood-brain barrier.

Guyuron B, Tucker T, Davis J (2002), Surgical treatment of migraine headaches. *Plastic and Reconstructive Surgery,* Vol 109, n. 7, pp. 2183-2189.

On entrapment of cranial nerves by CORRUGATOR SUPERCILII and possibly TEMPORALIS muscles, another link to the muscular origins of migraine. A letter from a physician suggests that favorable patient response to targeting these muscles is because migraine responds well to placebo effect. I would love to have had some placebo effect over the years.

Hack GD, and Hallgren RC (2004), Chronic headache relief after section of suboccipital muscle dural connections: a case report. *Headache,* Vol. 44, pp. 84-89.

Chronic headache relieved by cutting the connection betweena hypertrophied ally RECTUS CAPITIS POSTERIOR MINOR and the dura mater. See also Edeling H and others (1998). For mages available on-line in the NIH database, see: www.nlm.nih.gov/research/visible/vhp_conf/hack2/hack2.htm

__, Koritzer RT, Robinson WL, Hallgren RC, Greenman PE (1995), Anatomic relation between the rectus capitis posterior minor muscle and the dura mater. *Spine,* Vol. 20, n. 23, pp. 2484-2486.

The previously unreported connection between RECTUS CAPITIS POSTERIOR MINOR and the dura mater of the spinal cord and brain, the link between muscle contraction headaches and *migraines* via the pain-sensitive dura mater. See also Kimmel (1961).

Hamilton, Alyssa (2009), *Squeezed: What You Don't Know About Orange Juice* (Yale Agrarian Studies Series), Yale University Press, 288 pp.

Hammond, Corydon D (2007), *LENS: The Low Energy Neurofeedback System.*Routledge, 120 pp.

Hampton KK, Esack A, Peatfield RC, Grant PJ. (1991), Elevation of plasma vasopressin in spontaneous migraine. *Cephalalgia,* Vol. 11, n. 6, pp. 249-250.

Harries M (1997), Ice cream headache occurred during surfing in winter. *British Medical Journal,* Vol. 315, no. 7108, p. 609.

Hedaya, Robert J (2000), *The Antidepressant Survival Program*: Crown Publishers, 304 pp.

Notice the long list of nutrients with "depression" as the first sign of deficiency.

Helseth EK, Erickson JC (2008), The prevalence and impact of migraine on US Military officer trainees. *Headache,* Vol. 48, n. 6, pp. 883-889.

Holmes DR Jr, Cohen H, Katz WE, Reeder GS (2004), Patent foramen ovale, systemic embolization and closure. *Current Problems in Cardiology,* Vol. 29, n. 2, pp. 56-94.

A review of PFO diagnosis and treatment, and their safety profiles for migraineurs.

Hong CZ (1989), Eagle syndrome manifested with chronic myofascial trigger points in digastric muscle. *Archives of Physical Medicine and Rehabilitation* Vol. 70: A-19.

__ and Simons DG (1994), Considerations and recommendations regarding myofascial trigger point injection: *Journal of Musculoskeletal Pain,* Vol. 2, n. 1, pp. 29-59.

House AA, Eliasziw M, Cattran DC, Churchill DN, Oliver MJ, Fine A, Dresser GK, Spence JD (2010), Effect of B-vitamin therapy on progression of diabetic nephropathy: a randomized controlled trial. *Journal of the American Medical Association,* Vol. 303, n. 16, pp. 1603-1609.

Houlihan J, Thayer K, Klein J (2003), EWG finds heated Teflon pans can turn toxic faster than DuPont claims. *EWG Research,* on-line at: www.ewg.org/reports/toxicteflon.

Hulihan J (1997), Ice cream headache: no need for abstinence. *British Medical Journal*, Vol. 314, n. 7091, p. 1364. On-line: www.ncbi.nlm.nih.gov/pmc/articles/PMC2126629/pdf/9161304.pdf

Humphreys BK, Kenin S, Hubbard BB, Cramer GD (2003), Investigation of connective tissue attachments to the cervical spinal dura mater. *Clinical Anatomy*, Vol. 16, n. 2, pp. 152-159.

An investigation of the "dural bridge" between the RECTUS CAPITUS POSTERIOR MINOR muscle and the dura mater of the brain, found to be standard, sturdy, and visible on MRI.

Janis JE, Dhanik A, Howard JH (2011) Validation of the peripheral trigger point theory of migraine headaches: single-surgeon experience using botulinum toxin and surgical decompression. *Plastic and Reconstructive Surgery*, Vol. 128, n. 1 (Jul), pp. 123-131.

__, Hatef DA, Reece EM, McCluskey PD, Schaub TA, Guyuron B (2010), Neurovascular compression of the greater occipital nerve: implications for migraine headaches. *Plastic and Reconstructive Surgery*, Vol 126, n. 6 (Dec), pp. 1996-2001.

___, Hatef DA, Ducic I, Ahmad J, Wong C, Hoxworth RE, Osborn T (2010), Anatomy of the auriculotemporal nerve: variations in its relationship to the superficial temporal artery and implications for the treatment of migraine headaches. *Plastic and Reconstructive Surgery*, Vol. 125, n. 5, pp. 1422-1428.

Jansen SC, van Dusseldorp M, Bottema KC, Dubois AE (2003), Intolerance to dietary biogenic amines: a review. *Annals of Allergy Asthma Immunology*, Vol. 91, n. 3, pp. 233-240.

Jolly F (1902), Ueber Flimmersktom und Migräne. *Berl Klin Wochenschr*, Vol. 42, pp. 973-6.

Jowett NI, Robinson CG (1996), The tight pants syndrome—a sporting variant. *Postgraduate Medical Journal*. Vol. 72, n. 846, pp. 239-240.

Karacalar A and Karacalar S (2003), Hair transplantation and headaches. *Plastic and Reconstructive Surgery*, Vol. 111, p. 2103.

Responding to articles by Guyuron and others on surgical treatment of migraines, the authors observe that severity and frequency of chronic headaches were also reduced following hair transplants. This procedure involves injecting the supraorbital, temporal, and occipital areas with bupivacaine to block the supraorbital, auriculotemporal, and occipital nerves.

Kerrigan, Casey (1998) Knee osteoarthritis and high-heeled shoes: *Lancet*, Vol. 351, pp. 1399-1401.

Kessler L, Imperial J, Penev PD (2009), Exposure to recurrent sleep restriction in the setting of high caloric intake and physical inactivity results in increased insulin resistance and reduced glucose tolerance. *Journal of Clinical Endocrinology and Metabolism,* Vol. 94, n. 9, pp. 3242-3250.

Kimmel D (1961), Innervation of the spinal dura and the dura mater in the posterior cranial fossa. *Neurology*, Vol. 11, pp. 800-809.

Koperer H, Deinsberger W, Jodicke A, and Boker DK (1999), Postoperative headache after the lateral suboccipital approach: craniotomy versus craniectomy. *Minimally Invasive Neurosurgery*, Vol. 42, n. 4, pp. 175-178.

Kramarenko AV and Tan U (2003), Effects of high frequency electromagnetic fields on human EEG: A brain mapping study. *International Journal of Neuroscience*, Vol. 113, n. 7, 1007-1019.

In adults, just 20-40 seconds of cell phone use slowed frontal and temporal brainwaves on the opposite side of the head down to 2.5-6.0 Hz (delta and theta frequencies). The slowing lasted about 1 second, but reoccurred every 15-20 seconds for the duration of the call. In children, slow waves appeared sooner, had higher amplitude and lower frequencies (1.0-2.5 Hz, firmly in the delta range), reappeared at shorter intervals and lasted longer.

Koiwai EK (2002), Deaths Allegedly Caused by the Use of "Choke Holds" (*Shime-Waza*). Article on-line at: www.judoinfo.com/chokes5.htm

Langevin HM and Yandow JA (2002), Relationship of acupuncture points and meridians to connective tissue planes. *The Anatomical Record*, Vol. 269, n. 6, pp. 257–265.

Traditional acupuncture points compared with meat cuts and verified with sonography. Available at: www.onlinelibrary.wiley.com/doi/10.1002/ar.10185/full

Levy, Andrew (2009), *A Brain Wider Than the Sky: A Migraine Diary*. Simon and Schuster, 289 pp.

Levis S, Strickman-Stein N, Ganjei-Azaret P, Xu P, Doerge DR, Krischer J (2011), Isoflavones in the prevention of menopausal bone loss and menopausal symptoms" *Archives of Internal Medicine*, Vol. 171, n. 15, pp. 1363-1369.

Results do not support claims that soy helps slow osteoporosis.

Lindgren KA, Manninen H, Rytkönen H (1995), Thoracic outlet syndrome — a functional disturbance of the thoracic upper aperture? *Muscle Nerve*, Vol. 18, n. 5, pp. 526-530.

Loch C, Fehrman P, Dockhorn HU (1990), [Studies on the compression of the external carotid artery in the region of the styloid process of the temporal bone]. *Laryngorhinootologie* Vol. 69, n. 5, pp. 260-266. Article in German.

On the entrapment of the external carotid artery (and sometimes the posterior auricular artery) by the POSTERIOR DIGASTRIC muscle *alone* — with no calcification of styloid or digastric tendons.

Loomis, Chauncy C (2000), *Weird and Tragic Shores: The Story of Charles Francis Hall, Explorer.* Alfred A. Knopf, 392 pp.

Lopez-Art, Kenji (2010), The Best Beef Stew. *Cooks Illustrated* (Jan-Feb), p. 8-9.

Lustig RH (2008), Hypothalamic obesity: causes, consequences, treatment: *Pediatric Endocrinology Review,* Vol. 6, n. 2, pp. 220-227.

Malkan, Stacy (2007), *Not Just a Pretty Face: The Ugly Side of the Beauty Industry.* New Society Publishers, 192 pp.

Marcus DA, Bernstein C, Rudy TE (2005), Fibromyalgia and headache: an epidemiological study supporting migraine as part of the fibromyalgia syndrome. *Clinical Rheumatology,* Vol. 24, pp. 595-601.

Chronic headache was reported by 76% of treatment-seeking fibromyalgia patients, with 84% reporting substantial or severe impact from their headaches.

Maté, Gabor (2010) *In the Realm of Hungry Ghosts: Close Encounters with Addiction.* North Atlantic Books, 520 pp.

Mauskop A, Altura BT, Altura BM (2002), Serum ionized magnesium levels and serum ionized calcium/ionized magnesium ratios in women with menstrual migraine. *Headache,* Vol. 42 n. 4, pp. 242-248.

McGee SR, Boyko EJ (1998), Physical Examination and Chronic Lower-Extremity Ischemia: A Critical Review. *Archives of Internal Medicine,* Vol. 158, no. 12, pp. 1357-1364.

McNab I (1964), Acceleration injuries of the cervical spine. *Journal of Bone and Joint Surgery,* Vol. 46, pp. 1797-1799.

McPartland JM and Brodeur, RR (1999), Rectus capitis posterior minor: a small but important suboccipital muscle. *Journal of Bodywork and Movement Therapies,* Vol. 3, n. 1, pp. 30-35.

___ , and Hallgren RC (1997), Chronic neck pain, standing balance, and suboccipital muscle atrophy: a pilot study. *Journal of Manipulative and Physiological Therapeutics,* Vol. 20, pp. 24-29.

Milde-Busch A, Blaschek A, Borggräfe I, Heinen F, Straube A, von Kries R (2010), Associations of diet and lifestyle with headache in high-school students: results from a cross-sectional study. *Headache,* Vol. 50, n. 7, pp. 1104-1114.

Mishra NK, Rossetti AO, Ménétrey A, Carota A (2009), Recurrent Wernicke's aphasia: migraine and not stroke! *Headache,* Vol. 49, no. 5, pp. 765-768.

Mitchell J (2007), Doppler insonation of vertebral artery blood flow changes associated with cervical spine rotation: Implications for manual therapists.*Physiotherapy Theory and Practice.* Vol. 23, n. 6, pp. 303-313.

Monastra V, Monastra D, George S (2002), The effects of stimulant therapy, EEG biofeedback, and parenting style on the primary symptoms of attention-deficit/hyperactivity disorder. *Applied Psychophysiology and Biofeedback,* Vol. 27, no. 4. pp 239-249.

Study comparing patients treated with medications only, with patients treated with EEG only. Only the biofeedback group showed lasting changes in EEG.

Monro J, Carini C, and Brostoff J (1984), Migraine is a food-allergic disease. *Lancet,* Sept. 29; 2(8405): pp. 719-721.

Mora CV, Davison M, Wild JM. and Walker MM (2004), Magnetoreception and its trigeminal mediation in the homing pigeon, *Nature,* Vol. 432, pp. 508-511.

Morgenstein KM, and Krieger MK (1980), Experiences in middle turbinectomy. *Laryngoscope,* Vol. 90, p. 1596.

Moskowitz MA (1984), The neurobiology of vascular head pain. *Annals of Neurology,* Vol. 16, p. 157.

Mosser SW, Guyuron B, Janis JE, and Rohrich RJ (2004), The anatomy of the greater occipital nerve: implications for the etiology of migraine headaches. *Plastic and Reconstructive Surgery,* Vol. 113, n. 2, pp. 693-697.

On the course of the nerve and its variations in 20 adult cadavers investigating points where the it might be subject to entrapment and compression. Updated in 2010 with Janis JE as first author.

Muth OH and Allaway WH (1963), The relationship of white muscle disease to the distribution of naturally occurring selenium. *Journal of the American Veterinary Medical Association,* Vol. 142, p. 1380.

On selenium deficiency and toxicity in soils, with US map.

Myers, TW (2008), *Anatomy Trains: Myofascial Meridians for Manual and Movement Therapists.* Churchill Livingstone, 440 pages.

Vastly expanded text, illustrations, and training materials. Website: www.anatomytrains.net

National Geographic (2008), *Stress: Portrait of a Killer.* 50 minutes.

Documentary on the work of Robert Sapolsky, studying stress in wild baboons and unfortunate similarities found in members of the British Civil Service. How stress injures, kills, and even alters DNA.

Naficy ST and Panchanathan K (2008), *Buffy the Vampire Dater.*
Available on-line at: buddha.bol.ucla.edu/papers/Buffy.pdf

Nedeltcheva AV, Kilkus JM, Imperial J, Schoeller DA, Penev PD (2010), Insufficient sleep undermines dietary efforts to reduce adiposity. *Annals of Internal Medicine,* Vol. 153, pp. 435-441.

Nelson DV and Esty ML (2010), Neurotherapy for TBI: A CAM intervention. *Brain Injury,* Vol. 24, n. 3, p. 366.

__ and Esty ML, (2009). Neurotherapy for Chronic TBI/PTSD Symptoms in Vietnam Veterans. *Journal of Head Trauma Rehabilitation,* Vol. 24, n. 5, p. 403.

__ and Esty ML: Neurotherapy for pain in veterans with trauma spectrum disorders (2009), *Journal of Pain,* Vol. 10, n. 4, Supplement, p. S18.

Netter, Frank H. (2010), *Atlas of Human Anatomy.* Saunders, 624 pp.

Neuschwander TB, Cutrone J, Macias BR, Cutrone S, Murthy G, Chambers H, Hargens AR (2010), The Effect of Backpacks on the Lumbar Spine in Children: A Standing Magnetic Resonance Imaging Study. *Spine,* Vol. 35, pp. 83–88.

Newman LC and Lipton RB (2001), Migraine MLT-down: an unusual presentation of migraine in patients with aspartame-triggered headaches. *Headache,* Vol. 41, n. 9, pp. 899-901.

Newton KM, Grady D (2011), Soy isoflavones for prevention of menopausal bone loss and vasomotor symptoms. *Archives of Internal Medicine,* Vol. 171, n. 15, pp. 1369-1370.

Nezvalová-Henriksen K, Spigset O, Nordeng H (2010), Triptan exposure during pregnancy and the risk of major congenital malformations and adverse pregnancy outcomes: Results from the Norwegian Mother and Child Cohort Study. *Headache* Vol. 50, n. 4, pp. 563-575.

Oleski SL, Smith GH, Crow WT (2002), Radiographic evidence of cranial bone mobility. *Cranio,* Vol. 20, n. 1, pp. 34-38.

Do cranial bones shift and move? X-rays before and after osteopathic cranial manipulation showed mean angles of change as Atlas: 2.58°, mastoid: 1.66°, malar line: 1.25°, sphenoid: 2.42°, temporal line: 1.75°. Yes they do. See Ueno T for NASA's opinion.

Orlov, Melissa C. (2010) *The ADHD Effect on Marriage: Understand and Rebuild Your Relationship in Six Steps.* Specialty Press, 233 pp.

Behavioral therapy and coping strategies are essential for partners in ADD and migraine and may be needed to unpack years of resentments. Website: www.adhdmarriage.com

Parker-Pope, Tara (2011) Celiac Disease Becoming More Common. *The New York Times,* Health Section, Tuesday, July 5. Online at: www.well.blogs.nytimes.com/2009/07/02/celiac-disease-becoming-more-common/

Perreau-Linck E, Beauregard M, Gravel P, and others (2007), In vivo measurements of brain trapping of C-labeled alpha-methyl-L-tryptophan during acute changes in mood states. *Journal of Psychiatry and Neuroscience,* Vol. 32, pp. 430-434.

Plotnikoff GA, Quigley JM (2003), Prevalence of severe hypovitaminosis D in patients with persistent, nonspecific musculoskeletal pain. *Mayo Clinic Proceedings,* Vol. 78, n. 12, pp. 1463-70.

Podoll, Klaus and Robinson, Derek (2009), *Migraine Art: The Migraine Experience from Within.* North Atlantic Books, 400 pp.

300 illustrations and paintings by migraine sufferers around the world provide a unique window into visual disturbances, pain and impact of migraine on the artists' lives. Text includes detailed descriptions of visual and somatic experiences with technical commentary.

Ponikowski, P (2010), Clinical safety and efficacy of overnight transvenous unilateral phrenic nerve stimulation. *Berlin Heart Failure Conference 2010; Late Breaking Clinical Trial Session 2.*

Poole CJ, Lightman SL (1988), Inhibition of vasopressin secretion during migraine. *Journal of Neurology, Neurosurgery and Psychiatry.* Vol. 51, n. 11, pp. 1441-1444.

Porterfield JA and DeRosa Carl (1995), *Mechanical Neck Pain: Perspectives in Functional Anatomy.* W. B. Saunders Company.

On the muscular relationships to neck pain and resulting cervicogenic headache.

Prudden, Bonnie (1980 / 2002), *Pain Erasure the Bonnie Prudden Way.* M. Evans and Co., 274 pp.

Trigger points for laymen, based on the work of Travell & Simons. See also Davies, Clair (2004).

Rajalakshmi R, Ranade A, Nayak S, Rajanigandha V, Pai M, Krishnamurthy A (2008), A study of anatomical variability of the omohyoid muscle and its clinical relevance: *Clinics* Vol.63, n.4, pp. 521-524.

In 35 male cadavers, one had a double OMOHYOID, three arose directly from the clavicle, two merged with the STERNOHYOID muscle, and one had additional slips from the sternum. The muscle attaches to the fascia of the jugular vein, slowing venous return from the brain.

Ramprasad M, Alias J, Raghuveer AK (2010) Effect of backpack weight on postural angles in preadolescent children.*Indian Pediatrics.* Vol. 47, n. 7, pp. 575-580.

Rask, Michael R (1984), The omohyoideus myofascial pain syndrome: report of four patients. *Journal of Craniomandibular Practice,* Vol. 2, pp. 256-262. Online at: www.sarapin.com/myofascial.html.

Raskin NH, Howard MW, Ehrenfeld WK (1985), Headache as the leading symptom of the thoracic outlet syndrome. *Headache: Journal of Head and Face Pain,* Vol. 25, n. 4, pp. 208 - 210.

Ray BS, Wolff HG (1940), Experimental studies on headache: pain sensitive structures of the head and their significance in headache. *Archives of Surgery,* Vol. 41, pp. 813-856.

This heavily illustrated review of pain-producing structures in head and brain became a chapter in early editions of the classic headache textbook, *Wolff's Headache and Other Head Pains.* Editions from the 1980's on (with invention of MRI) reduced this material to a few pages of bibliographic citations and no pictures at all. For update on dural pain, see Koperer (1999).

Reid TR (1999), The official inventory of the crown jewels of Britain's royal family: *The Washington Post,* Monday, Jan 4, 1999, A16.

Ripley, Amanda (2010), *The Unthinkable: Who Survives When Disaster Strikes and Why.* Crown Publishers, 266 pp.

Rocabado M, Iglarsh ZA (1991), *Musculoskeletal Approach to Maxillofacial Pain.* J. B. Lippincott Co., 500 pp.

Superb review of head and neck musculature with directions for palpation and evaluation.

Rolf, Ida P (1989) *Rolfing: Reestablishing the Natural Alignment and Structural Integration of the Human Body for Vitality and Well-Being.* Healing Arts Press, 304 pp.

Rubenowitz-Lundin E, Hiscock KM (2005), Water Hardness and Health Effects, *in Essentials of Medical Geology: Impacts of the Natural Environment on Public Health* (Chapter 13), pp. 331-345, Elsevier Academic Press (Olle Selinus. Ed.)

Sahrmann, Shirley A, (2003), *Diagnosis and Treatment of Movement impairment Syndromes*

While myofascial therapists tend to concentrate on pain due to muscle *shortening,* Sahrmann emphasizes the relatively ignored issue of pain due to muscle *overlengthening.*

Samuels, Adrienne (1999), The Toxicity / Safety of Processed Free Glutamic Acid (MSG): A Study in Suppression of Information. *Accountability in Research,* Vol. 6, pp. 259-310.

A disturbing review of the food industry defense of MSG and other excitotoxins. Available on-line at: www.truthinlabeling.com/l-manuscript.html.

Sapkota AR, Berger S, Vogel TM (2009) Human Pathogens Abundant in the Bacterial Metagenome of Cigarettes: *Environmental Health Perspectives,* 2009 | doi:10.1289/ehp.0901201, U.S. National Institute of Environmental Health Sciences, National Institutes of Health.

Sapone A, Lammers KM, Casolaro V, Cammarota M, Giuliano MT, De Rosa M, Stefanile R, Mazzarella G, Tolone C, Russo MI, Esposito P, Ferraraccio F, Cartenì M, Riegler G, de Magistris L, Fasano A. (2011), Divergence of gut permeability and mucosal immune gene expression in two gluten-associated conditions: celiac disease and gluten sensitivity. *BMC Medicine,* Vol. 9, n. 23. Article on-line at: www.ncbi.nlm.nih.gov/pubmed/21392369.

Schleip R, Klingler W, Lehmann-Horn F (2006), Active fascial contractility: Fascia is able to contract and relax in a smooth muscle like manner and thereby influence biomechanical behavior. *Acta Physiologica* Vol. 186, Supplement 1, p. 247.

Schoenberger N, Shiflett SC, Esty ML, Ochs L, Matheis RJ (2001). Flexyx Neurotherapy System in the treatment of traumatic brain injury: An initial evaluation. *Journal of Head Trauma Rehabilitation.* Vol. 16, n. 3, pp. 260-274.

A study done at Kessler Rehabilitation Hospital with patients who had suffered closed head injury at least 12 months earlier. The general belief is that how you are a year later is as good as you're going to get, yet depression, fatigue, and cognitive function improved for these patients.

Schulte-Mattler WJ., Wieser T, and Zierz S (1999), Treatment of tension-type headache with botulinum toxin: a pilot study. *European Journal of Medical Research,* Vol. 4, p. 183.

Scopp A (1991), Monosodium glutamate and hydrolyzed vegetable protein induced headache: review and case studies. *Headache,* Vol. 31, n. 2, pp. 107-110.

Case studies in which elimination of MSG decreased headache frequency.

Seelig, Mildred (2003), *The Magnesium Factor.* Avery, 376 pp.

The late Mildred Seelig was a leading authority on magnesium in biological systems and health. See Cohen JS (2004) for an extensive review of magnesium in migraine and vascular aberrations.

Seletz E (1958) Headache of extracranial origin. *California Medicine,* Vol. 89, n. 5, pp. 314-317. Citation at www.PubMed.com includes link to full article.

An excellent review of contributions to migraine headaches by trigeminal and greater occipital nerves in concert with other structures in the cervical spine.

Sikdar S, Shah JP, Gebreab T, Yen R-H, Gilliams E, Danoff J, Gerber LH (2009) Novel applications of ultrasound technology to visualize and characterize myofascial trigger points and surrounding soft tissue.*Archives of Physical Medicine and Rehabilitation*, Vol. 90, pp. 1829-1838.

Silberstein SD, and Lipton RB (1993), Epidemiology of Migraine: *Neuroepidemiology*, Vol. 12, p. 179.

Simons DG, Travell JG, and Simons Lois S (1999), *Travell & Simons' Myofascial Pain and Dysfunction: The Trigger Point Manual* (Vol.1: Upper Half of Body, Second Ed.)

The second edition greatly expands the original Vol. 1. In this update, Dr. Simons discarded the original spasm model of muscle pain. The Bible of myofascial pain and what to do about it.

__(1996), Clinical and etiological update of myofascial pain from trigger points. In: *Clinical Overview and Pathogenesis of Fibromyalgia Syndrome, Myofascial Pain Syndrome, and Other Pain Syndromes.* Hayworth Medical Press, pp. 93-121.

Simpson, K (1940), Shelter deaths from pulmonary embolism. *Lancet,* Vol. 2, n. 744, 1940.

Singh S and Kumar A (2007) Wernicke encephalopathy after obesity surgery: a systematic review. *Neurology,* Vol. 68 n. 11, pp. 807-811.

Cases of severe thiamine deficiency after bariatric surgery. On losing more than weight.

Sjaastad O and Bakketeig LS (2006), Hydrogen sulphide headache and other rare, global headaches: Vågå study. *Cephalalgia,* Vol. 26, n. 4, pp. 466-476.

Skrtic, Lana (2006), Hydrogen Sulfide, Oil and Gas, and People's Health. Master's thesis, University of California, Berkeley, 78 pp.

Available online at: www.earthworksaction.org/pubs/hydrogensulfide_oilgas_health.pdf

Sola AE, Rodenberger ML, Gettys BB (1955), Incidence of hypersensitive areas in posterior shoulder muscles. *American Journal of Physical Medicine*, Vol. 34, pp. 585-590.

Soumekhetal B, Levine SC, Haines JJ, Wulf JA (1996), Retrospective study of postcraniotomy headaches in suboccipital approach: diagnosis and management. *American Otolaryngology*, Vol. 17, pp. 617-619.

On causes and prevention of post-surgical headaches. See Koperer H (1999) on differences between discarding the occipital bone versus putting it back where it belongs.

Streeter CC, Whitfield TH, Owen L, Rein T, Karri SK, Yakhkind A, Perlmutter R, Prescot A, Renshaw PF, Ciraulo DA, Jensen JE (2010), Effects of yoga versus walking on mood, anxiety, and brain GABA levels: a randomized controlled MRS study. *Journal of Alternative and Complementary Medicine*, Vol. 16, n. 11, pp. 1145-1152.

Sztajzel R, Genoud D, Roth S, Mermillod B, Le Floch-Rohr J (2002), Patent foramen ovale, a possible cause of symptomatic migraine: A study of 74 patients with acute ischemic stroke. *Cerebrovascular Diseases*, Vol. 13, n. 2, pp. 102-106.

A study of the relationship between migraine and stroke due to paradoxical embolism.

Sun-Edelstein C, Mauskop A (2009) Foods and supplements in the management of migraine headaches. *Clinical Journal of Pain*, Vol. 25, no. 5, pp. 446-452.

Identifying food triggers with the help of food diaries. Also reviews treatment with magnesium, *Petasites hybridus,* feverfew, coenzyme Q10, riboflavin, and alpha lipoic acid.

Kuhn, Cynthia, Swartzwelder, Scott, and Wilson, Wilkie (2008), *Buzzed: The Straight Facts About the Most Used and Abused Drugs from Alcohol to Ecstasy.* W. W. Norton & Co., 368 pp.

Theoharides TC, Donelan J, Kandere-Grzybowska K, Konstantinidou A (2005), The role of mast cells in migraine pathophysiology. *Brain Research, Brain Research Reviews*, Vol. 49, pp. 65-76.

On vasodilation involved with migraine and its relation to allergy.

Tietjen GE, Brandes JL, Digre KB, Baggaley S, Martin V, Recober A, Geweke LO, Hafeez F, Aurora SK, Herial NA, Utley C, Khuder SA (2007), High prevalence of somatic symptoms and depression in women with disabling chronic headache. *Neurology*, Vol. 68, pp. 134-140.

Tietjen's study suggests that muscle pain, stomach upsets, chronic headache and a greatly elevated rate of depression are strongly related, possibly through the serotonin system.

Travell JG and Simons DG (1983), *Myofascial Pain and Dysfunction: The Trigger Point Manual* (Vol. 1, Upper Body).

__(1992), *Myofascial Pain and Dysfunction: The Trigger Point Manual* (Vol. 2: The Lower Extremities). Lippincott, Williams & Wilkins.

Ueno T, Ballard RE, Macias BR and others (2003), Cranial diameter pulsation measured by non-invasive ultrasound decrease with tilt. *Aviation, Space and Environmental Medicine*, Vol. 74 n. 8, pp. 882-885.

__, Ballard RE, Shuer LM, Yost WT, Cantrell, Hargens AR (1998). Noninvasive measurement of pulsatile intracranial pressure using ultrasound. *Acta Neurochir.* [Suppl] 71, pp. 66-69.

In summary, the NASA research team stated, "Although the skull is often assumed to be a rigid container with a constant volume, many researchers have demonstrated that the skull moves on the order of a few μm in association with changes in intracranial pressure."

__, Ballard RE, Cantrell JH, and others (1996), Noninvasive estimation of pulsatile intracranial pressure using ultrasound. *NASA Technical Memorandum* 112195.

Underwood, Anne (2003), Fibromyalgia: not all in your head. *Newsweek*, May 19, 2003, p. 53.

A history of fibromyalgia research, from imaginary disease ("these women are crazy!") to progress in understanding and treatment. Migraines are frequently concurrent with fibro.

Upledger JE and Vredevoogd JD (1983), *Craniosacral Therapy*, Eastland Press, 367 pp.

Usha PR and Naidu MU (2004) Double-blind, parallel, placebo-controlled study of oral glucosamine, methylsulfonylmethane and their combination in osteoarthritis. *Clinical Drug Investigation*, Vol. 24, n. 6, pp. 353-363.

Glucosamine combined with MSM relieved pain and reduced inflammation in osteoarthritis. Results were best in combination than as individually.

Utiger D, Eichenberger U, Bernasch D, Baumgartner RW, Bärtsch P (2002), Transient minor improvement of high altitude headache by sumatriptan. *High Altitude Medical Biology.* Vol. 3, n. 4, pp. 387-393.

Valtonen EJ (1969), The omohyoid syndrome. *Lancet*, Nov. 15, p. 1073.

A case report of omohyoid spasmSee Wilmot (1969), Zachary (1969), and Rask (1984).

Vincent MB and Hadjikhani N (2007), Migraine aura and related phenomena: beyond scotomata and scintillations. *Cephalalgia*, Vol. 27, pp. 1368-1377.

Volkow ND, Wang GJ, Newcorn J, Telang F, Solanto MV, Fowler JS, Logan J, Ma Y, Schulz K, Pradhan K, Wong C, Swanson JM (2007), Depressed dopamine activity in caudate and preliminary evidence of limbic involvement in adults with attention-deficit / hyperactivity disorder. *Archives of General Psychiatry*, Vol. 64, n. 8, pp. 932-40.

This study confirmed that depressed dopamine activity in various areas of the brain was associated with the inattention of ADD and the pattern of craving for drugs linked with ADD / ADHD.

Wade N (2010), Scientists Cite Fastest Case of Human Evolution: *New York Times*, July 2, p. A7.

On evolutionary changes at high altitude on the Tibetan Plateau.

Weiss AB (2010), Absolutely the last word on physical diagnosis: Not! *Proceedings* (Baylor University Medical Center), Vol. 23, n. 3, pp. 301–303.

Article available on-line at: www.ncbi.nlm.nih.gov/pmc/articles/PMC2900986/

Wheeler AH (1998), Botulinum Toxin A, adjunctive therapy for refractory headaches associated with pericranial muscle tension. *Headache*, Vol. 38, n. 6 (June), p. 468.

Case histories of intractable migraine unresponsive to medications including trigger point injection, treated with Botox A (BXTA). One of the first reports of Botox in dealing with headache, giving rise to the awareness of the relationship between migraine and muscles.

Wilmot TJ (1969), The omohyoid syndrome. *Lancet*, Dec. 13, pp. 1298-1299.

Omohyoid strain by lifting cement blocks. See also Rask (1984).

Wilmshurst PT, Nightingale S, Walsh KP, Morrison WL (2005), Clopidogrel reduces migraine with aura after transcatheter closure of persistent foramen ovale and atrial septal defects. *Heart*. Vol. 91, n. 9, pp. 1173-1175.

__, Pearson MJ, Nightingale S, Walsh KP, Morrison WL (2004), Inheritance of persistent foramen ovale and atrial septal defects and the relation to familial migraine with aura. *Heart*, Vol. 90, pp. 1315-20

__, Nightingale S, Walsh KP, Morrison WL (2000), Effect on migraine of closure of cardiac right-to-left shunts to prevent recurrence of decompression illness or stroke or for haemodynamic reasons. *Lancet*, Vol. 356, n. 9242, pp. 1648-1651.

Wise, David and Anderson, Rodney (2008), *A Headache in the Pelvis: A new understanding and treatment for prostatitis and chronic pelvic pain syndromes (5th Ed.)*: National Center for Pelvic Pain Research, Occidental, CA.

Myofascial issues behind the symptoms known as "interstitial cystitis," "prostatitis," "vulvodynia," and a host of other names with a common origin — trigger points and myofascial dysfunction.

Young, SN (2007), How to increase serotonin in the human brain without drugs. *Journal of Psychiatry and Neuroscience*, Vol. 32, pp. 394-399.

Zachary RB, Young A, and Hammond JDS (1969), The omohyoid syndrome. *Lancet*, pp. 104-105.

# Index

ergotamines 234
naproxen 30
NSAIDs 30
opioids 234
Paxil 50, 161
Prozac 50, 161
Viagra 241
drunk tank and migraine / stroke 111
dura mater 8, 40, 43, 44, 89, 179, 185, 270, 271
dural bridge 8, 274
dysmenorrhea (menstrual cramping) 165

**E**

Ebers Papyrus 2
Electrolytes
  blood testing 9
  calcium and magnesium 11
  Exatest 106, 153, 238
electromyography (EMG)
  See sEMG 32
epineurium 40
Estrogen 5, 11, 156
  and hypothyroid 160
  contraceptives and clotting 106
  endocrine disruptors 11
  in hair straightener 163
  in pellagra 176
  in sex change therapy and migraines 5
  Phyto- and Xeno-estrogens 160, 161
eye pain 54

**F**

facial nerve (CN VII). See Cranial Nerves
fascia 39-44
FDA 143, 162, 165, 203
fibromyalgia 13, 86, 150, 151, 154, 156, 221
Food Sensitivities 6, 13, 137, 183, 197, 267
  and gluten 31
  and PFO 104
  top 8 items 31
foramen magnum 43, 120
formaldehyde 162, 186, 196, 207, 212, 252
  in carpet 212
frontalis. See Muscles.
frowning as headache trigger 54, 55
Functional effect of
  formaldehyde 162
  sulfites 203

**G**

Genes 122, 197
  and celiac disease 9
  and Circle of Willis 100
  and familial hemiplegic migraine 9
  and gluten sensitivity 31
  and iron absorption 155
  and PFO 104

and vitamin D requirements 10
  Factor V Leiden 106
glossopharyngeal nerve (CN IX). See Cranial Nerves
gluten sensitivity 31
goiter belt 156
Greek foot. See Morton Foot 187

**H**

hamstring flexibility 41
Head Injury 11
Headache Types
  chronic migraine 4, 7
  cluster 6, 10, 14, 107, 133
  episodic migraine 3, 4
  general list of 14
  hangover and ice-cream 7
  in children 5
  in men 5
  migraine and risk factors 4
  migraine, tension, and dural bridge 8
  muscle contraction headache 4, 14
  sinus 5, 8, 14, 22, 49, 50, 51, 52, 54, 55, 107 182, 218, 237
Head-Forward posture 193, 218, 220
hematoma, subdural 10
hoarding and brain injury 225
hyperventilation 169
hypoglossal nerve (CN XII). See Cranial Nerves
hypoglycemia 32, 183
Hypothyroid 11, 26, 31, 144, 163
  and anti-depressants 161
  and estrogen 160
  and thiamine 144

**I**

ibuprofen 30
infections 11, 30

**J**

Judo 264
  and carotids 91, 101, 274
  and Feldenkrais 264
jugular foramen 117, 118, 119, 120
jugular vein. See Blood vessels.

**L**

Light 111, 146, 173
  as nutrient 9, 145, 172, 177
  sensitivity (photophobia) 5, 12, 13, 15, 21, 149
  and optic nerve 113

**M**

MAST (Medical Anti-Shock Trousers) 93-94

Fibromyalgia 278
Horner's 55
Irritable Bowel (IBS) 13, 198
Jugular Foramen (Vernet's) 119
Metabolic 129
Movement Impairment 277
Myofascial Pain 158
Pelvic Pain 279
Piriformis 265
Post Traumatic Stress (PTSD) 129, 223, 263
Pre-Menstrual (PMS) 11, 149, 234
Pseudo Disc 68
Restless Leg (RLS) 41, 64, 92, 139
Rotator Cuff 265
Scalenus Anticus 62
Scapulocostal 61
Sick Building 9, 14
Subclavian Steal 96
Subclavian Steal (SSI) 102
Thoracic Outlet (TOS) 21, 25, 57, 58, 62, 63
Tight Pants 216

# T

Temporo-mandibular joint. See TMJD.
tentorium 43, 44
thrombus 106
Thyroid
    function 144, 156
    Temperature Measurement Protocol 159
TMJD 11, 51, 117, 181, 182, 183, 184, 236, 237, 267
    testing 183
Traumatic Brain Injury (TBI) 194, 223, 238, 260, 262, 263, 266, 270
trigeminal nerve (CN V). See Cranial Nerves
trigeminal neuralgia 8, 133

trigemino-vascular system 13, 30
triptans 116, 154, 233, 234
trochlear nerve (CN IV). See Cranial Nerves
TSH 31, 157, 158
tunica adventitia 40
Tylenol 30, 207
tyramines 179, 196

# U

UL (Upper Level of Tolerable Intake) 174
urination 111, 138

# V

vagus nerve (CN X). See Cranial Nerves
Veins. See Blood vessels.
vestibulocochlear nerve (CN VIII). See Cranial Nerves.
violin, TOS, and migraine 37, 62, 72, 97, 220, 267

# W

Wallet Butt 218
Water
    balance (osmoregulation) 110
    intake 135
    wells and acid drainage 136

# Y

yawning as migraine prodrome 9
yoga 265

# Z

zinc 148, 154, 160, 171, 172